Overcoming Dyslexia in Children, Adolescents, and Adults

THIRD EDITION

Dale R. Jordan

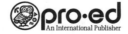

8700 Shoal Creek Boulevard
Austin, Texas 78757-6897
800/897-3202 Fax 800/397-7633
www.proedinc.com

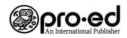
An International Publisher

© 2002, 1996, 1989 by PRO-ED, Inc.
8700 Shoal Creek Boulevard
Austin, Texas 78757-6897
800/897-3202 Fax 800/397-7633
www.proedinc.com

Library of Congress Cataloging-in-Publication Data

Jordan, Dale R.
 Overcoming dyslexia in children, adolescents, and adults / Dale R. Jordan.—3rd ed.
  p. cm.
 Includes bibliographical references and index.
 ISBN 0-89079-879-6
 1. Dyslexia—Popular works. 2. Learning disabilities— Popular works. I. Title.

RC394.W6 J67 2002
616.85'53—dc21

                                    2001048731

This book is designed in Italia and New Century Schoolbook.

Printed in the United States of America

1 2 3 4 5 6 7 8 9 10   06 05 04 03 02

Overcoming
Dyslexia in Children,
Adolescents, and Adults

To
Josef Sanders—
A loving and faithful friend
who encouraged and guided me
to publish what I know
about dyslexia and other
classroom learning problems

Contents

Preface

My classroom teaching career began in 1957 when I was hired, not for my teaching skills, but because the middle school needed a young man strong enough to deal with rowdy teenagers. Only a few of those students could read. None of them could spell correctly. All of them expressed hatred for school as they openly said to me: "I hate this place. You can't make me learn!" On that first intimidating day of my teaching career, my newly completed master's degree in elementary education ran out during the first 10 minutes, leaving me inadequately on my own before those surly youngsters. Nothing in my college studies had prepared me for such a challenge.

Instinctively I knew that those teenagers were not "dumb," as they self-consciously called themselves and each other. Although their oral language was uneducated, the stories they told were colorful and intelligent. Only when they were forced to focus attention on books and writing tasks did they call themselves "dumb."

As if responding to a forgotten voice from childhood, I began to read to those reluctant learners. I brought them action stories filled with suspense and mystery. To my amazement, those youngsters who "hated school" settled into eager, thoughtful listening. They came indoors early from the playground, begging me to read some more. We followed those eager listening experiences with class discussion. Soon the students agreed to work in small groups to develop their own stories to share with others. From this oral language beginning came a library of homemade books that were lovingly illustrated by nonreaders who had come to me believing that they were "dumb."

Every year of my classroom teaching career was spent with such reluctant learners. Each year I welcomed the nonreaders whom no other teacher wished to have in class. Finally I returned to graduate school to find answers for why such bright children have difficulty learning to read, write, and spell adequately. The required graduate courses for my doctorate in educational psychology and reading education provided no answers.

But several years of research with nonreaders in the military, in state and federal prisons, and throughout the workplace set me on the trail of defining dyslexia.

Throughout the 43 years of my career working with struggling learners, I wondered why I felt a natural kinship with the thousands of nonreaders I have known. Why have I always been drawn to this portion of our culture? Why have I always felt comfortable and in sympathy with those who cannot function well within mainstream education? Finally the answer came in the spring of 2000 when my family had to move my elderly mother into a skilled nursing center. While helping her sort through lifelong keepsakes, I discovered a dusty box that had not been opened in many years. Inside that box I found a collection of my childhood school papers that had been saved with maternal affection. I discovered that as a child, I had been a struggling learner like countless ones I have met.

Figure P.1 shows an example of my handwriting when I entered fourth grade. Today we recognize readily this LD signature in a bright but struggling child: awkward penmanship; inconsistent letter formations; inability to keep the writing level on the lines; frequent overwriting to correct mistakes; obvious insecurity and uncertainty during the writing task; frequent erasing to change what was written first; ragged, uneven spacing between words; inconsistent use of capital letters and punctuation marks; failure to bump the left margin; inability to judge the writing space correctly.

As I pondered this forgotten classroom moment from my childhood, I understood my career choice and my attraction to those who struggle to read and write. All my life I have had to cope with moderate dyslexic patterns that never were identified or described for me or my family. Through constant lifelong effort, I overcame dyslexia enough to succeed. In an important way, this book is the story of my life, showing the several faces of dyslexia that I have overcome.

The following chapters describe numerous faces of dyslexia that frustrate classroom learning for as many as 12 out of every 100 learners in our culture. Chapter 1 summarizes remarkable new information about how genetic codes determine brain development from the moment of conception into adolescence. Chapter 1 also describes how differences in brain structure cause dyslexia. Chapter 2 explains the perceptual and emotional

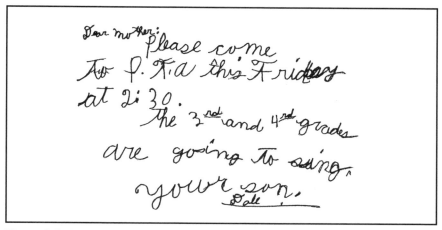

Figure P.1. My dyslexic handwriting when I was 9 years old.

nature of dyslexia. Chapter 3 describes the problems of poor central vision for reading and attention deficit disorders that often exist beneath the surface of dyslexia. Chapters 4 through 6 describe the four most common subtypes of this learning difference: visual dyslexia, auditory dyslexia, dysgraphia, and dyscalculia. Chapter 7 describes the emotions, feelings, and moods that trip up struggling learners with failure and low self-confidence. Chapter 8 tells about the NVLD (nonverbal LD) and SELD (social–emotional LD) that often accompany dyslexia. Chapter 8 also presents strategies for developing effective social skills and learning to live independently. Chapter 9 tells dynamic victory stories of how eight prominent adults overcame dyslexic challenges in their lives. Finally, the appendices provide assessment techniques to help teachers and parents identify types of dyslexia, attention deficits, and other kinds of differences that make classroom learning and social success difficult for 20% of our population.

How the Brain Prepares for Learning

1

The 20th century ended with mixed messages for educators who work with those who struggle to read. On one hand, the century closed with enthusiastic hope as the Decade of the Brain revealed inspiring new information about how the human brain functions in learning—or in failing to learn. Through several genome projects, an international consortium of scientists unlocked genetic secrets to read the biological codes that tell genes and chromosomes how to build new offspring. Using new generations of brain mapping, such as fMRI (functional magnetic resonance imaging), neuroscientists discovered astonishing details about how the brain develops and learns, or fails to learn. New chapters opened in our understanding of how inherited tendencies blend with cultural experience to mold the "hardwiring" of the maturing brain. The Decade of the Brain added new knowledge of the plasticity of the brain throughout life. We learned that certain types of stimulus continue to change brain structure into advanced old age. Also, scientists documented unfortunate lifelong consequences of failing to give a young child's brain the right kinds of stimulation for learning (Bandler & Shipley, 1994; Birren & Shaie, 1990; Brothers, 1997; Charness & Bosman, 1992; Chugani, 1999; Damasio, 1994, 1999; Eliot, 1999; Fisher, 1992; Hooker, 1992).

On the other hand, the American culture continues to face the fact that several million children, adolescents, and adults are illiterate. On the eve of the new millennium, the National Institute of Child Health and Human Development (NICHD) published this statement:

> At least 20 percent of all children have difficulty due to learn-ing disabilities. The first casualty is self-esteem. They soon grow ashamed as they struggle with a skill their classmates master easily. (NICHD, 1998)

As the new millennium began, the *Jordan Dyslexia Assess-ment/Reading Program* summarized the social challenge that illiteracy continues to impose on the American culture:

> Being illiterate in our culture is a devasting condition. Enor-mous emotional problems develop early in nonreaders who suf-fer from low self-esteem and anger over being isolated from the rest of society. Being illiterate spawns disruptive behavior that often leads desperate individuals into addictions, emotional im-balance, or even mental illness. Being illiterate is degrading and a constant source of shame. (Jordan, 2000a, p. 1)

Brain Structure and Dyslexia

This chapter reviews current knowledge about how the human brain prepares for learning, along with new information about why certain individuals do not learn to read, write, or spell. Knowing how the brain develops gives educators increased power to discover new ways to stimulate brain regions to read. Step by step, this chapter explains brain development from the moment of conception into childhood, showing how differences in brain for-mation contribute to learning difficulties. The goal of this chapter is to focus the reader's attention first on how brain development controls classroom learning, and second on how knowledge of brain functions guides new teaching strategies that bring hope to struggling learners. Through understanding the brain, educators are equipped to deal more successfully with dyslexia and other types of learning struggles described in later chapters.

The Role of Genetic Codes

It is nothing new to say that who we are at birth and who we be-come as adults are largely determined by inherited family char-acteristics. For centuries we have known that physical traits such as tallness, left or right handedness, color of eyes, shape of ears, or how one smiles often are passed down family lines so that grandchildren may closely resemble grandparents. Human tradition has assumed that certain talents "run in families," as when several children of Johann Sebastian Bach also became musicians. During the 1920s Samuel Orton's research of dyslexic families (described in Chapter 2) convinced him that dyslexia is inherited (Orton, 1925, 1937). However, Orton had no way to prove his hypothesis. During the 1960s Norman Geschwind and Walter Levitsky at Harvard School of Medicine discovered predictable differences in how dyslexic brains are structured, adding to the belief that genetics plays a major role in passing dyslexia from one generation to the next (Geschwind & Levitsky, 1968). Finally in 1991 a research team at the University of Colorado discovered that dyslexia is genetically transmitted by chromosomes 6 and 15 (DeFries, Olson, Pennington, & Smith, 1991). As instructors work with struggling readers, knowing that these individuals cannot help being dyslexic removes temptation to blame them or shame them for not trying harder.

During the Decade of the Brain neuroscientists learned that approximately 97% of brain formations are predetermined by genetic codes that are activated at the moment of conception. From that moment onward, neurons appear and interconnect according to specific genetic blueprints. Axons follow preset genetic plans in building connections between neurons, both in persons who are gifted readers and in those who inherit a dyslexic block that prohibits reading. Dendrites and synapse junctions sprout from neurons according to inherited genetic commands (Damasio, 1994, 1999; Eliot, 1999; O'Rahilly & Muller, 1996). The remainder of this chapter guides the reader step by step through how the brain develops during gestation and how differences in brain structure cause such learning difficulties as *learning disability* (LD), *dyslexia, attention deficit disorder,* or *delayed language development.*

The First Stage of Brain Development

Synaptogenesis

At the moment of fertilization, the impregnated ovum receives the urgent genetic command to grow and multiply at a mind-boggling speed of cell reproduction. Between the moment of conception and the birth of a full-term infant 9 months later, the initial fertilized single cell multiplies into several trillion cells that make up the body of the newborn child. New cells emerge at astonishing speed. For example, at the 25th day of gestation, a highly specialized process called *synaptogenesis* begins in the embryonic spinal cord. Between the 4th week of pregnancy and age 2, synaptogenesis produces new synapse junctions at the unbelievable rate of 1.8 million per second (Carlson, 1994; Eliot, 1999; Huttenlocher, 1990; Jacobson, 1991). Yet building new offspring at such incredible speed is not a random process. Nearly every developmental step between conception and birth is guided by preset genetic codes that persist from one generation to the next. When genetic codes for dyslexia exist, some of the earliest neuronal pathways develop differently so that when higher brain regions begin to process language, the child struggles to hear speech sounds, imitate speech patterns, and comprehend the meaning of oral language.

How Genetic Codes Build a Brain

To construct a brain, nature uses a variety of predesignated parts, much as a construction crew erects a building from predesigned girders, boards, and insulating materials. A human brain is made from as many as 100 billion nerve cells, each of which plays an individual role. Each nerve cell is called a *neuron,* as Figure 1.1 shows. When neurons first appear, they resemble newly sprouted seeds with a simple root at one end and a short stem at the other. The roots of the neuron are called *dendrites.* Their purpose is to bring new information into the neuron from other cells. At the opposite end of the neuron grows a stem-like structure called an *axon.* The purpose of each axon is to pass information on to connecting neurons. Most axons are extremely short, sometimes only a millimeter or so in length. Some specialized axons are several inches long in order to connect distant body regions to the brain. When dyslexia exists, many neurons fail to develop completely, leaving gaps along axon pathways that interfere with brain activity. These gaps are similar to bridges out along a highway system. To think through a mental task from start to finish, dyslexic individuals are forced to exert much more brain energy than those who are not dyslexic. These gaps in neuron structure require the dyslexic brain to spend precious energy and extra time seeking detours around missing links along axon pathways.

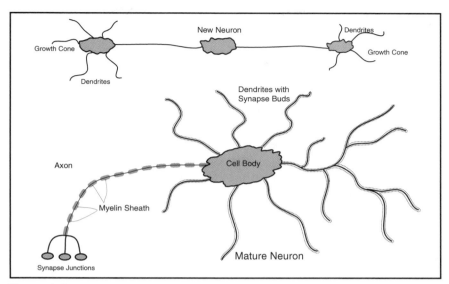

Figure 1.1. During the 9 months of gestation, new neurons emerge at the rate of 250,000 per minute. Many neurons require several years of physical maturation and stimulus to become fully mature.

Neurogenesis

Shortly after the fertilized ovum grows into an embryo, a process called *neurogenesis* becomes active. As the embryo grows older, neurogenesis causes each neuron to develop new features that look like a plant with roots, a stem, buds, and branches (see Figure 1.1). Neuroscientists often use the term *dendrite tree*. The brain is made of billions of neurons whose branches (dendrites and axons) interconnect to form an incredibly complex electrical system. By the time a baby is born, the brain contains most of the basic neurons that the central nervous system will use for the rest of that person's life. However, many years of physical maturation are required before neurons become fully developed. Genetic codes dictate that by birth, the brain must contain approximately 100 billion neurons. To reach this amazing goal, neurogenesis is genetically driven to create new neurons at the rate of 250,000 per minute during the 9 months of gestation. When LD, dyslexia, or attention deficits exist in the family line, many neurons are stunted and only partially developed at these early stages of development. Later in the child's life, too many neurons remain underdeveloped to allow the brain to build rapid, fluent habits of processing new information accurately.

Growth Cones

The neurons that emerge during gestation are at first very simple in shape and structure (see Figure 1.1). At the tip of each dendrite is a *growth cone*. Genetic codes create an aggressive "seeking out" activity that causes new dendrites to grow toward other neurons. The goal of the growth cones is to form connections that link neurons into tiny communication clusters called *nuclei*. Immediately after each neuron pops into existance, it begins to migrate to its final location by following the "tugging effect" of the growth cones. Each growth cone is genetically programmed to follow particular chemical signals coming from other newborn neurons. Genetic codes trigger production of chemicals that bond preselected neurons into countless neuronal networks that eventually make up the white matter and gray matter of the mature brain.

Science has not learned yet why certain neurons find their way to specific regions of the brain. Why does a new neuron migrate to the retina to become part of the complex system that gives us sight? Why do other neurons migrate to the middle ear or the auditory cortex to give us hearing? Neuroscientists have discovered that the final destination of migrating neurons is determined mostly by genetic codes (nature) and partly by the quality of stimulus (nurture) the developing brain receives. In the 1980s, Albert Galaburda (1986) and Veronika Grimm (1986) discovered that when the fetus is predisposed to being dyslexic, early neuron development is interrupted by imbalances in body chemistry. For these pregnancies, the mother's body chemistry is allergic to the fetus. Most of these pregnancies are marked by pronounced morning sickness. This biochemical struggle between mother and fetus interrupts normal development of neurons in the fetal brain. During childhood, these babies experience delayed language development that later is diagnosed as dyslexia.

Synapses and Neurotransmitters

Every part of the brain communicates through electrical energy that fires down dendrite pathways, along with specialized chemicals that squirt across synapses from one axon or dendrite to the next. Starting at the 8th week of gestation, synaptogenesis introduces a new feature of neuron development that prepares the emerging spinal cord and brain stem for rapid information processing. As axons mature, they sprout new sequences of spaced segments called *synapses*. During peak dendrite growth, new synapses emerge at the rate of 1.8 million per second. Chemical bundles called *neurotransmitters* squirt across synapse junctions, carrying the brain's information from sending axons to receiving dendrites.

Brain research has identified several dozen neurotransmitters that perform specialized communication tasks throughout the brain. Four neurotransmitters are responsible for most of an individual's learning, memory, and emotional well-being. *Dopamine* regulates the alertness, or arousal, of the higher brain where logic and commonsense reasoning occur. Dopamine is the key brain regulator for paying attention. Well-balanced dopamine also creates a sense of self-satisfaction and tells the brain when the person has had enough. Poorly balanced dopamine contributes to attention deficit disorder and social–emotional LD, as described in Chapters 3 and 8. *Serotonin* stays in charge of strong emotions and feelings that want to "do it now, not later." Serotonin enables the brain to wait rather than yield to impulse. Not enough serotonin triggers depression, anxiety, and impulsivity. Too much serotonin fosters aggression and violent behavior. *Acetylcholine* is a key regulator in developing accurate short-term and long-term memory. Low levels of acetylcholine prevent the higher brain from building permanent memory of classroom skills. *Norepinephrine* teams with serotonin and dopamine to stabilize emotions and feelings in order to avoid depression or too much anxiety. Lack of norepinephrine sets into motion the habits of tantrums, emotional outbursts, rapid mood swings, and insatiable demands.

In most individuals with learning disabilities, these neurotransmitters are out of balance. Along with reading problems, dyslexic students often are troubled by mood swings, cycles of depression, overwhelming anxiety, and fear of failure caused by neurotransmitters that became out of balance even before birth.

Myelination

The brain can be compared with a computer that transmits information through electrical energy carried by pulsing electrons along connecting wires. The brain does function through electrical energy, but instead of sending a prolonged electron flow along axon pathways, the brain fires bundles of ionized chemical particles along neuron pathways. This rapid flow of ions creates the brain's "fluidlike electrical flow" that can be measured as electrical energy (Calvin & Ojemann, 1980; Damasio, 1994, 1999; Llinas, 1993). As chemical ion bundles travel along neuron pathways, they leak. This causes brain activity to lose power and focus. To avoid ion leakage, the brain develops a fatty insulation material called *myelin* that coats each neuron segment the way insulation covers wires within electrical circuits. The process of covering axon segments with myelin is called *myelination*. The primary purpose of myelin is to speed up the rate at which axons and dendrites transfer information throughout the brain. As myelination builds insulation around axon and dendrite fibers, the brain develops faster rates of processing (Eliot, 1999; Huttenlocher, 1990; Llinas, 1993).

Figure 1.1 shows the myelin bundles that insulate axons to preserve brain energy between sending and receiving cells. Incomplete myelin development is largely responsible for attention deficits, dyslexia, and a slow rate of mental processing. When myelin formation is incomplete, the individual cannot speed up his or her rate of processing, nor can the person keep on paying attention.

Diet and Brain Development

Genetic codes (nature) determine when myelination should begin in different regions of the brain. However, the mother's diet (nurture) controls how well myelination occurs. For example, the developing fetus must receive ample amounts of fat, folic acid (vitamin B_1 complex), iron, iodine, and vitamin B_{12} to produce complete myelination. If the mother fails to eat adequate amounts of these building block foods, the myelin of an undernourished fetus will be too thin with many gaps that fail to insulate neuron pathways adequately. If the mother's diet is too low in calories or lacks enough protein, growth of the developing brain will be stunted with too few neurons to form complete linking pathways. Such a malnourished brain cannot acquire the fully developed neuronal structures required for good language development and long-term memory (Eliot, 1999; Jordan, 1998; Rogan & Gladen, 1993). Babies born to young teenage mothers are likely to be low-birthweight infants whose mothers had poor diets during gestation. These newborns are at very high risk for having delayed language development, reading disabilities, and attention deficits.

Pruning

The Decade of the Brain documented the irony that the young brain produces far more dendrites, axons, and synapses than the mature brain can use effectively. Between the 8th month of gestation and age 2, the new brain develops a tangled thicket of surplus neurons, as shown in Figure 1.2. From the moment of birth, fierce competition occurs inside this mass of neuron structures. The most frequently used neurons survive this competition, but

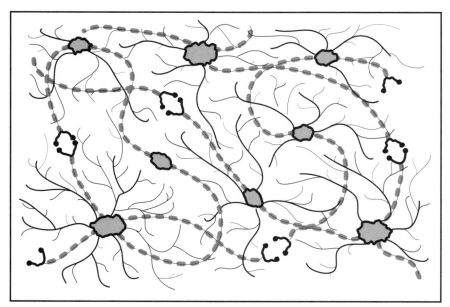

Figure 1.2. Between the 8th month of gestation and age 2, several billion neural pathways emerge like a tangled thicket. If all of these neural clusters survived, it would be impossible for the brain to become organized and efficient.

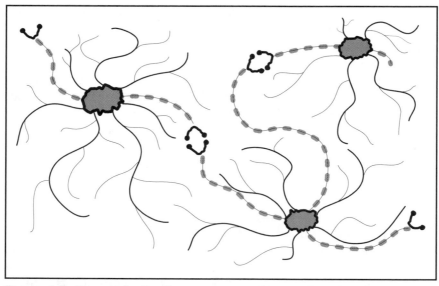

Figure 1.3. Repeated stimulus causes certain neural pathways to become strong and dominant, whereas other pathways that are not stimulated melt away through a process called *pruning*.

those used least melt away in a process called *pruning*. As time goes by, excess neurons are pruned so that only the most efficient ones remain, as Figure 1.3 shows. The surviving dendrites and axons become the permanent, lifelong pathways that connect brain regions and govern future learning and long-term memory.

When genetic tendencies for dyslexia or attention deficit disorder exist, too little pruning takes place. This leaves too many brain pathways, making it impossible for the person to stay focused and alert or to build long-term memory for literacy skills. These students are classroom underachievers and poorly functioning workers who rarely perform to their full potential.

The Three-Part Brain

Emotions and Feelings: Descartes' Error

New information from the Decade of the Brain has pressed educators and mental health providers to reconsider how the brain functions in learning and building long-term memory. For more than 300 years, most curriculum models in Western cultures have assumed that the duty of teachers is to stuff the higher brain with facts and information largely through passive listening and reading. Educators have believed that the duty of learners is to absorb reams of facts and data, then return that knowledge through exams to show how much the brain has learned. This model of education was based largely on the philosophy of the 17th-century French mathematician, René Descartes, who taught that formal learning must be kept free from emotions and feelings. Descartes insisted that the best learners are those who leave their emotions and feelings outside the classroom experience. Descartes believed that the brain is a living machine that processes new information the way a mathematician solves algebraic equations through unemotional logic. This point of view has molded most of the Western world's attitudes toward how the brain works while learning and remembering.

In 1994 Antonio Damasio, an imaginative neuroscientist at the University of Iowa School of Medicine, challenged Descartes' ideas in the book *Descartes' Error: Emotion, Reason, and the Human Brain.* By incorporating new knowledge gleaned through brain imaging science, Damasio demonstrated that historically we have gone about teaching and learning backwards. Several specialists have described the critical role that emotions and feelings play in all learning experiences (Damasio, 1994, 1999; Denckla, 1991a; Jordan, 1998, 2000a, 2000b; Ratey & Johnson, 1997; Schacter, 1996).

Is This Safe?

As our culture enters the new millennium, we have realized that learning does not happen first in the higher brain, as Descartes insisted. Instead, learning and memory result from filtered information that first must pass the brain stem's test question: "Is this safe?" If new events and data are harmless and safe, then the higher brain receives that information with calm emotions and feelings so that logic prevails and long-term memory occurs. However, if new data threaten the individual with unsafe consequences, the "fight-or-flight" reflex is triggered throughout the brain. Deciding whether to run away, or stay and fight, is where the brain begins to learn. Facts come later after the three-part brain has filtered new information for the issue of emotional comfort (safety). When the genetic tendency for dyslexia or attention deficit exists, the individual is vulnerable to overly charged emotions and feelings that interfere with learning. One of the most time-consuming tasks of instructors is to help struggling learners remain calm in their emotions and feelings. It is impossible to teach new skills to students who are overly afraid or feel threatened by possible failure.

The Three-Part Human Brain

From the time of Leonardo da Vinci in the 15th century, scientists have known that the human brain is not a single solid structure. Da Vinci's anatomical research revealed that the brain is made of many parts, some of which we see but others are hidden inside thick layers of "gray matter." In the final decades of the 20th century, neuroscientists discovered developmental sequences that govern how regions of the brain work together for learning.

Basal Brain

The first step in learning occurs within the long ignored brain region called the *reptilian brain,* the *ancient brain,* or the *basal brain.* The first part of the basal brain to emerge in a developing embryo is the spinal column (see Figure 1.4). Nestled safely inside this structure is the *spinal cord* that, for the rest of the person's life, is the point of entry for all new data the higher brain receives (Damasio, 1994, 1999; Eliot, 1999; Jordan, 1998, 2000a, 2000b). By the end of the 4th week of gestation, genetic programs have guided specialized neurons to form what soon becomes the *spinal column.* At this stage of fetal development, new neurons emerge at the rate of 250,000 per minute. The emerging spinal column is the primitive brain that controls movement and sensory reactions of the embryo before it develops into the fetus. Figure 1.5 shows the specialized motor and sensory neurons that surround the spinal cord. Later these neurons connect with the motor cortex and somatosensory cortex in the higher brain (see Figure 1.8 later in this chapter). Five weeks after conception, emerging eyelids react with a flutter to being touched by currents in the amniotic fluid. The four limb buds that soon become tiny arms and legs begin to twitch and rotate. Already the primitive

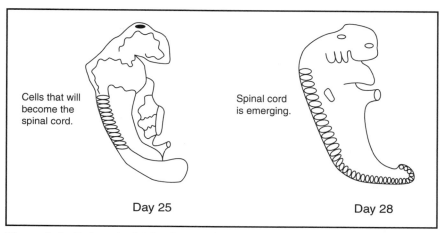

Cells that will become the spinal cord.

Spinal cord is emerging.

Day 25

Day 28

Figure 1.4. Before the higher brain emerges, the embryonic spinal cord begins to filter incoming data. This is the first step in the brain's lifelong work of dealing first with feelings and emotions, then with facts. By day 28, the emerging spinal cord starts its task of monitoring new sensations. (Based on research by Carlson, 1994; Eliot, 1999; Hill & Mistretta, 1990; and Larsen, 1993.)

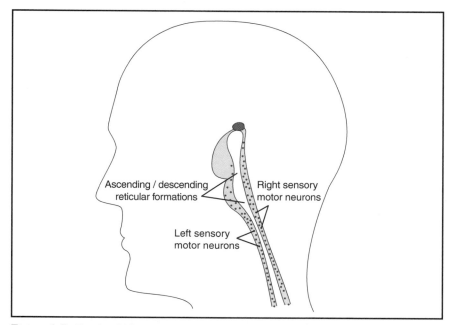

Ascending / descending reticular formations

Right sensory motor neurons

Left sensory motor neurons

Figure 1.5. By the fifth week of gestation, the spinal cord's left and right sensory and motor neurons, along with the emerging reticular formations, begin to send movement signals to the limb buds that will become the baby's arms and legs.

tongue can taste chemical elements in the amniotic fluid. These very early actions and reactions are governed by the motor and sensory neurons within the spinal column (Carlson, 1994; Eliot, 1999; Hill & Mistretta, 1990; Larsen, 1993). For the rest of the individual's life, these spinal cord motor and sensory neurons will play critical roles in governing automatic reponse to environmental stimuli. At this early stage of fetal development, it is possible to detect chronic hyperactivity that will become a source of social conflict and frustrated learning during childhood.

Brain Stem

Between the 1st and 7th months of gestation, the fetus achieves a fully developed basal brain, as shown in Figure 1.6. Atop the

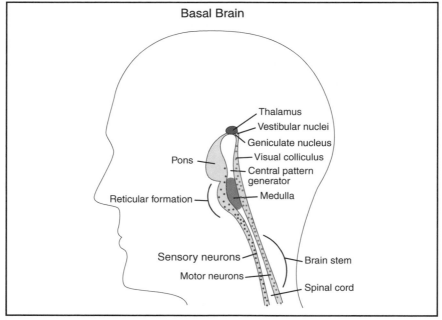

Figure 1.6. By the end of the 6th month of gestation, the basal brain is fully formed. For the rest of this person's life, these basal brain regions will filter all new data before any new information reaches the higher brain. The basal brain stands guard over the fight-or-flight reflex that protects the person from emotional danger. At the same time, these regions of the basal brain control all of the body's autonomic activities, such as breathing, digestion, heart beat, and blood pressure.

spinal column grows the *brain stem* that performs critical life-long functions that keep the individual well balanced, feeling safe, and skilled at motor tasks. Within the brain stem are several specialized regions that work automatically in teams to regulate essential body functions.

Sensory Neurons. Along the right side of the emerging spinal column are strings of specialized neurons that filter sensations from touch, which is the first body sense to emerge. By the 9th week of gestation, these sensory neurons have formed axon links to the cells that will become the chin, eyelids, and arms. By the 10th week, sensory neurons connect with emerging legs. By the 12th week, these spinal cord sensory neurons are connected with the entire body surface of the fetus. Toward the end of the second trimester of gestation, spinal cord sensory neurons begin to communicate with the thalamus for the lifelong purpose of regulating emotional reactions to touching and being touched. In most developing fetuses, these early sensory reactions become rhythmical, steady, and safe. However, when genetic tendencies for attention deficits exist, the fetus remains overly sensitive and "touchy." During childhood these youngsters have difficulty learning socialization skills. They are difficult children who overreact to normal events that involve physical contact with others.

Motor Neurons. By the 7th week of gestation, other specialized neurons along the left side of the spinal cord begin to control movement in the developing head and four limb buds. These are the *motor neurons* that later will link with the higher brain motor cortex to regulate muscle movements throughout the body. When a fetus inherits genetic codes for dyslexia, these early motor neurons develop differently. Later on the child tends to be awkward and behind schedule in achieving normal motor coordination.

Central Pattern Generator. One of the first motor control regions of the early brain is the *central pattern generator* (CPG) that emerges in the brain stem toward the end of the first trimester of gestation. The CPG is a cluster of motor neurons that becomes the lifelong control center of rhythmical muscle movements anywhere in the body. As the limb buds develop, the CPG regulates sweeping, rotating movements of the emerging arms and legs. As the eyes develop, the CPG regulates back-and-forth and up-and-down eye motions called *nystagmus*. During the second and third trimesters of gestation, the CPG controls rapid eye movements (REM) as the fetus enters sleep/wake cycles. Throughout an individual's lifetime, the CPG regulates all rhythmical muscle activity, such as chewing, breathing, walking, running, hopping, skipping, or swimming. In many children who inherit dyslexia, the CPG and other motor coordination centers of the brain do not reach complete development, causing the child not to learn how to do things rhythmically.

Medulla. Figure 1.6 shows the lower region of the brain stem called the medulla. The medulla is the first part of the brain to challenge new data with the emotional question: "Is this safe?" Toward the end of the first trimester of gestation, the medulla sets into motion the fight-or-flight reflex that will govern how the individual responds to new events (Calvin & Ojemann, 1980; Damasio, 1994, 1999; Eliot, 1999; Jordan, 1998, 2000a, 2000b; Schacter, 1996). Children who have learning difficulties tend to remain overly fearful and anxious all their lives. In these LD individuals, the medulla does not become mature enough to carry out its job of safeguarding the whole brain from fight-or-flight reactions.

Reticular Formation. As the brain stem emerges, a neuron cluster called the reticular formation takes shape above the medulla. The *reticular formation* plays a key lifelong role in how the individual perceives and responds to the external environment. The reticular formation filters and organizes the first sensations of pleasure and pain. As internal organs emerge within the fetus, the reticular formation governs the rhythms of the heart, lungs, and digestive tract. As the fetus enters higher levels of development, the reticular formation participates in taste, as well as in cycles of wakefulness and deep sleep. Finally, the reticular formation becomes the regulator for the lifelong balance among essential body functions called *homeostasis*. As the brain reaches full maturity during childhood and adolescence, the reticular formation takes charge of keeping emotions, feelings, sensations, and perceptions evenly balanced. For the rest of the individual's life, the reticular formation plays a critical role in the person's sense of well-being.

Chapter 2 describes the physical differences seen in many individuals who are dyslexic. A major problem for dyslexic persons is lifelong discomfort in the digestive tract, especially the lower intestine. Regardless of how diet is changed or controlled, dyslexic individuals live with chronic "gut ache" called gastritis. This physical problem is linked to incomplete development of the reticular formation during gestation.

Pons. By the beginning of the second trimester, a prominent bulge forms at the top of the brain stem. This dense cluster of neurons rapidly builds axon links to the spinal cord, central pattern generator, reticular formation, and basal ganglia. The *pons* is a major participant in regulating the body's physical activity. The pons also plays a key role in sleep. As the higher brain falls asleep, the pons fires a command that paralyzes all of the larger muscles. This is called *sleep paralysis,* which occurs as the brain slips into deep sleep cycles. During sleep paralysis, the higher brain engages in dreaming, which often involves episodes of aggressive, hyperactive body activity. If the pons fails to complete its sleep paralysis job, dream energy "leaks" into large muscles, causing the sleeping person to thrash about, cry out, sleepwalk, or act out part of the dream content. Individuals who inherit attention deficits or dyslexia often have lifelong sleep disturbance because the pons does not achieve full development.

Thalamus. During the 15th week of gestation, the top of the brain stem grows into a divided formation called the *thalamus* that becomes the relay station between the basal brain and higher brain regions. Incoming sensory data are filtered by the thalamus, then fired up to the somatosensory cortex in the left- and right-brain hemispheres. At the same time, the left region of the thalamus filters and preorganizes verbal data that are transferred to the parietal and temporal lobes for processing. The right region of the thalamus filters and preorganizes visual and spatial information that is fired to appropriate regions of the higher brain.

Vestibular Nuclei. In the top region of the brain stem are clusters of specialized neurons called the *vestibular nuclei.* These neurons are the first step in hearing. During the third trimester of gestation, the developing vestibular organs within both ears begin to hear sound patterns, such as mother's voice, certain decibel ranges of environmental sound and noise, and certain ranges of musical tone. The vestibular nuclei become part of the lifelong fight-or-flight filtering system by checking the safety of all new sounds and noise. When family genetic lines transfer dyslexia or attention deficits to new generations, it is not unusual to find several blood relatives who overreact to sounds. These individuals are "jumpy" and nervous. All their lives they are too easily startled, react to sound with exaggerated protests, and rarely feel comfortable with or safe from environmental noise.

Visual Colliculus. During the third trimester of gestation, the eyes become sensitive to light. This primitive visual response is processed by the *visual colliculus* in the brain stem. As vision develops during infancy and childhood, the visual colliculus becomes part of the visual system described in Chapter 3. Difficulties in visual perception often begin when neurons are underdeveloped within the visual colliculus. A major earmark of dyslexia is lifelong difficulty interpreting what the person sees. Neurons within the visual colliculus fail to reach full maturity, which contributes to inaccurate visual perception throughout the person's life span.

Geniculate Nucleus. Nestled close to the thalamus is a cluster of specialized neurons called the *geniculate nucleus.* During infancy and early childhood, the geniculate nucleus plays a critical role in how the individual sees and hears. If neurons in the lateral geniculate nucleus fail to develop fully, visual perception problems such as scotopic sensitivity syndrome may emerge to create "word blindness" in which print patterns swirl, move sideways, or merge into dark smudges. Underdeveloped neurons within the medial geniculate nucleus may distort how the person perceives oral language. This causes the poor auditory perceptual dysfunction called *central auditory processing disorder,* or the "tone-deaf" condition called *auditory dyslexia.*

Midbrain

During the second trimester of gestation, the *midbrain* emerges, as shown in Figure 1.7. The midbrain also is called the *limbic system.* As brain development continues, the midbrain becomes one of the master control centers for the three-part brain. Clustered together in the limbic system are the major controls for strong emotions and feelings. Several regions of the limbic system filter incoming verbal and nonverbal information, then determine what data reach the higher brain. Some of the midbrain members regulate the many enzymes, hormones, and neurotransmitters

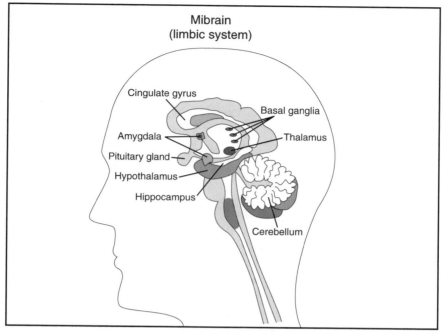

Figure 1.7. During the second trimester of gestation, these regions of the midbrain (limbic system) emerge. The limbic system becomes one of the brain's master control centers that regulates strong emotions, filters new verbal and nonverbal information, and maintains balance of brain chemistry. (Based on research by Calvin & Ojemann, 1980; Damasio, 1994, 1999; Eliot, 1990; Hampton-Turner, 1981; Jacobson, 1991; and Purves & Lichtman, 1985.)

that make up body chemistry. Contrary to what Descartes and other philosophers believed, the process of blending information into learning and memory begins in the midbrain.

Cerebellum. One of the first midbrain structures to emerge is the *cerebellum*. This part of the limbic system contains half of all the neurons in the entire brain. Lise Eliot (1999) has compared the cerebellum to the air traffic control tower that regulates aircraft movements at a busy airport. The main job of the cerebellum is to interpret for the higher brain every type of movement attempted by large and small muscles. The cerebellum determines the best possible integration of body movement, vision, and hearing. It would be impossible for the body to walk, lean, run, stand, or turn corners without the cerebellum's constant monitoring. Martha Denckla (1985, 1991b, 1993) at Johns Hopkins School of

Medicine has been a pioneer in observing the role that the cerebellum plays in paying full attention, preventing random muscle movement, and organizing whole body behavior.

The cerebellum also regulates a vital process called *proprioception*. Within the cerebellum specialized neurons called *proprioceptors* form a sensory loop that links the spinal cord with the higher brain. This proprioceptor network is similar to an antilock braking system that keeps vehicles from skidding on slick pavement. Many times per second the vehicle computer adjusts how much pressure the braking system applies to each wheel. In milliseconds each wheel receives slightly more or less pressure to stop. This constantly changing braking pressure keeps wheels from locking, which would send the vehicle skidding out of control. In a similar way, the proprioceptor neurons adjust the extension and retraction movements of muscle fibers all over the body. The cerebellum is the command center that "fine-tunes" all muscle action to keep the body well balanced.

Individuals who inherit attention deficit disorder or dyslexia often have incomplete neuron development throughout the cerebellum. This triggers disruptive behavior that involves excessive restlessness, poor attention, irregular motor coordination, and nonstop overflow of energy that normally would be contained by the proprioceptor system.

Basal Ganglia. During the second trimester of gestation, twin neuron clusters appear near the thalamus. The *basal ganglia* are the first brain regions to distinguish between voluntary and involuntary muscle movements. The body's muscle coordination team consists of motor neurons, the central pattern generator, the cerebellum, the motor cortex, and the basal ganglia. As the basal ganglia mature, the person gains fluency of volunteer muscle movement for such activities as walking, running, lifting, turning, swimming, handwriting, and keyboard writing. The basal ganglia provide a feedback circuit that instantaneously informs the whole brain of what muscle systems are doing. A major problem for many dyslexic individuals is awkwardness in writing, walking, running, hopping, and playing active games. When dyslexia is inherited, many blood-related family members behave in this awkward way.

Cingulate Gyrus. Like a walkway encircling a park, following curves and hills and valleys, the *cingulate gyrus* surrounds much of the limbic system. This long portion of the midbrain plays a key role in integrating and coordinating body motion, speech, and emotional expression. For most individuals, these are the core elements of personality that distinguish each person from all others. The cingulate gyrus teams with the hypothalamus and thalamus to create a "self-map" of who each of us is as an individual. Often this is called the *proto-self* that, like a self-portrait, allows us to know ourselves for who we really are. The cingulate gyrus also filters sensory data and emotions that are linked to pain and pleasure. Chapter 8 describes personality disorders, such as Asperger's syndrome, SELD (social–emotional LD), and NVLD (nonverbal LD), that are partly caused when neurons within the cingulate gyrus fail to develop fully. When this occurs, individuals do not develop the ability to see themselves accurately. In these developmentally delayed individuals, the proto-self is distorted and incomplete. When underdeveloped neurons within the cingulate gyrus produce a warped or twisted proto-self, delusional syndromes such as schizophrenia and paranoia emerge to prevent the individual from perceiving reality.

Amygdala. Toward the end of the second trimester of gestation, twin clusters of neurons called the *amygdala* emerge within the limbic system. The amygdala becomes a vital crossroads of neurons that connect the brain stem and the higher brain. Most of the linking neurons in the brain pass through the amygdala terminals. The amygdala regulates automatic decision making that does not require conscious thought, such as reflexes that pull us away from being burned, falling off a cliff, or stepping into the path of speeding vehicles. The twin lobes of the amygdala team with the prefrontal cortex in the higher brain to blend unconscious decisions with logic and commonsense reasoning.

A major function of the amygdala is control of fear. When the neurons of the amygdala develop fully, the person learns to read danger signals in the environment. The amygdala enables the higher brain to develop a stable emotional balance (homeostasis) that keeps fear and anxiety under control. The amygdala is the midbrain center of social behavior, enabling individuals to suppress inappropriate social impulse, avoid inappropriate social habits, and learn how to balance positive and negative emotions. The amygdala controls strong emotions such as rage, terror, hatred, urge to kill, lust, and desire for revenge. The amygdala modifies impulsive urges so that individuals learn to wait. Chapter 8 describes the irregular lifestyle of Asperger's syndrome, also called "social dyslexia," that is caused when incomplete neurons within the amygdala fail to control inappropriate social habits and behaviors. When the amygdala does not develop fully, there may be no sense of fear or no fight-or-flight reflex to keep the person safe.

Hypothalamus and Pituitary Gland. Two parts of the midbrain work together to regulate how the body responds to stress. The *hypothalamus* and the *pituitary gland* keep constant vigil over external and internal stress signals. The moment an individual experiences stress or anxiety, the hypothalamus and pituitary gland transform neural electrical energy into chemical signals that trigger production of stress control hormones. These stress regulation hormones squirt across synapse junctions to control surges of fear, anxiety, or panic. The hypothalamus and pituitary gland stand constant watch over strong emotions. These midbrain members govern the fight-or-flight reflex. They also regulate the autonomic system that controls involuntary body functions such as heart beat, breathing, intestinal action, and blood pressure. The hypothalamus and pituitary gland cooperate with the amygdala to govern strong negative emotions such as sadness, depression, anger, fear, and despair. These limbic system members help the cingulate gyrus to maintain a positive protoself that fosters positive self-esteem. The hypothalamus and pituitary gland help the higher brain maintain full attention with full arousal of thinking processes (Calvin & Ojemann, 1980; Damasio, 1994, 1999; Eliot, 1999; Hampton-Turner, 1981; Jacobson, 1991; Purves & Lichtman, 1985).

Higher Brain

By the end of the second trimester of gestation, the higher brain has emerged, as Figure 1.8 shows. However, several more years will pass before all of the higher brain regions become fully functional. The higher brain is enclosed in a tough membrane called the *dura.* Beneath the dura is the *cerebrum,* the outer surface of the brain that includes all of the folds (fissures) and crevices (sulci) that create the brain's distinctive appearance. The paper-thin outer layer of the cerebrum is the *cerebral cortex* where most of the brain's thinking, learning, and remem-

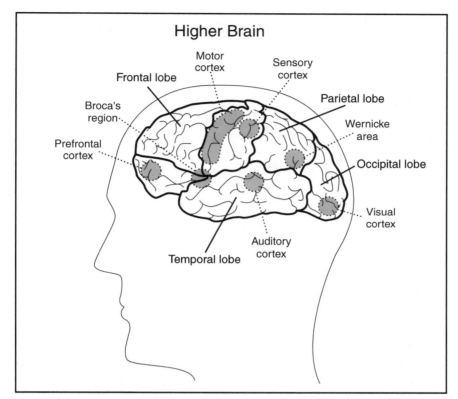

Figure 1.8. By the end of the second trimester of gestation, these regions of the higher brain have emerged. However, the higher brain will not become functional until early childhood. For the rest of this person's life, cultural stimulus will govern neuron pruning that will establish which talents and skills this individual will achieve.

bering occur. The cerebral cortex is made of three layers of neurons only 3 millimeters thick, less than the distance between two typewriter spaces. At the end of the third trimester of gestation, only a few neurons within the cerebral cortex are fully myelinated. As the infant's head squeezes through the birth canal, a new cycle of neuron development is triggered. This birth canal stimulus starts rapid myelination of higher brain neurons. Between birth and age 7, hundreds of millions of new dendrites and synapse junctions emerge throughout the higher brain at the rate of 250,000 per minute. Rapid myelination prepares the higher brain neurons for their work of developing control of body functions, speech, motor skills, language usage, socialization skills, and readiness for formal school learning (Calvin & Ojemann, 1980; Damasio, 1994, 1999; Eliot, 1999).

Chapters 3 through 6 describe how incomplete neuron formation in the cerebrum causes learning disabilities such as dyslexia, attention deficits, and delayed language development. When these learning differences are genetic in origin, whole families often display similar or identical patterns in struggling to read, write, spell, or pay full attention.

Right-Brain and Left-Brain Hemispheres

The higher brain is made of two hemispheres almost equal in size. In most individuals, the right-brain hemisphere is somewhat larger than the left because of extra neurons. In individuals who are dyslexic, both brain hemispheres are of equal size (Galaburda, 1983; Geschwind, 1984). The right and left hemispheres are connected by the *corpus collosum,* a thick bundle of neurons that links the brain halves for instant communication. Each hemisphere includes the regions shown in Figure 1.8. The brain is constructed so that the right hemisphere controls the left side of the body, whereas the left hemisphere controls the right side of the body. As neurons mature during early childhood, each brain hemisphere develops specialized abilities.

Right-Brain Hemisphere. If the young child receives safe, culturally rich stimulus during the first 2 years of life, the right brain becomes the control center for positive emotion-based thinking, intuition, and nonlanguage problem solving. The right brain is illiterate. It does not learn to read, write, or spell. However, in most individuals a specialized region within the right parietal lobe learns how to monitor the left brain's language processing. Erin Zaidel at the University of California at Los Angeles has described the right brain's "oooops center," which tells the left brain when it has made a mistake in speaking, spelling, reading, handwriting, or math computation (Zaidel & Zaidel, 1979). The major business of the right brain is to imagine, think, plan, create, and make decisions based on feelings, emotions, and hunches (intuition). The right brain is the home of nonverbal talents, such as higher mathematics reasoning, engineering, artistic creation, athletics, and mechanical skills. Also, the right brain teams with the left brain to create and perform music.

Thanks to Zaidel, parents and instructors have reason to appreciate the gift of self-correction as it emerges in children. When a child's higher brain is maturing on schedule, he or she begins to self-correct mistakes during kindergarten or first grade. This is when children begin to erase and change their original writing. This milestone of developing the "Ooops!" response is a signal that learning is on schedule. An earmark of delayed brain development is that dyslexic persons often do not reach this self-correcting milestone. They become adults still not spotting their errors or knowing how to correct them.

Left-Brain Hemisphere. The left brain specializes in logical thinking, commonsense reasoning, and factual thinking. Through the executive function of the prefrontal cortex, the left brain maintains whole brain organization, develops lifelong habits of being methodical, and enables the individual to wait instead of yielding to impulses. In four out of five individuals, the left brain is the language center that has the capacity to learn to read, write, and spell. In one out of five persons who have specific language dysfunctions such as dyslexia, the left brain does not become skilled at reading, handwriting, or spelling (Jordan, 1996a, 1996b, 2000a; Kirsch, Jungeblut, & Campbell, 1992; Lyon, 2000; McGuinness, 1997). If the young child's developing brain is stimulated by cultural emphasis on socialization skills, the left brain becomes the center of higher feelings and emotions, such as patience, kindness, gentleness, and contentment.

Motor/Somatosensory Cortex. The first regions of the higher brain to become active are the *motor cortex* and the *somatosensory cortex*. These centers work together to control muscle behavior and to interpret sensations that are reported by the brain stem and midbrain. As Figure 1.9 shows, motor and sensory control regions develop sequentially, starting with the mouth (tongue and lips), then the face, next the hands and arms, then the trunk of the body, and finally the legs.

As each of these motor cortex regions matures, the child gains control of bathroom functions while learning to tie shoes, open and close zippers, and button or unbutton clothing. By age 6 most children have gained enough motor cortex maturity to learn how to write with a pencil and stay inside the lines with crayons. However, youngsters who have inherited tendencies for delayed language development, dyslexia, or attention deficit

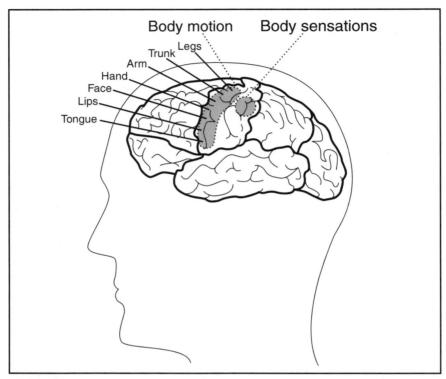

Figure 1.9. By the end of the third trimester of gestation, these sensory and motor control regions of the higher brain are ready to emerge. The more movement, touching, tasting, and smelling the newborn infant enjoys, the faster these motor milestones will be achieved.

often do not follow this developmental schedule. Many of these LD children are significantly behind schedule in bathroom control, zipping, buttoning, using silverware, coloring with crayons, and writing with a pencil.

Parietal Lobes

Toward the back of each brain hemisphere is the parietal lobe that plays several important roles in the person's life. A major function of the parietal lobes is to receive new data from the midbrain and distribute this information to specialized brain regions for final processing. The parietal lobes guide the higher brain in blending previously learned data with new information. The parietal lobes edit and condense new data as they enter long-term memory. When neurons fail to develop fully within the parietal lobes, youngsters are confused by new information and have constant difficulty with long-term memory. What they learn has trouble integrating with what they already know.

Right Parietal Lobe. A major function of the right parietal lobe is to regulate how individuals perceive their own bodies. This physical self-perception is linked to the work of the cingulate gyrus that generates the proto-self, or the self-image each person achieves through repeated emotions and feelings. The right parietal lobe participates in higher math reasoning that does not rely on words. Most of the higher brain's interpretation of the environment, how and where things are placed, and how physical objects relate to each other is done by the right parietal lobe. This region of the brain governs vivid imagination in artistic expression, such as composing music, creating a play, making a movie, designing new clothing, sculpting a statue, or filling a canvas with a painted scene. The right parietal lobe regulates body-in-space activities, such as moving about safely inside one's home or driving a vehicle. Putting on or taking off clothing is governed by how fluently the right parietal lobe coordinates where body parts go. The right parietal lobe plays a critical role in visual perception by assembling all parts of visual images, such as seeing a complete clock face, the shape of a tree, or details of outdoor scenes. Finally, the right parietal lobe regulates how a person fits parts together into whole structures, as in rebuilding an automobile engine, tailoring a new garment, or constructing a new building.

Left Parietal Lobe. Two major functions of the left parietal lobe are math calculation and arithmetic computation, especially division and subtraction. The left parietal lobe guides the verbal process of labeling and naming math symbols while also governing a person's sense of direction (left or right). The first steps in reading occur as the left parietal lobe interprets printed or written language symbols, then takes the first step in connecting sounds to letters. In Chapter 4, Figure 4.1 shows the critical role that the left parietal lobe plays in learning to read.

A major characteristic of learning disability, especially dyslexia, is the struggle to blend new data with what the person already knows. Often it is hard for a dyslexic individual to learn directionality, such as left/right and top/bottom. These LD students have difficulty naming objects, especially geometric shapes such as square, triangle, and rectangle. An earmark of dyslexia is having lopsided talents, such as very high nonverbal skills (artistic creativity, athletics, mechanical skills) compared with very low verbal abilities (poor reading, trouble expressing ideas, tangled speech in telling).

Occipital Lobes. At the back of the head are the right and left *occipital lobes* where vision occurs. Within each occipital lobe is the visual cortex. These specialized brain regions work together to govern how individuals see. The major work of the occipital lobes is to blend countless bits of visual data into whole images. Neuroscientists often compare the occipital lobes to a wall that is covered by computer screens, each of which shows a tiny portion of a whole image. At a distance, such a mosaic is seen as a whole image. It is the job of the occipital lobes to blend visual bits into whole mosaics of what the person sees.

The occipital lobes regulate the process of developing new visual images as light energy is transformed into electrical impulses. The occipital lobes supervise constantly changing images of what the eyes see from one millisecond to the next. Specialized neurons throughout the visual cortex interpret contrasting variations between dark and light, fluctuations in movement, differences in form and shape, distances between objects, and the space context (figure/ground perception) of where objects are.

The right visual cortex specializes in recognizing human faces, pictures, designs, and nonverbal images in the environment. The left visual cortex specializes in interpreting language symbols, such as alphabet letters, segments of words, and arithmetic numerals. Chapter 3 describes several kinds of visual perception problems that emerge when dyslexia is inherited. When neurons and axons are underdeveloped within the occipital lobes, individuals see a distorted world in which details do not fit together.

Frontal Lobes. The left and right *frontal lobes* team together to govern the expression of oral and written language. The frontal lobes team with the cingulate gyrus (see Figure 1.7) in determining how the proto-self (self-image) is expressed and presented to others. The frontal lobes regulate the flexibility, spontaneity, and adaptiveness of personality as individuals interact with others. Also, the frontal lobes determine how individuals interact with the environment. How neurons develop within the frontal lobes governs how active or passive persons become in social behavior. A major characteristic of many LD persons is their inflexibility in relating to others. Chapter 8 presents the social awkwardness of Asperger's syndrome, often seen in conjunction with dyslexia. Within families in which LD tendencies move down genetic lines, many relatives may be awkward socially with poor ability to establish flexible or adaptable relationships.

Temporal Lobes

Above the ear on each side of the brain are the temporal lobes that govern language processing, interpretation of sound, time awareness, and how a person perceives the environment. The *right temporal lobe* works with the right frontal and parietal lobes to interpret visual/spatial relationships. The right brain governs complex movements required to drive a vehicle, play athletic games, use tools and machinery, work at a computer, and play musical instruments. The right temporal lobe is the center of time awareness, such as the chronological sequence of seasons and life events. Also, the right temporal lobe distinguishes between music and environmental noise. This region of the right brain processes musical tone, loudness of sound, and volume of noise within the environment. When the right and left temporal lobes work together, a person hears and responds to musical rhythms and tonal changes. If the right temporal lobe fails to do this teamwork, the person has a monotone perception of music without the richness of tonal variations and changes in musical pitch. He or she speaks in a rather loud monotone voice that lacks normal inflection and language rhythms.

The *left temporal lobe* is the center for language. Figure 1.8 shows the "auditory arch" that links *Broca's region, auditory cortex,* and *Wernicke area* where the brain processes oral language. At the front of the left temporal lobe is *Broca's region,* named after the French neurologist Paul Broca who first defined this left brain speech center. The Broca region links the frontal lobe (also called the *basal forebrain*) and the temporal lobe to process segments of speech. This portion of the left brain controls a person's use of words and phrases. At the opposite end of the left temporal lobe is the *Wernicke area,* named after the German neurologist Karl Wernicke who first described how this brain region controls fluency in talking, use of grammar, and creativity in word usage. This three-part temporal lobe team controls spelling, phonetics (sounding out words), oral reading and speaking, and syntax (sentence structure). Also, the left temporal lobe governs a person's thoughts of morality, religion, and serious reflection. The left temporal lobe teams with the cingulate gyrus in self-criticism that requires clear awareness of one's proto-self. Finally, the left temporal lobe is the brain's music center where harmony, tonal variations, and musical beauty originate.

Prefrontal Cortex

Just above the left eye within the left frontal lobe is a highly specialized region called the *prefrontal cortex*. This region of the higher brain is the command center for logic, patience, and commonsense reasoning. The governing role of the prefrontal cortex is called the *executive function*. As an executive stays in charge of how an organization functions, so the prefrontal cortex governs the work of the whole brain. The prefrontal cortex is one of the last higher brain regions to reach maturity. Between birth and age 7, the neurons of the prefrontal cortex gradually become myelinated. If the child grows up in a rational, organized, peaceful environment, the prefrontal cortex becomes the center of socially constructive emotions and feelings, such as patience, kindness, gentleness, tolerance, and contentment. A major function of the prefrontal cortex is to ensure that the person learns how to wait, not yield to impulse.

Cell Firing. The prefrontal cortex stays in command of the whole brain through a process called *cell firing*. When neurons are well developed, brain energy pulses along axons and dendrites in regular bursts that last 1/1,000 of a second. These energy pulses, called brain waves, are 1,000 times weaker than household electrical current. The fuel for this brain energy is glucose. As glucose is oxidized within brain cells, each neuron is charged or recharged (Calvin & Ojemann, 1980; Damasio, 1994, 1999; Llinas, 1993). Cell firing permits the prefrontal cortex to carry out its executive function in two ways. To communicate with specific brain regions, direct signals are fired along selected axon pathways that link the prefrontal cortex with certain parts of the brain. This is similar to an individual dialing a specific phone number for a personal call. At the same time, the prefrontal cortex fires generalized brain waves that sweep the whole brain, as radar waves sweep outward from a sending station. All regions of the brain answer these signals either by sending back a direct line message or by returning a sweeping surge of brain energy.

Neurotransmitters and Cell Firing Rhythm. As pulses of brain energy reach synapse junctions, tiny chemical bundles called *neurotransmitters* squirt across synapse spaces to be absorbed by the other side of the synapse junction. To do its work, the prefrontal cortex relies on the neurotransmitter *dopamine* that regulates the rate of cell firing. To maintain executive function, the prefrontal cortex must fire in a consistently regular rhythm. If cell firing is too fast, the brain receives overstimulating signals that trigger static-like interference between brain regions. This "hyperactive" state is called *overarousal* or *attention surplus*. If cell firing is too slow, the prefrontal cortex loses control by becoming "drowsy." This is called *underarousal* or *attention deficit*. Dopamine stays in charge of the level of arousal by creating homeostasis in the prefrontal cortex.

Early in the Decade of the Brain, Rodolfo Llinas (1993) at the Massachussetts Institute of Technology estimated that to maintain full executive control, the prefrontal cortex must fire at the rate of 40 cycles per second. This steady rate of cell firing permits the prefrontal cortex to stay in communication with all regions of the brain. Dopamine is the key to maintaining the cell firing rhythm of 40 cycles per second. The chemical influence of dopamine is similar to a simple computer that automatically increases or decreases energy flow within an electrical system.

Nature and Nurture in Brain Development

Approximately 97% of brain development is governed by genetic codes that command neurons, dendrites, and axons to grow in certain ways. Obviously, genetic predispositions play a key role in brain development. How regions of the brain develop also is determined by what happens to the fetus, the infant, or the child. In fact, recent research has discovered that some parts of the brain continue to change into old age according to what happens to the individual (Birren & Shaie, 1990; Charness & Bosman,

1992; Craik & Salthouse, 1992; Damasio, 1994, 1999; Eliot, 1999; Hooker, 1992; Kogan, 1990; Park, 1992; Ramachandrian, 1993; Schieber, 1992).

The brain is amazingly plastic, not a fixed solid structure. As long as a person lives, regions of his or her brain respond to cultural pressure, stress, and stimulus. When neurons are subjected to prolonged stress, they undergo changes in dendrite structures and how neurotransmitters function across synapse gaps. Too much stress causes neurons to shrink in size and stop doing their essential work. Too little stress causes neurons to atrophy and lose their ability to communicate within their nuclei groups. Too much fear or threat of failure can overload the hypothalamus and pituitary glands so that they no longer can trigger production of safeguarding hormones. On the other hand, prolonged success that is surrounded by praise and acceptance can generate new neuron activity within the cingulate gyrus, amygdala, and frontal lobes to replace shame with hope. When lifelong threat is replaced by safety, changes occur in vital brain regions to awaken dormant abilities that had atrophied under the weight of chronic stress.

The Nature of Dyslexia

Reading Is Not a Natural Process

Programmatic research over the past 35 years has not supported the view that reading development reflects a natural process that children learn to read as they learn to speak, through natural exposure to a literate environment. . . . If learning to read were natural, there would not exist the substantial number of cultures that have yet to develop a written language, despite having a rich oral language. If learning to read unfolds naturally, why does our literate society have so many youngsters and adults who are illiterate?

—G. Reid Lyon, January/February, 2000

We have just reviewed 5,500 years of evidence to show that writing systems are inventions, and that humans do not spontaneously and effortlessly develop writing systems or find it easy to learn them. We have seen that the alphabet is a particularly "nonnatural" writing system. Reading is definitely not a biological property of the human brain.

—Diane McGuinness, 1997

What Is Dyslexia?

For more than 100 years, the issue of dyslexia has been a source of controversy among educators and neuroscientists. In 1884 the German ophthalmologist Reinhold Berlin coined the term *dyslexia* from Greek words that mean "poor reading" or "poor skill with words." In his clinical work with intelligent persons who were illiterate, Berlin observed reading difficulty that included reversed letters, scrambled sound sequences inside words, poor spelling, and very poor handwriting. He devised the label "word blind" to describe a mysterious inability to see black print on white paper in spite of having 20/20 visual acuity. When "word blind" individuals looked at printed pages, they saw moving, twisting, blurring images that made it impossible for them to read. The British scientists James Hinshelwood (1896, 1900) and William Broadbent (1872) validated Berlin's conclusions as they studied poor readers in England and Scotland. By 1915 the concepts of dyslexia and word blindness had spread across Europe and Britain.

During his European military service in World War I, the American neurologist Samuel T. Orton encountered European interest in dyslexia. Following the war, Orton brought the concept of dyslexia to the United States where he continued to study this literacy problem in children, adolescents, and adults. Orton was intrigued by the question: "Is dyslexia a brain-based disability?" He speculated that a portion of the left brain called the *angular gyrus* might be the cause for dyslexia. Orton was the first to study families of dyslexic individuals (Orton, 1925, 1928, 1937).

The first scientific effort to find the cause for dyslexia occurred during the 1960s at Harvard Medical School. Norman Geschwind and Walter Levitsky (1968) undertook a comprehensive study of adults who were poor readers. Through the Armed Forces Institute of Pathology, they performed anatomical studies of 100 adult brains. During the 1970s Thomas Kemper and Albert Galaburda expanded the Geschwind–Levitsky research by performing dissections of 16 brains from dyslexic males who were not brain injured (Galaburda, 1983). Those studies revealed specific, predictable differences in left brain neuron formation of all 16 brains. Kemper and Galaburda concluded that brain injury and dyslexia are separate issues (Galaburda, Sherman, Rosen, Aboitiz, & Geschwind, 1985). During the 1980s genome research at the University of Colorado led to the discovery that dyslexia is genetic. Dyslexia is linked to chromosomes 6 and 15 in the DNA heredity chain (DeFries et al., 1991).

Dyslexia Rises from Differences in Brain Development

Much of the research into how dyslexic brains function has been done with individuals who have had some type of trauma to the brain. This research examined lesions that damage neuron pathways anywhere in the brain. Lesions are like bruises or cracks in myelin that allow brain energy to leak or to be scattered instead of sent forward along axons and dendrites. Neuroscientists call these lesions *knockout points,* an analogy to what happens when power lines are "knocked out" by storms. Although dyslexia seldom is caused by brain lesions, many of the symptoms of dyslexia are similar to the knockout patterns seen in persons who have lost neurological functions. When brain scans are done with individuals who are dyslexic, lesions seldom are seen along neuron pathways. However, language processing skills show knockout behaviors that require special treatment. Brain scans of dyslexic brains show differences in how dendrites, neurons, and axons are formed rather than lesions that contribute to brain damage.

Can Dyslexia Be Defined Through Scientific Method?

From the time of Berlin's first discussions of dyslexia, a persistent question has been raised in scientific circles: "Is there such a thing as dyslexia? Or is this a notion from those who don't think scientifically?" As our culture enters a new millennium, two schools of thought dominate professional opinion regarding the nature of dyslexia. On one hand, many scientists insist that if dyslexia exists, it can be measured on standard tests and described through statistical models that yield the same results each time dyslexia is studied. This point of view insists that if dyslexia cannot be measured by scientific models, then it does not exist despite the claims of those who say it does.

For example, among scientists holding this view are British reading specialists Michael Rutter and William Yule. During the 1970s they conducted exhaustive research with students in London and on the Isle of Wight. Their purpose was to see if two types of poor reading exist within typical student populations: *group 1,* poor readers whose reading test scores show a wide discrepancy between age/IQ and actual reading skill (called *specific reading retardation,* or dyslexia), and *group 2,* poor readers with below-normal IQ and low scores from reading tests. To Rutter and Yule's dismay, test results from group 1 refused to follow normal distribution on a bell-shaped curve. Far too many students with high IQ scored very low on reading tests. This failure to establish statistically reliable norms to identify dyslexia from test scores led Rutter and Yule (1975) to conclude,

> There has been a complete failure to show that the signs of dyslexia constitute any meaningful pattern. It may be concluded that the question of whether specific reading retardation is or is not dyslexic can be abandoned as meaningless. (p. 194)

Can Dyslexia Be Defined Through Observation?

> We the people of the United States, in order to form a more perefect urion, to establish Justice, insure domest tranqualley, provide for the comon definse, pormote the general wellfare, insure the blesing of libert to ourseves, and are postety, do ordain that establish this Constution of the United States of America

(Copied slowly and laboriously by a bright 15-year-old boy who is dyslexic)

A point of view opposite to that of Rutter and Yule (1975) is held by many educators and neuroscientists who see dyslexia from a broad lifestyle perspective. This school of thought acknowledges that reading, spelling, and handwriting are inventions, not natural biological abilities. These specialists do not define dyslexia according to results from standard tests or statistical research. Instead, dyslexia is defined by observing the overall behaviors of those who struggle with reading, writing, and spelling. This school of thought recognizes dyslexia as a comprehensive condition that involves a great deal more than reading difficulty.

For example, Margaret Byrd Rawson (1988) spoke for many when she defined dyslexia as follows:

> Dyslexia, or the ineptitude in acquisition of one's native tongue, shows itself in many ways. . . . It becomes thus not only language difficulties that concern us, but the entire symbolic aspect of life. (p. ix)

From my 40-year career of diagnosing and remediating dyslexia in all ages from many cultures, I have summarized the nature of dyslexia as follows:

Dyslexia is the inability of an intelligent person to become fluent in the basic skills of reading, spelling, and handwriting in spite of prolonged teaching and tutoring. Math computation may also remain at the level of struggle. Dyslexia means that the person will always struggle to some degree with reading printed passages, writing with a pen or pencil, spelling accurately from memory, and developing sentences and paragraphs with correct grammar and punctuation. Dyslexia also may include difficulty telling oral information accurately. No matter how hard the person tries, certain types of errors continue to appear in reading, writing, and spelling. Dyslexia is a brain-based dysfunction that often is genetic. It tends to run in families. Through certain kinds of remedial training, dyslexic patterns can be partly overcome or reduced, but dyslexia cannot be completely eliminated. It is a lifelong, brain-based condition that most dyslexics can learn to compensate for successfully. (Jordan, 2000b, pp. 3–4)

Dyslexia Is Lack of Neurological Talent for Literacy Skills

Early in the Decade of the Brain, Martha Denckla, pediatric neurologist at Johns Hopkins University School of Medicine, presented the concept of *neurological talent for reading*. Denckla (1991b) insists that IQ has little to do with reading ability. "If we must have an IQ score," she has stated, "let's assign everyone IQ 100, then get on with figuring out why many bright students don't learn to read." Denckla has devoted much of her career to studying neuron formations in the brain regions that control emotional stability and language processing (described in Chapter 1). She has concluded that children enter formal education with a wide range of neurological talent for reading. Denckla pointed out that our culture does not expect uniformity in athletic skill, musical ability, or math aptitude. The Western world awards star status to those who have exceptional gifts and talents on playing fields, in concert halls, and in research laboratories, but those who lack such talents are regarded as perfectly normal. "Why, then," Denckla (1991b) asks, "do we expect all children to have neurological talent for reading? Why do we not acknowledge different levels of talent for becoming competent readers?"

The Pathology of Superiority

Dyslexia imposes limited neurological talent for reading, spelling, and handwriting. Genetic predisposition for dyslexia "hardwires" brain pathways differently so that typical language processing does not always emerge. Furthermore, dyslexia seldom is caused by brain damage (Denckla, 1993; Galaburda et al., 1985; Geschwind, 1982; Jordan, 1998, 2000a, 2000b). Usually dyslexia brings the gift of superior right-brain abilities that often are obscured by the struggle to read. Geschwind (1982) summarized his years of research by concluding that although dyslexia occurs mostly in the left brain, the right brain in most dyslexic individuals compensates by expanding nonlanguage talent beyond typical levels. Geschwind called this "the pathology of superiority." He concluded that when left-brain language processing centers are inadequate, right-brain nonverbal centers compensate by developing outstanding spatial perception talents. As Chapter 1 described, if dyslexic youngsters grow up in caring, nurturing environments, their proto-self (self-image) becomes strong and confident. This fosters nonlanguage thinking that leads to outstanding intuition, creative thinking, and problem solving. Geschwind believed that all individuals have natural right-brain talents that tend to go undeveloped when the left brain is fluent at reading and other language processing skills.

Range of Severity of Dyslexia

To understand the impact of dyslexia, it is important that a certain point of view be maintained. No two dyslexic persons display exactly the same patterns, and not all of these individuals show the same level of severity. Clusters of dyslexic patterns must be seen along a continuum from mild to severe. Many individuals who are dyslexic show only mild or moderate problems, whereas others are severely disabled. Diagnosticians and counselors use a severity scale to show the approximate level of dyslexic struggle.

1	2	3		4	5	6	7		8	9	10
	mild					moderate				severe	

Mild Level of Severity

Most individuals have a few dyslexic-like "blips" in their literacy and mathematics skills. It would be reasonable to say that each of us is dyslexic at levels 1 or 2. Few persons have perfect literacy skills without some area of deficit. This poses no problem so long as perceptual blips do not create costly mistakes on the job. Adults typically choose professions or occupations that permit them to bypass whatever minor deficits exist in spelling, rapid recall of details, or mathematics processing. Mild dyslexia causes uncertainty in recalling certain kinds of details, need for extra time, inconsistent spelling, somewhat ragged style of reading, apology for substandard handwriting, and so forth. Mild dyslexia is more a nuisance than a problem.

Moderate Level of Severity

Dyslexia becomes a problem when it begins to interfere with classroom performance, academic success, or accuracy in job performance. An individual at the low moderate level of severity (level 4 or 5) continually makes mistakes in spelling, punctuation, and use of capital letters. Grammar errors are heard in the person's speech and are seen in the individual's writing. This person always has had trouble compehending the full meaning of what he or she reads. Many level 4 or 5 dyslexic persons stumble over arithmetic computation and math processing. They never are comfortable with writing assignments whether they write brief notes or develop complex written projects. They rely on computer spell check programs to find their spelling errors. They must rewrite original work two or three times before original mistakes have been corrected. With enough time and effort, level 4 or 5 dyslexic individuals can make top grades and be listed on the honor roll. However, they must maintain a high level of self-discipline to compensate for moderate dyslexia.

When dyslexia is at the high moderate level of severity (level 6 or 7), a major struggle occurs in all areas of academic performance along with creating problems on the job. Spelling always is filled with mistakes, and textbook reading is slow and labored. Much more time than usual is required to finish assignments, and a high level of personal frustration is experienced. Persons at level 6 or 7 reach burnout before they can finish any academic task. They must deal continually with strong negative emotions triggered by a sense of failure. It is possible for intelligent individuals with high moderate dyslexia to earn top grades in certain classes where they have neurological talent for that subject. Sometimes level 6 or 7 individuals win academic honors or achieve awards for job performance. It is possible for these dyslexic learners to finish college programs, including master's or doctoral degrees. But to do so, enormous effort must be made along with having great courage and self-discipline.

Severe Dyslexia

When dyslexia is severe (level 8 or 9), academic achievement often is impossible unless instructors modify the curriculum to accommodate dyslexic tendencies. Individuals at level 8 or 9 remain several years below grade level in academic skill achievement. Spelling skills always will be primitive, reading always will be a struggle, and handwriting always will be messy and partly illegible. Severely dyslexic individuals require two to three times longer than normal to finish assignments and process new information. It is virtually impossible for these learners to attain independent study skills. They must have continual tutoring and coaching to prepare for tests, do assignments, master new information, and fill in gaps in their skills and knowledge. If severely dyslexic persons are taught to write using a word processor, they can bypass enough problems to turn out good work through a keyboard. However, all academic work will be labored, slow, and deeply frustrating.

Occasionally an individual is at level 10 on the severity scale. At this level of severity, it is impossible for the brain to learn how to read, spell, or write. Level 10 dyslexia is called *alexia* (Jordan, 1996b, 2000a; Lichteim, 1885).

Forms of Dyslexia

Most of the professional controversy about dyslexia is caused by misunderstanding as to which form of this learning difference one is referring. The three general forms of dyslexia are *acquired dyslexia, deep dyslexia,* and *developmental dyselxia.* It is critically important that these different forms of dyslexia be recognized. If only one form is acknowledged by those who discuss this issue, then it becomes impossible for professionals to deal effectively with dyslexia. Also, the level of severity must be taken into account when dyslexia is discussed across lines of professional concern.

Acquired Dyslexia

As a rule, dyslexia is not related to brain injury. However, some types of trauma to the brain can create dyslexic patterns that are not inherited and did not exist before the traumatic event. Approximately 3 individuals out of 1,000 acquire dyslexia through traumatic events that damage language structures within the left brain (Jordan, 1996a). Acquired dyslexia seldom is seen outside the populations involved with rehabilitation therapy or in assisted living organizations.

Chapter 1 described the extremely rapid development of neuron structures during the 9 months of gestation. During the first trimester of fetal development, emerging neuron pathways are especially vulnerable to trauma that can impair the child's ability to learn to read, write, or spell. Childhood accidents involving closed head injury to the occipital lobe or left temportal cortex can create dyslexic struggle with literacy skills. Head injuries incurred in athletic events, traffic accidents, or workplace mishaps can leave the individual with dyslexic struggle that did not exist before brain trauma occurred.

Drug overdose sometimes injures enough brain pathways to create acquired dyslexia. Diseases that infect the central nervous system often create dyslexic struggle where none existed before the illness. As individuals enter old age, deterioration of brain pathways often brings on dyslexia, to the surprise of those who knew the person when there was no dyslexic activity.

Deep Dyslexia

Lifelong Struggle with Literacy Skills

The term *deep dyslexia* refers to deep-seated, lifelong trouble with literacy skills, such as reading comprehension, using phonetic rules to sound out words, writing legibly, spelling accurately, and correctly using grammar and punctuation. Many individuals with deep dyslexia also struggle with arithmetic computation. Deep dyslexia does not decrease or improve with age. At age 50, persons with deep dyslexia still read below fourth-grade level and have spelling skills below third-grade level. Yet they may be successful entrepreneurs or specialists in vocations that do not require reading ability.

Genetic Predisposition

Deep dyslexia is linked to chromosomes 6 and 15 in the genetic chain (DeFries et al., 1991). This form of dyslexia usually occurs in males. Deep dyslexia is seen approximately nine times more often in males than in females (Jordan, 1996a, 1998, 2000a). Deep dyslexia can skip a generation if passed along by the mother. A grandfather and his male relatives can be dyslexic, but his daughter may not show significant signs of dyslexia. Yet her son (third generation) can have deep dyslexia and pass the pattern on down the family line. Yet, individuals with deep dyslexia are well above average in intelligence (Jordan, 1996a, 1998, 2000a, 2000b; Rawson, 1988; Weisel, 1992, 2001).

Deep Dyslexia Involves the Whole Body

As he studied families of dyslexic individuals, Orton (1925, 1928, 1937) documented how the whole body is involved when deep dyslexia exists in families. He concluded that approximately 5% of all individuals have deep dyslexia that does not improve as the person grows up. Orton observed that most dyslexic individuals are above average in intelligence if their mental ability is not judged solely by standard IQ test scores. He described a range of physical patterns that are seen in members of dyslexic families. For example, a majority of the blood relatives of deep dyslexic persons begin to show gray or white streaks in their hair during their late teens or early 20s. Many are gray or white haired by age 30. Approximately 13% of dyslexic family members are left handed, compared with 3% of the general population. Dyslexic families display many more allergies than nondyslexic groups, including allergic sensitivity to the environment, food substances, and beverage ingredients. In particular, individuals with dyslexia tend to be highly allergic (cytotoxic) to whole milk. This condition of lactose intolerance creates intense gastric distress along with swelling of the brain. Many persons with dyslexia are allergic to wheat gluten, resulting in unwell symptoms that include swelling of joints and inflammation of large muscle neurons.

Dyslexic families include increased numbers of relatives with autoimmune disorders, such as lupus in women and arithritis and fibromyalgia in men. Most dyslexic individuals live with gastritis that keeps the lower intestinal tract in a state of irritation (irritable bowel syndrome or colitis). Dyslexic individuals and their blood relatives are prone to develop Crohn's disease with polyps protruding into the digestive tract. Most persons with deep dyslexia have lifelong problems with flatulence (gas build-up within the small intestine) caused by lack of digestive enzymes in the lower bowel. As Chapter 3 describes, more than half of all dyslexic individuals also have scotopic sensitivity, the "word blindness" documented by Berlin during the 19th century. Orton (1925, 1928, 1937) concluded that dyslexia is a whole body issue that causes lifelong discomfort and borderline poor health in most persons who inherit the predisposition for dyslexia.

Developmental Dyslexia

The third form of dyslexia is called *developmental dyslexia* because it decreases in severity as individuals pass through puberty and early adulthood. This form of dyslexia also may be passed down family lines, although it can appear when no other relatives have the symptoms. Developmental dyslexia is seen in 12% to 15% of the general population and appears five times more often in males than in females. A child who at age 7 is at level 7 in severity of dyslexic symptoms may be down to level 5 by age 14, then down to level 3 by age 25. As brain development continues through childhood and adolescence, left-brain neurons involved with literacy skills become "hardwired" to cope more successfully with reading, spelling, and writing.

Research by Norman Geschwind (1972), Albert Galaburda (1983), and Veronika Grimm (1986) has linked developmental dyslexia to allergic reactions between the mother's body chemistry and the fetus during the first trimester of gestation. Pregnancies of those who will be dyslexic often are marked by biochemical struggle by the mother's body to discharge the fetus as "foreign tissue." Excessive morning sickness signals the internal battle waged between the emerging fetus and the mother's body chemistry.

Further biochemical activity marks the emergence of a fetus that likely will have developmental dyslexia. Toward the end of the first trimester, the embryonic gonad cells of the fetus produce a surge of the male hormone testosterone. At this stage of fetal development, the higher brain is just starting to take shape (see Figure 1.4). Groups of neurons that later become the right-brain and left-brain hemispheres are migrating upward toward the developing head of the fetus. The surge of testosterone slows down development of the left-brain cells while the right-brain cells continue to develop on schedule. Developmental dyslexia begins when the testosterone surge slows down the growth rate of the left brain. Years later during puberty, the left-brain neurons start to catch up in maturity as the left brain finally attains normal size. This "late bloomer" brain activity allows youngsters with developmental dyslexia to catch up in literacy skills that were impossible to achieve in early years (Barkley, 1990; Damasio, 1995; Denckla, 1993; Galaburda, 1983; Grimm, 1986; Jordan, 1996a, 1998, 2000a, 2000b; Levine, 1999; Pennington et al., 1991; Weis & Hechtmann, 1993; Weisel, 1992, 2001).

The Signature of Dyslexia

Instead of depending on test scores to identify dyslexia, many educators and neuroscientists document the overall signature of dyslexia as it inhibits childhood language development, frustrates fine motor coordination for handwriting, prohibits fluency in reading, and disables one's memory for spelling. Rawson's concept of "the many faces of dyslexia" provides a broad view of the various ways in which dyslexia affects classroom learning and communication skills (Denckla, 1972, 1985, 1991a, 1991b, 1993; Irlen, 1991; Jordan, 1972, 1996a, 1996b, 1998, 2000a, 2000b; Rawson, 1998; Weisel, 1992, 2001).

Dyslexia Creates Awkward Speech

An unfortunate social consequence of dyslexia is the tendency for the tongue to twist speech sounds, scramble the order of words, and fail to say what the person is thinking. Figure 1.6 shows the geniculate nucleus within the midbrain. Everything the ears hear comes first to the *medial geniculate nucleus* where speech sounds are separated from noise and nonlanguage sounds. Chapter 5 describes the condition called *auditory dyslexia* that occurs when neurons within the geniculate nucleus fail to develop completely. When auditory dyslexia exists, young children fail to comprehend oral language accurately. This auditory processing deficit often is called "tone deafness" because the person cannot "hear" the soft/slow speech particles called vowels and soft consonants. This makes it impossible for youngsters to mimic speech correctly. They cannot learn to say what they do not hear. Consequently, dyslexic individuals tend to mispronounce or scramble words as they speak.

For example, a prominent civic leader in the American Southwest was noted for the dyslexic signature of his speech. One day he met a relative of someone who recently had died. "Was that you or your brother who was killed in that wreck?" he asked. Another time this dyslexic man said, "I can see the writing on the handwall." One day he posted a notice in his workplace: "There will be no before drinking till after the job." At a company party he commented to a friend, "That guy over there keeps watching me like I was a hawk." At a dinner party he noticed a woman who was somewhat overdressed for the occasion: "She ain't exactly no fried chicken," he said to a friend. One day he amazed his office staff when he said, "If the phone answers for me, tell them for a few minutes that I've gone for down the street coffee."

This awkward speech signature of dyslexia emerges early as children learn to talk. For example, a bright but "tone-deaf" girl with auditory dyslexia bewildered her family by constant mispronunciations of familiar words. In learning to manage personal hygiene, she needed a "tallow" to dry herself after a bath. Her grandparents lived in "Mervont" that was not far from "Mass-too-shets." An intelligent dyslexic boy always said that he was "very tryer" after playing hard. He often complained about "falling updown the stairs." His creative right brain continually originated "new ideals" about how certain things could be done better. These kinds of dyslexic tongue twisters persist after reading skills become established. Listening to a dyslexic person speak often reveals underlying language differences that are not revealed by test scores.

Dyslexia Confuses One's Sense of Direction

Individuals who are dyslexic seldom are sure about where their bodies are in space. Spatial orientation never feels quite right. These individuals are unsure about north or south, east or west. Under pressure to act in a hurry, they reverse left and right, causing them to move in the opposite direction. Dyslexic individuals feel lost in new places until they have time to memorize place markers. Few persons who are dyslexic follow mental images of which direction to turn or in which direction places are located. Instead of thinking "turn right" or "turn east," dyslexic individuals depend on visual markers such as a large tree, a familiar building, or other permanent place signals. Once permanent memory is anchored to visual guideposts, persons with dyslexia are easily confused and frustrated when familiar markers are changed. It is especially difficult for them to function well in new places. All their lives they must compensate for poor directionality.

Dyslexia Confuses Printed Language Symbols

Chapter 4 describes *visual dyslexia,* which causes printed symbols to turn backward, flip upside down, or "jump" to different positions within words. As dyslexic persons try to read, copy, or write, alphabet symbols and numbers continue to change. Figure 2.1 shows the visual dyslexia signature of a bright 8-year-old boy.

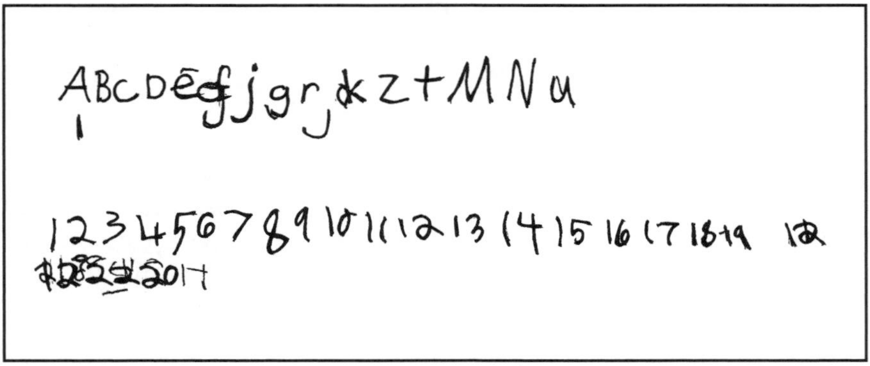

Figure 2.1. For 3 years in school, this 8-year-old boy has practiced writing the alphabet and numbers 1 through 20. No matter how hard he tries, his dyslexic tendencies make this task impossible.

Into his fourth year of formal education, he struggles to write the alphabet and number line from memory. Figure 2.2 shows this student's struggle to remember which way alphabet letters and numbers should face. No matter how hard he tries, he cannot stop these reversing, scrambling perceptions every time he tries to read.

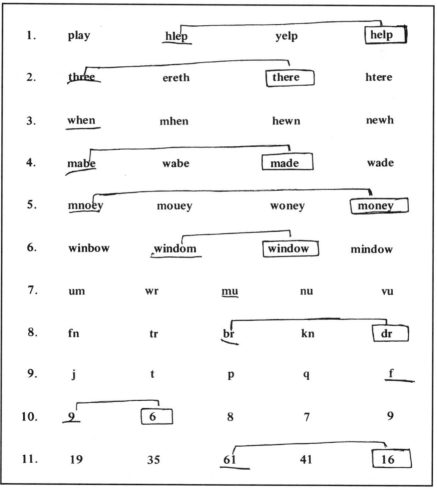

Figure 2.2. This 8-year-old boy struggles with symbol sequence and direction-ality as he matches words in daily school activities. *Note.* From *Slingerland Screening Tests for Identifying Children with Specific Language Disability,* Form B, by B. H. Slingerland, 1984, Cambridge, MA: Educators Publishing Service. Copyright 1984 by Educators Publishing Service. Reprinted with permission.

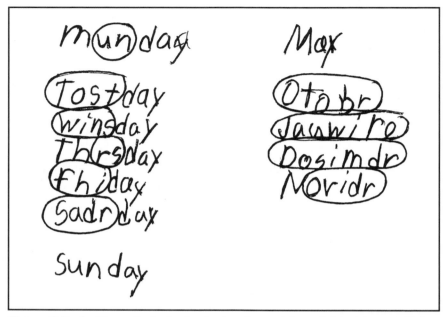

Figure 2.3. Auditory dyslexia frustrates the writing of this 10-year-old boy who cannot build permanent memory for how to spell familiar words.

Dyslexia Prevents Correct Spelling

Chapter 5 describes *auditory dyslexia,* or "tone deafness," which keeps the individual from comprehending the soft/slow sounds of speech. These individuals identify only parts of words they hear and speak. This dyslexic condition makes it impossible for the brain to build accurate permanent memory for familiar words the person hears and says. Figure 2.3 shows the written signature of auditory dyslexia as a highly intelligent 10-year-old boy tried to write the days of the week and months of the year from memory. Figure 2.4 shows a 9-year-old dyslexic child's struggle to write words and phrases from dictation.

Dyslexia Often Prevents Legible Handwriting

Chapter 6 describes *dysgraphia,* which makes legible handwriting impossible to achieve. Figure 1.9 shows the sequence of motor skills that normally develop during early childhood. When a child is dyslexic, the motor cortex region that controls hand-

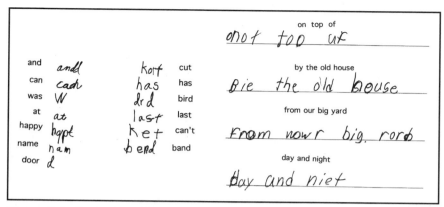

Figure 2.4. Dyslexia makes it impossible for this 9-year-old girl to write from dictation. Her writing is very slow and labored with heavy pencil pressure. *Note.* The lower example is from the *Slingerland Screening Tests for Identifying Children with Specific Language Disability,* Form B, by B. H. Slingerland, 1984, Cambridge, MA: Educators Publishing Service. Copyright 1984 by Educators Publishing Service. Reprinted with permission.

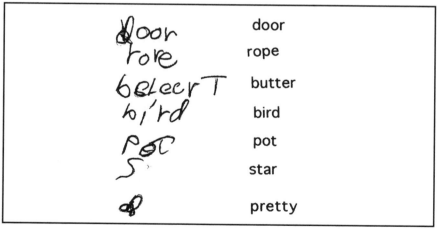

Figure 2.5. In spite of having superior intelligence, this severely dyslexic 11-year-old girl cannot write simple, familiar words from dictation.

writing fails to develop fully. The result is a lifelong struggle to write clearly. Handwriting has an irregular, stressful, and "messy" appearance that humiliates the writer and frustrates those who attempt to read the writing. Figure 2.5 shows the struggle of an 11-year-old girl to write some familiar words from dictation. Figure 2.6 shows how difficult it is for this dysgraphic girl to copy or draw simple geometric shapes. Figure 2.7 illustrates the struggle dysgraphic students face when they cannot control handwriting while doing daily assignments.

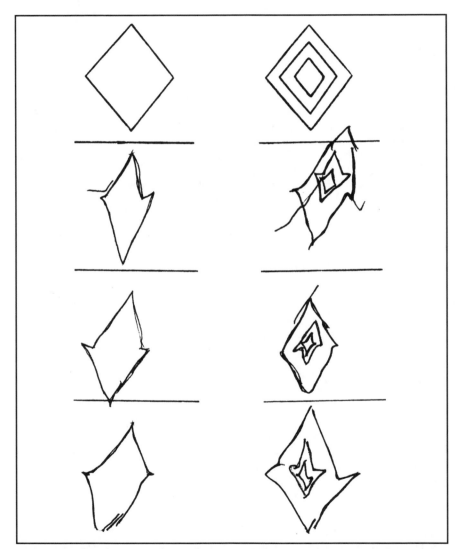

Figure 2.6. Dysgraphia makes it impossible for this intelligent 11-year-old girl to copy or draw diamond shapes accurately. As her pencil reaches each corner, her brain gives a reversed signal that causes her fingers to turn the opposite direction. Then she corrects her directional error, which produces "ears" at the corners.

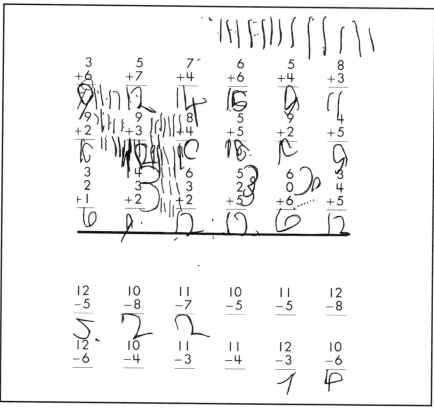

Figure 2.7. Dysgraphia makes it impossible for students to produce neat, legible written work, even in math. This 13-year-old dysgraphic boy becomes intensely frustrated doing math assignments.

Dyslexia Often Causes Dyscalculia

Figure 2.8 shows the regions of the brain where arithmetic computation and math reasoning occur. Many dyslexic individuals do not have the neurological talent for success with math. This genetic condition is called *dyscalculia*. No matter how long they practice basic arithmetic computation skills, these students do not develop permanent memory for math facts. Dyscalculia often produces half-finished assignments along with a great deal of rehearsal on scratch paper trying to figure out correct answers. Figures 2.9 and 2.10 show the written signature of dyscalculia in the work of a 12-year-old student.

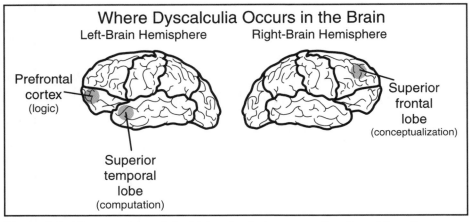

Figure 2.8. These regions of the higher brain team together for arithmetic computation and higher math reasoning. When neural clusters fail to prune excess dendrites, these brain regions cannot do math thinking or processing. This incomplete brain formation is called *dyscalculia*.

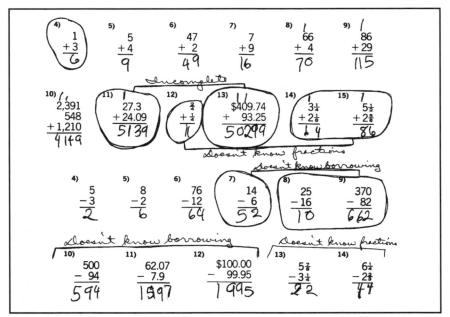

Figure 2.9. Dyscalculia is a serious handicap for this bright 12-year-old boy who cannot build permanent memory for arithmetic facts and procedures. No matter how many times he practices number functions, his brain cannot develop long-term memory for math information.

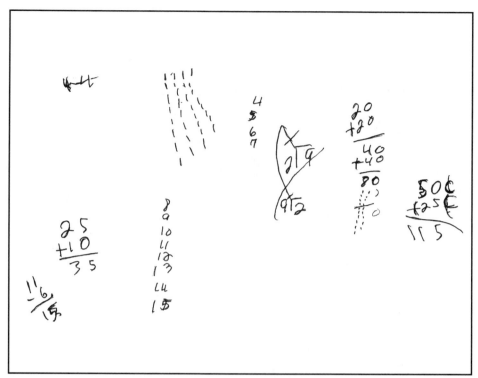

Figure 2.10. This 12-year-old student cannot work math problems unless he experiments with trial-and-error strategies on scratch paper. This was part of his scratch paper work to do the problems shown in Figure 2.9.

Untreated Dyslexia Triggers Social Conflict

A major part of the dyslexia signature is lifelong potential for social conflict when others do not understand the challenges that dyslexic persons face. Figure 2.11 is an example of strong conflict between a 15-year-old dyslexic boy and his teachers who did not understand why his work failed to meet their standards. Shortly after he was forced to write this apology, this adolescent acted out the bitterness expressed in his writing by dropping out of school and running away from home. Chapter 7 describes the overwhelming emotions and feelings of dyslexic individuals whose learning differences are not recognized or accommodated.

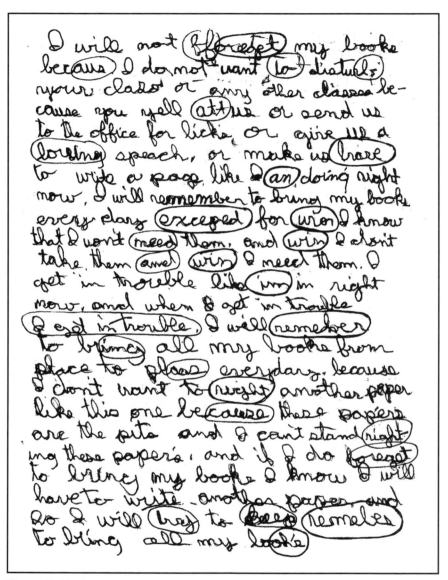

Figure 2.11. Unrecognized dyslexia and dysgraphia caused this frustrated 15-year-old boy to drop out of school. When he was forced to write this essay that is filled with bitter feelings toward school, he decided that he could no longer tolerate being punished for mistakes he could not help making. His deep shame from years of school failure overwhelmed all other considerations.

Dyslexic Failure Produces Shame

Chapter 7 begins by discussing the devastation of shame that emerges when individuals try to do their best, but their best never is good enough to satisfy adult expectations. Dyslexic children especially are vulnerable to feeling shame everytime adults scold by saying, "You could do better, but you just won't try," or "Don't you ever listen to what I say?" Over time such criticism implants negative self-image in intelligent youngsters who do their best to listen and do things correctly. Yet in spite of their good intentions, they never seem to get it right. These individuals are at high risk for depression, which leads to a lifestyle of conflict, failing more than succeeding, and believing that he or she is not worth much.

Checklist Signature of Dyslexia

The following checklist includes the nine areas of classroom effort in which dyslexic students struggle hardest. As an observer checks several items in more than one of these areas, a dyslexia signature emerges that shows specific ways in which the student struggles in classroom learning.

Symbol Reversal

_____ Certain letters or numbers are made backwards.

_____ Certain letters or numbers are made upside down.

_____ Whole words or parts of words are written backwards.

_____ Reading often is backwards (right to left).

_____ Writing often is backwards (right to left).

Poor Sense of Direction

_____ Can't remember main directions: north, south, east, west.

(continues)

_____ Must use a memory crutch to recall directions, such as "Never Eat Sour Watermelon" for north/east/south/west.

_____ Can't remember left and right.

_____ Turns pages the opposite way.

_____ Is continually confused about where to start on work pages.

_____ Can't remember which way to turn when someone says "Turn right" or "Turn left."

Loss of Sequence

_____ Can't remember details in sequence: alphabet, days, months, math facts, phone numbers, addresses, etc.

_____ Loses the sequence after starting to get it right.

_____ Can't tell things in the right order. Becomes mixed up telling things.

_____ Can't work math problems in the right direction.

_____ Can't keep track of several things to be done.

_____ Can't follow directions when he or she must turn corners.

_____ Gets sequence of instructions out of order while doing tasks.

Poor Listening

_____ Can't keep track in listening. Misunderstands. Frequently asks "What? Huh? What do you mean?"

_____ Misinterprets what is heard. Remembers it differently.

_____ Can't take notes. Writing can't keep up with listening.

_____ Continually says, "You didn't tell me that" or "I never heard you say that."

_____ Stops listening. Starts doing something else or begins to daydream.

Poor Writing

_____ Handwriting is messy and poorly organized.

_____ Pencil cuts down through the line, then floats above the line.

_____ Mixes capital letters with lowercase letters.

_____ Mixes manuscript print with cursive writing.

_____ Quality of writing deteriorates rapidly.

_____ Size of writing is too large or too small for work space.

_____ Columns zigzag or drift away from the left margin.

_____ Writing hand soon cramps. Must stop writing to shake or rub hand.

_____ Lays head down on left wrist with eyes close to the paper.

_____ Turns paper and head at different angles while writing.

Poor Phonics

_____ Can't remember which sounds go with which letters.

_____ Word sounding is very slow and labored.

_____ Frequently pauses to whisper each sound before saying the word.

_____ Says "Wait!" or "Hold it!" while trying to sound out words.

_____ Can't blend syllables together in longer words.

_____ Scrambles the sequence of sounds inside words.

Poor Spelling

_____ Spells words the way they sound. Can't remember spelling rules.

_____ Reverses inside patterns: *gril* for *girl, Apirl* for *April, bran* for *barn, form* for *from.*

_____ Misspells words while copying and rewriting.

_____ Memorizes words for a test but can't remember them later.

_____ Can't hear soft/slow speech sounds (vowels and soft consonants). Is "tone deaf" to soft/slow speech sounds.

(continues)

Short Attention Span

_____ Attention darts or drifts away into daydreaming while doing schoolwork or routine job work.

_____ Changes the subject without finishing what was started.

_____ Interrupts others while they are talking.

_____ Asks a question, then doesn't finish listening to the answer.

_____ Body is restless and disruptive. Can't sit still or stay still during quiet time.

Poor Central Vision for Doing Sustained Close Work

_____ Eyes quickly become too tired to keep on reading, writing, copying, or working with a computer screen.

_____ Eyes soon begin to ache or hurt behind, above, below, or at the inside corner of each eye.

_____ Eyes start to burn and water.

_____ Headache starts across the forehead, over the temples, or at the back of the head.

_____ Printed details start to pulse in and out of focus.

_____ Small details or whole words start to double briefly, then become clear (off and on in pulsing cycles).

_____ Begins to complain about headache, eyes hurting, or not feeling well after working for a while.

_____ Continually moves around, turns head to see from different angles, leans back, then leans forward again.

_____ Begins to squint eyes and rub at eyes.

_____ Starts to yawn frequently.

_____ Glances away instead of looking steadily at work.

_____ Is bothered by bright overhead light. Tries to shade the page by leaning over it. Wants to wear bill cap indoors with the bill down over the eyes.

_____ Wants to read or work in dim "twilight."

Learning Problems in the Shadow of Dyslexia

3

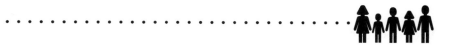

Dyslexia Rarely Comes Alone

Since the 19th century when Berlin first coined the label *dyslexia,* teachers and diagnosticians often have felt frustrated trying to see dyslexic patterns clearly. Many have complained that dyslexia is too elusive and indistinct to be defined. It is not unusual for diagnosticians and teachers to give up trying to identify or describe dyslexia. This is especially true when narrow limits are imposed on definitions of dyslexia, or when research to explore this learning difficulty is too narrowly defined. Is dyslexia a condition that turns letters backwards and upside down? Often, but not always. Does dyslexia make it impossible for individuals to learn to read? Sometimes, but not always. Does dyslexia mean that a person spells poorly? Usually, but not always. Does dyslexia include difficulty with handwriting and math computation? Frequently, but not always. Do dyslexic individuals have poor eyesight for reading? Quite often, but not always. Is attention deficit part of being dyslexic? Usually, but not always. With this degree of variability, is it possible to separate dyslexia from other types of learning difficulty? Yes, if other types of learning problems in the shadow of dyslexia are clearly defined.

Identifying Layers of Learning Difficulty

Rarely does any type of learning difficulty (LD) exist alone. In most instances, several kinds of learning struggle overlap like layers of an onion. Seeing dyslexia clearly requires teachers and diagnosticians to peel away each layer of LD, give it an appropriate name, and define its characteristics. This process of separating the layers of LD brings into clear focus the overlapping factors that make classroom learning difficult. Before dyslexia can be defined correctly, it must be separated from other patterns that tend to hide in its shadow (Barkley, 1990, 1995; Denckla, 1985; Geiger & Lettvin, 1987; Irlen, 1991; Jordan, 1996a, 1996b, 1998, 2000a, 2000b; Rawson, 1988; Weisel, 1992, 2001).

Word Blindness

In 1884 Reinhold Berlin described what he called *word blindness* that existed in most of the dyslexic individuals he met in his practice of ophthalmology. He was perplexed by this reading impediment in persons who had normal vision acuity (20/20), yet who could not "see to read." When those struggling readers looked at black print on white paper, their eyes felt overwhelmed by glare from the white background. Those poor readers saw continual motion of letters, words, and lines of print. Portions of the printed page moved back and forth, up and down, or swirled in a twisting motion. Words stacked atop each other, then separated. As words spread apart, rivers of changing space cascaded down the page. At times those struggling readers saw things fall off the edge of the page. Often dark smudges appeared on the page as words merged, then separated. Sometimes inner portions of words faded in and out in a pulsing rhythm.

Berlin discovered that most of the visual distortions stopped momentarily if a card were held below each line, if the reader swept a finger below each line, or if a slot were cut in a card to show only one line of print while masking the rest of the page. Framing each word between two fingers often stopped print distortion for a while. No one in Berlin's time could explain what caused word blindness, nor could they find a remedy for this reading problem (Berlin, 1884, 1887; Hinshelwood, 1900; Lichteim, 1885).

Following World War I, the American neurologist Samuel Orton studied word blindness in children whom he identified as being dyslexic. Orton (1925, 1937) also saw the kinds of print distortions that Berlin reported. However, Orton's research did not explain the cause for this type of reading disability, nor could he find a remedy that alleviated word blindness for dyslexic readers.

Scotopic Sensitivity, or Irlen Syndrome

During the 1970s the first effective treatment for word blindness was developed by Helen Irlen, an educational psychologist at Long Beach Community College in California. While tutoring a group of dyslexic adults, Irlen discovered that laying colored stage light filters on printed pages often caused word blind distortions to disappear. When Irlen's struggling readers found their best color, most of them no longer saw movement on the page. By adding the right color, many struggling readers no longer were "blinded" by glare from the white page background. When print stood still without background glare, Irlen's dyslexic students began to read normally. At first Irlen called this phenomenon *scotopic sensitivity syndrome*. Later this reading disability pattern was named *Irlen syndrome* (Irlen, 1991).

Dyslexia and Scotopic Sensitivity

Dyslexia and scotopic sensitivity are found together in more than half of those who struggle to read (Eden, 1996; Irlen, 1991; Jordan, 1998, 2000a, 2000b; Weisel, 2001). During the Decade of the Brain, three research teams discovered what causes word blindness, scotopic sensitivity, or Irlen syndrome (Eden, 1996; Lehmkuhle, Garzia, Turner, Hash, & Baro, 1993; Livingstone, Rosen, Drislane, & Galaburda, 1991). Figure 3.1 shows the *magnicellular pathway* that links the retina to the *lateral geniculate nucleus* in the midbrain. These highly specialized portions of the midbrain play a critical role in how the higher brain interprets visual images. We see by light that is reflected from objects around us. In reading and in general seeing, reflected light is absorbed by thousands of *photoreceptors* in the retina. Each photoreceptor is like a tiny camera that takes a snapshot of part of what we see. Photoreceptors change these tiny snapshots of visual information into fast and slow particles of electrical energy. These fast/slow energy bundles are passed along the magnicellular pathway by

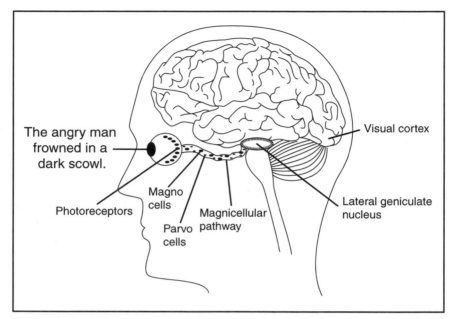

Figure 3.1. Between the retina of each eye and the visual cortex, where the brain interprets what the eyes see, is the magnicellular pathway. This visual pathway contains pairs of cells that work together to pass visual data from the eyes to the brain. Incomplete neural development within the magnicellular pathway causes the brain to see distorted images, especially black print on white paper. These twisting, moving, blurring visual images are called scotopic sensitivity syndrome, or Irlen syndrome.

pairs of specialized neurons called *magno cells* and *parvo cells.* The larger magno cells transfer fast visual chunks from the retina to the midbrain. Magno cells process light impulses for luminance contrast, space, depth perception, movement, motion, and position in space. The smaller parvo cells transfer slower visual particles related to color, shape, curvature, form, and still images. The lateral geniculate nucleus is designed to blend these bundles of fast/slow visual information into mental images that the brain can recognize.

Figure 3.1 shows the neural pathway that links the retina of each eye with the visual cortex. Scotopic sensitivity (Irlen syndrome) is caused by two neurological deficits along this visual pathway. First, the magno cells along the magnicellular pathway are incompletely developed. This makes it impossible for the midbrain to receive accurate fast-vision data. Second, neurons within the lateral geniculate nucleus are underdeveloped, making it impossible for fast/slow vision particles to become blended correctly. Thus the higher brain receives incomplete, unstable visual images that are distorted in the patterns shown in Figures 3.2, 3.3, 3.4, and 3.5.

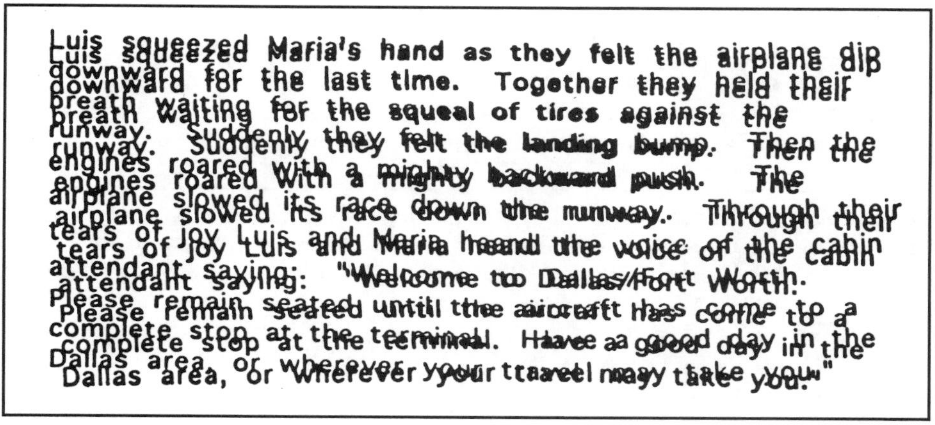

Figure 3.2. Swirl effect. As the eyes focus on a particular word, lines begin to swirl like a rotating wheel. *Note.* From *Attention Deficit Disorder: ADHD and ADD Syndromes* (p. 127), by D. R. Jordan, 1998, Austin, TX: PRO-ED. Copyright 1998 by PRO-ED. Reprinted with permission.

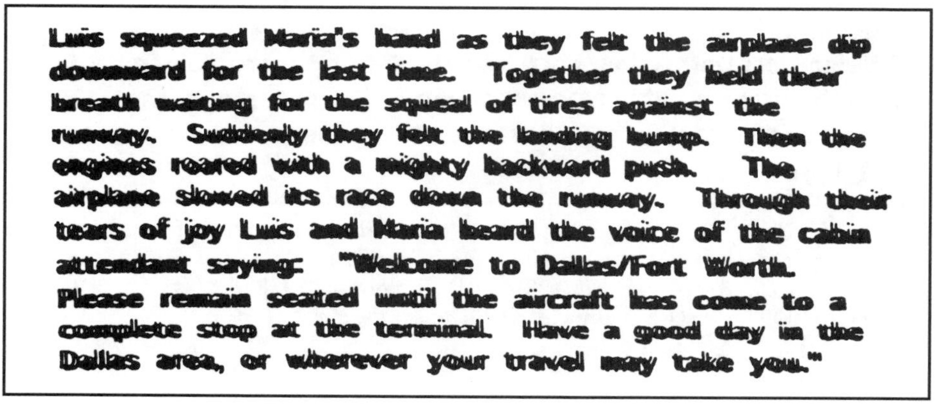

Figure 3.3. Smudge effect. Letters and words move sideways and stack atop each other, then move apart. The page is filled with moving black smudges that are impossible to read. *Note.* From *Attention Deficit Disorder: ADHD and ADD Syndromes* (p. 128), by D. R. Jordan, 1998, Austin, TX: PRO-ED. Copyright 1998 by PRO-ED. Reprinted with permission.

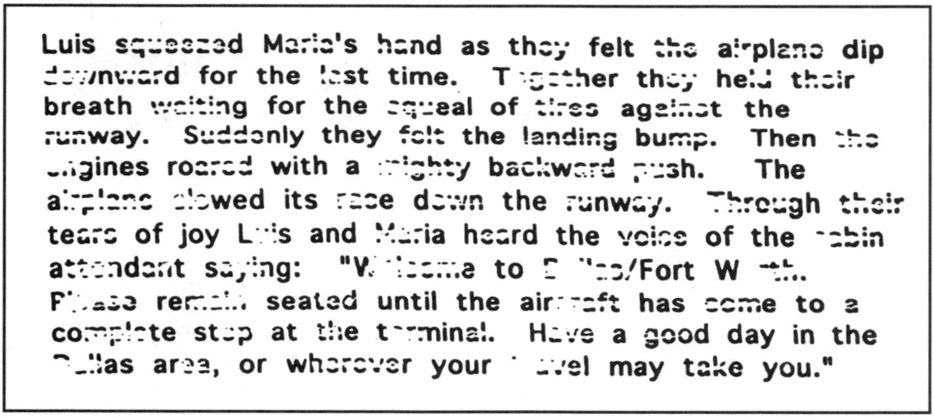

Luis squeezed Maria's hand as they felt the airplane dip
downward for the last time. Together they held their
breath waiting for the squeal of tires against the
runway. Suddenly they felt the landing bump. Then the
engines roared with a mighty backward push. The
airplane slowed its race down the runway. Through their
tears of joy Luis and Maria heard the voice of the cabin
attendant saying: "Welcome to Dallas/Fort Worth.
Please remain seated until the aircraft has come to a
complete stop at the terminal. Have a good day in the
Dallas area, or wherever your travel may take you."

Figure 3.4. Fade in/fade out effect. Inside portions of words begin to fade in and out
in a pulsing rhythm. *Note.* From *Attention Deficit Disorder: ADHD and ADD Syndromes* (p. 129), by D. R. Jordan, 1998, Austin, TX: PRO-ED. Copyright 1998 by
PRO-ED. Reprinted with permission.

Luis squeezed   Maria'shandasthey   felttheairplanedip
downwardfor   thelasttime.Together   theyheldtheir
breathwait   ingforthesqueal of tir   esagainstthe   runw
Suddenlythey   feltthelandingbump.   Thentheengi   nes
roaredwithamig   htybackward push.   Theairplaneslow
itsracedowntherun   way.Throughthe   irtearsofjoy   Luis
andMariaheard   thevoiceofthecabin   attendantsaying
"WelcometoDal   las/Fort Worth.Plea   seremainseated
untiltheaircr   afthascometoacom   pletestopatthe   ga
Haveagood   dayintheDallasarea,or   whereveryour   trav
maytake   you."

Figure 3.5. Cascading rivers effect. Words slide sideways, opening rivers of moving
space that cascade up and down the page. *Note.* From *Attention Deficit Disorder:
ADHD and ADD Syndromes* (p. 128), by D. R. Jordan, 1998, Austin, TX: PRO-ED.
Copyright 1998 by PRO-ED. Reprinted with permission.

Checklist Signature of Scotopic Sensitivity (Irlen Syndrome)

By observing the characteristics of scotopic sensitivity in struggling readers, it is not difficult to separate Irlen syndrome from dyslexia so that each type of learning difficulty is clearly defined. The following checklist provides a quick summary of scotopic sensitivity symptoms. Appendix A presents the Jordan Scotopic Sensitivity Assessment Scale, which provides comprehensive evaluation for the presence of this type of central vision deficit.

_____ Eyes begin to sting or burn while reading, writing, or copying.

_____ Eyes squint to shut out bright light.

_____ Eyes begin to ache or hurt after a few minutes of reading, writing, or copying.

_____ Student shades the page from bright light by leaning over it or holding a hand between the page and overhead light.

_____ Student shades eyes by wearing a bill cap or holding a hand above the eyes.

_____ Print begins to blur immediately after starting to read.

_____ Letters and words run together.

_____ Words and lines start to move or swirl on the page.

_____ Lines begin to merge (stack atop each other), then separate.

_____ Rivers of space cascade down the page so that words separate into chunks that don't make sense.

_____ Letters and words flicker, flash, or blink on and off.

_____ Portions of words begin to fade away, then come back.

_____ Words seem to fall or slide off the edge of the page.

_____ Letters and words become three dimensional as items rise up from the page while other items sink into the background.

(continues)

_____ Print begins to pulse in and out of focus.

_____ Student begins to lean down close to the page, then stretch back away from the page.

_____ Student begins to turn body, shoulders, and head in different directions to see from different angles.

_____ Headache develops first around the eyes, then spreads upward across the forehead and across the temples. Pain may move down the back of the head into the neck.

Aubert–Foerster Syndrome

In 1857 the German ophthalmologists Heinrich Aubert and Manfred Foerster discovered an eye structure difference that caused "symbol blindness" in individuals with normal eyesight (20/20 acuity). In many of the struggling readers they evaluated, the retina of each eye was shaped differently (Aubert & Foerster, 1857). In normal eye development, a specialized cluster of neurons called the *fovea* emerges at the center of the retina. Incoming light is bent by the lense to focus precisely on the fovea where light energy is transformed into electrical pulses. Aubert and Foerster documented how off-center foveal formation frustrates reading for many individuals who are dyslexic. It is impossible for them to integrate what they see straight ahead with what their eyes glimpse from the side. A major problem for these struggling readers is their impression that ascending or descending strokes on tall letters "swim" or "wave" back and forth while the peripheral field appears as a jumbled mass. This type of reading disability became known as the *Aubert–Foerster syndrome.*

Central and Peripheral Vision

It was not until 1987 that off-center foveal structure was linked to dyslexia. Following Aubert and Foerster's research, Gad Geiger and Jerome Lettvin at the Massachusetts Institute of Technology studied the visual patterns of dyslexic adults who struggled to read (Geiger & Lettvin, 1987). Their research explored the relationship between central vision and peripheral vision in dyslexic individuals. To see adequately, the brain must deal with two types of vision at the same time. As the eyes look straight ahead at specific objects (central vision), the eyes also see images around the edges of the visual field (peripheral vision). A critical developmental milestone in young children is when they learn to ignore what they see on the periphery in order to concentrate full attention on what is seen straight ahead. In fact, one of the red flag signals of delayed neuron maturity is the inability to "tune out" peripheral images while attending to what is central in the visual field (Brody, 1987; Hendrickson, 1993). Geiger and Lettvin discovered that many persons who are dyslexic struggle to separate central images from those seen at the outer edges of the visual field.

Saccadic Eye Movement in Reading

Aubert and Foerster were the first to describe the process of lateral masking that must be achieved if an individual is to learn to read. When the fovea of each eye is positioned in the center of the retina, the eyes work together as a team in scanning rhythmically along lines of print. Eye movements in reading are called *saccads*. Normal foveal development permits the eyes to learn how to focus together on a certain spot, then refocus smoothly together to the next focal spot again and again for long periods of time. This rhythmical, sweeping eye movement activity is called saccadic movement. Chapter 2 presented Denckla's concept of neurological talent for reading (see page 37). Struggling readers with off-center foveal structure cannot master rhythmic *saccadic movement* because they do not have neurological talent for reading.

Lateral Masking

Aubert and Foerster created the concept of *lateral masking,* which is a critical factor in reading successfully. They were the first to document what the eyes of a neurologically talented reader see as the eyes travel together along lines of print. Figure 3.6 illustrates the constantly changing peripheral image that occurs during reading. As the eyes make saccadic movements,

> Soon after midnight
> Juan and Daniella woke with
> fear. A giant <u>explosion</u> shook the house
> and rattled the windows very hard.
> Daniella screamed as Juan held
> her in his arms.

Figure 3.6. If the fovea is centered in each retina, the reader's eyes focus on the central word *explosion* while also seeing all of the other words surrounding this central point of focus. The brain learns to concentrate only on the central image while ignoring the periphery. The shape of the central visual field changes constantly with each saccadic movement that refocuses central vision on a new place on the printed page. Auber and Foerster named this ability to process central vision and peripheral vision at the same time *lateral masking.*

the shape and size of the peripheral field change. When both eyes focus on a particular word, central vision reads that word while peripheral vision sees but ignores other words on all sides. Lateral masking is the automatic process most individuals learn to do in blending central and peripheral vision while reading printed symbols on a page.

Using a Slotted Card Marker

When off-center foveal structure exists, it is impossible for the reader to see the whole text. Figure 3.7 shows the "mess" that occurs in off-center foveal reading. Auber–Foerster syndrome makes it impossible for the eyes to team together for smooth saccadic movement. Geiger and Lettvin (1987) demonstrated that masking the print on all sides of the point of focus eliminates symptoms of Auber–Foerster syndrome. Figure 3.8 illustrates the use of a slotted card to let the eyes see only the central image. The body of the card masks the periphery so that the brain does not receive conflicting impressions.

So fer dnht
Jan nd Danla wke ith
f r. gant eplson sh   the hse
and rtl he wdow vry had.
Dnel sremd a Ju hed
he nhi srm

Figure 3.7. Aubert and Foerster (1857) discovered that when foveal structure is off-center, the reader sees this kind of "mess." Off-center foveal development makes it impossible for the eyes to learn smooth saccadic rhythm. The brain receives incomplete images that do not make sense. Most individuals with this off-center foveal structure complain that "the print swims (or waves) back and forth." Lateral masking is impossible for these individuals to achieve.

A giant explosion

Figure 3.8. Geiger and Lettvin (1987) demonstrated how using a slotted card removes the conflict between central and peripheral vision. The slotted card is moved left to right along each line of print. This provides temporary lateral masking so that the individual can see words clearly enough to read successfully. As new segments of print appear in the slot, the reader is able to apply basic reading skills to decode the text.

Checklist Signature of Aubert–Foerster Syndrome

_____ Must touch printed information to read it.

_____ Frames words between two fingers.

_____ Frames lines of print by laying one hand above and the other hand below the line.

_____ Frames lines by laying the left hand above the line while sliding a finger beneath the line.

_____ Reads with a card marker below the line while laying the other hand above the line.

_____ Reads best with a slotted card that shows only a few words at a time.

_____ Upper body posture is changed constantly by leaning in different directions to look at the page from different angles.

_____ Leans down close to the page, then leans back away from the page again and again.

_____ Lays head down on left arm while looking sideways to see the printed page or to guide pencil in writing.

_____ Makes tripod with left hand, then props head against hand and looks sideways at the page.

_____ Frames distant objects with fingers in order to see specific information far away.

_____ Continually loses the place while copying from a chalkboard or overhead projection screen.

_____ Uses fingers to find small objects (screwheads, bolts, slots) instead of looking at them.

_____ Guides tools (screwdriver into screwhead slots, wrench to bolts) instead of using vision to guide tools.

_____ Views computer screen through many "sideways" glances instead of by looking straight ahead at the screen.

_____ Drives vehicles by constantly glancing side to side instead of looking straight ahead.

_____ Reads words correctly through a slot in a card but cannot read the same words without masking the periphery.

Attention Deficit Disorder

For more than 20 years Russell Barkley, Martha Denckla, Mel Levine, Dale Jordan, and others have tracked the relationship between attention deficit disorder and other types of classroom learning differences. This research has found that approximately half of those with hyperactive attention deficit (ADHD) also have dyslexia. It is rare for a struggling learner to have only dyslexia or only ADHD (Barkley, 1990, 1995; Denckla, 1985, 1991a, 1991b, 1993; Jordan, 1998, 2000a, 2000b; Levine, 1990, 1993). The issue of attention deficit disorder is one of the most controversial topics in the treatment of learning differences. A broad range of opinions about attention deficit disorder exist among professionals who treat inattention in children, adolescents, and adults. At one end of the opinion scale is the point of view presented by Thomas Armstrong's book *The Myth of the A.D.D. Child.* Armstrong (1995) expresses deep skepticism that there is such a problem as ADHD or ADD. This school of thought insists that although inattentive children may be socially or educationally disruptive, such behavior is normal and should not be treated as a medical or mental health problem.

On the opposite end of the opinion scale is the point of view that chronic inattention in children, adolescents, and adults is a brain-based difference that must be regarded as a medical and/or mental health challenge. An enormous body of research has documented differences in neurotransmitter functions, neuron formation, and genetic predisposition for ADHD (Attention-Deficit/Hyperactive Disorder) and ADD (Attention Deficit without Hyperactivity) (Barkley, 1990, 1995; Copeland, 1991; Hallowell & Ratey, 1994a, 1994b; Jordan, 1998; Parker, 1989; Warren & Capehart, 1995; Weiss, 1992, 1995). Brain imaging research has provided a scientific structure for understanding causes of inattention, as well as for seeing the link between attention deficit and dyslexia.

How the Brain Pays Attention

Figure 3.9 shows the nine regions of the brain that team together to create full attention. Chapter 1 described how the brain becomes organized to pay full attention. The prefrontal cortex is the executive in charge of brain functions related to

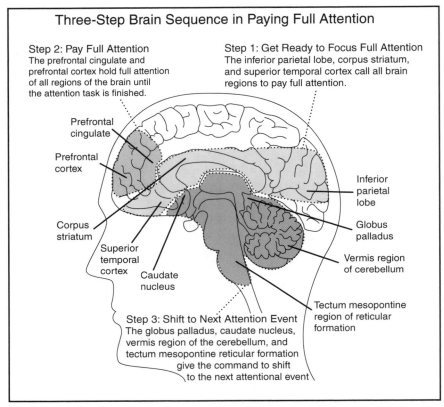

Three-Step Brain Sequence in Paying Full Attention

Step 2: Pay Full Attention
The prefrontal cingulate and prefrontal cortex hold full attention of all regions of the brain until the attention task is finished.

Step 1: Get Ready to Focus Full Attention
The inferior parietal lobe, corpus striatum, and superior temporal cortex call all brain regions to pay full attention.

Prefrontal cingulate

Prefrontal cortex

Corpus striatum

Superior temporal cortex

Caudate nucleus

Inferior parietal lobe

Globus palladus

Vermis region of cerebellum

Tectum mesopontine region of reticular formation

Step 3: Shift to Next Attention Event
The globus palladus, caudate nucleus, vermis region of the cerebellum, and tectum mesopontine reticular formation give the command to shift to the next attentional event

Figure 3.9. Countless times every day this three-step cycle is repeated as the brain pays attention. When any of these nine brain regions fails to play its role in this cycle, or when different brain regions fire too slowly or too rapidly, the brain loses its ability to keep on paying attention. Sometimes inattention is accompanied by hyperactivity, impulsivity, and other disruptive ADHD behavior. Sometimes inattention is masked by passive ADD behavior that involves daydreaming and make-believe thinking. (Based on research by Barkley, 1990, 1995; Damasio, 1994, 1999; Denckla, 1985, 1991a, 1993; Hampton-Turner, 1981; and Hinshaw, Henker, & Whalen, 1984.)

intelligence, language, and choice. The prefrontal cortex communicates continually with other brain regions through rhythmical flows of electrical and chemical energy.

To stay in charge as the brain's executive, the prefrontal cortex maintains a steady firing rhythm of 40 cycles per second. This rate of firing depends on a constant supply of two neurotransmitters: dopamine and serotonin. When the prefrontal cortex is firing steadily 40 times per second, the nine brain regions shown in Figure 3.9 stay in close communication and act together as a well-coordinated team. If any of these nine brain regions fires too slowly or too rapidly, the rhythm of the brain falters and attention is lost.

Basal Emotions Must Wait

Chapter 1 described how the brain must maintain a balance between socially disruptive emotions that originate in the midbrain and socially constructive emotions that originate in the prefrontal cortex. The main task of the executive function is to make sure that the brain waits before taking action. Waiting permits the brain to apply logic, consider cause-and-effect consequences, and think through possibilities and alternatives to make sure that actions do not place the individual in danger. This thoughtful higher brain process fosters commonsense thinking and mature, safe behavior. To maintain this pursuit of logic, the three-step sequence in paying attention (Figure 3.9) must occur without fail. Step by step, these brain teams command basal emotions to "Wait!" When dopamine and serotonin are well balanced throughout the brain, the executive function stays in charge through a type of dialogue: "What might happen if we choose to do this? What would be the consequences? Would this action create a threatening or unsafe situation?" Waiting before acting is the first responsibility of the higher brain.

What Is Attention Deficit Disorder?

Whether loss of attention is accompanied by hyperactivity (ADHD) or by passivity (ADD), attention deficit disorder means that the brain cannot wait. Impulsivity takes charge of decision making. Snap judgment replaces thinking things through before acting. Socially disruptive behavior erupts to interfere with socially constructive intentions. Attention deficit disorder means that the strong emotions from the limbic system overwhelm higher emotions within the executive function. If the inattentive person is hyperactive (ADHD), satisfying body sensations and indulging the urge to move take charge of brain activity. If the inattentive person is passive (ADD), he or she slips into a private, invisible world of make-believe, fantasy thinking, and daydreaming that disconnects the individual from reality. More than half of those who are dyslexic also have ADHD or ADD, which greatly complicates their academic performance and social success.

The Levine Principles for Full Attention

Early in the Decade of the Brain, pediatric neurologist Mel Levine (1990) proposed a model of how the brain pays attention. Levine's model names nine control systems, or "principles," within the brain that are disrupted when attention deficit disorder exists. When these nine principles of paying attention are fully developed, individuals become socially mature. The following passages have been paraphrased to simplify the technical language of Levine's original presentation.

1. *Focal control.* To pay attention fully, the brain must achieve focal control that regulates attention span. While the basal brain filters out (ignores) extraneous information, the higher brain focuses without being distracted. Attention deficit occurs when the higher brain cannot maintain focal control. Too much extraneous data enter thought streams, resulting in cluttered mental images and confused perception. This loss of focal control is called *short attention span* and triggers impulsive, random, disorganized behavior filled with mistakes and poor decisions.

2. *Sensory control.* Ignoring body feelings requires the brain to say "no" to impulses linked to moving about or to satisfying body feelings. Having sensory control means that individuals ignore body feelings in order to do tasks that require full attention. Mature sensory control allows the brain to ignore nearby sound, tune out nearby activity, decide not to respond to nearby conversation, and so forth. Attention deficit means that the person is controlled by "sensory distractibility" that interferes with learning and disrupts social relationships. Poor sensory control triggers poor listening, continual mistakes in comprehension, jittery/nervous mannerisms, inability to "stay plugged in" when full attention is required, obsessive habits, and compulsive behaviors.

3. *Associative control.* When a child's brain develops normally, he or she quickly learns how to concentrate on a thought without becoming distracted or sidetracked. The brain learns to finish tasks instead of leaving them unfinished. Attention deficit

disorder involves poor associative control. These individuals continually wander off on "mental rabbit trails" that lead them into daydreaming or fantasy thinking. Make-believe thinking takes the place of reality. Hyperactive inattention (ADHD) triggers body actions that act out fantasy thinking. Passive inattention (ADD) produces quiet, private episodes that separate the individual from what occurs in his or her world.

4. *Appetite control.* When the brain follows normal developmental patterns, children learn to wait. They develop self-control of urges for gratification. This often is called *delayed gratification.* Attention deficit disorder makes it impossible for a person to wait for gratification. He or she follows a lifestyle of "chosen restlessness" that disrupts others. Poor appetite control involves self-focus instead of seeing the needs of others. Individuals with poor appetite control do not share. They are overly concerned about themselves. They struggle against rules and regulations that require them to remain still, stay calm, and put off satisfying desires.

5. *Social control.* Our culture assumes that as children reach developmental milestones, they learn social control that enables them to "read" boundary signals that protect personal privacy. A major problem with ADHD is the compulsive behavior of invading the privacy of others. Poor social control provokes others and disrupts relationships because of intrusive, thoughtless invasions of privacy.

6. *Motor control.* A major goal of childhood development is to learn how to plan and think before acting. Motor control involves purpose and having a good reason for whatever the body does. Attention deficit includes poor motor control that triggers random activity with no real purpose. ADHD and ADD individuals are "socially inefficient." They do not follow goals or stay organized without supervision.

7. *Behavioral control.* Normal behavioral control produces self-control, ability to fit in with others, and the lifestyle of taking responsibility for what one does. Attention deficit disorder includes poor behavioral control. Behavior is impulsive and unplanned. ADHD or ADD individuals do not accept responsibility for mistakes and blunders. They blame others, deny their part in disruptive incidents, and continue to repeat inappropriate behavior without learning from mistakes.

8. *Communicative control.* When children develop normally, they learn the social principle of appropriate behavior. They learn

good manners and how to respect others. Attention deficit disorder includes inappropriate habits that embarrass others. ADHD individuals overreact with inappropriate emotional eruptions. They are too quick to argue, complain, and blame others. They do not understand why it is important to please others and why it is necessary not to offend others with rude or vulgar speech.

9. *Affective control.* As children reach developmental milestones, they learn to control emotions and not to be moody and unpleasant. Individuals with ADHD have poor affective control. They are prone to having mood swings that range from being deeply unhappy to being overly elated. Poor affective control causes disruptions in the classroom, in social groups, and in personal relationships.

Checklist Signature of Attention Deficit Disorder

The following checklist provides an overview of how individuals pay attention. Separating dyslexia from ADHD or ADD requires careful observation of lifestyle habits. Appendix B presents the Jordan Attention Deficit Scale, which provides a comprehensive assessment of attention deficit patterns.

_____ *Hyperactivity.* Excessive body activity. Cannot ignore what goes on nearby. Cannot say "no" to impulses. Cannot leave others alone. Cannot be alone without feeling nervous and left out. Cannot leave things alone. Cannot keep still or stay quiet. Cannot stay calm.

_____ *Passivity.* Below-normal body activity. Spends long periods of time off in own private world of make-believe/fantasy thinking and daydreaming. Is reluctant to become part of group activities. Avoids answering questions. Does not volunteer information. Uses fewest possible words when required to talk. Prefers to be alone while avoiding group activities.

_____ *Short attention span.* Cannot keep thoughts focused or concentrated longer than 60–90 seconds. Continually is off on "mental rabbit trails." Must continually be called back to finish tasks. Drifts or darts away from tasks and personal interaction.

_____ *Loose thought patterns.* Cannot maintain organized mental images. Continually loses important details. Cannot remember a series of events, facts, or details. Cannot do a series of things without starting to make mistakes and losing the sequence. Must have help to tell what has happened. Cannot follow a series of instructions without being reminded. Cannot remember assignments or responsibilities over time. Cannot remember game rules, names of people, names of places, and names of things.

_____ *Poor organization.* Cannot keep life organized without help. Continually loses things. Cannot stay on a schedule without supervision. Lives in a cluttered space. Cannot straighten up own room or work space without help. Cannot do homework without supervision. Cannot stay on time schedules or meet deadlines without supervision

_____ *Change of first impression.* First impressions do not stay the same. Mental images change immediately. While writing or copying, he or she continually erases and changes. Has the impression that others "play tricks" because things seem to shift and change. Printed words, spelling patterns, and math problems seem to change.

_____ *Poor listening comprehension.* Continually says "What?" or "Huh?" or "What do you mean?" Cannot get the full meaning of what others say. Cannot follow oral instructions without hearing them again. Needs oral information to be repeated and explained again. Does not keep on listening. Attention drifts or fades away before others finish speaking. Later insists "You didn't say that" or "I didn't hear you say that." Later cannot remember what a speaker said.

(continues)

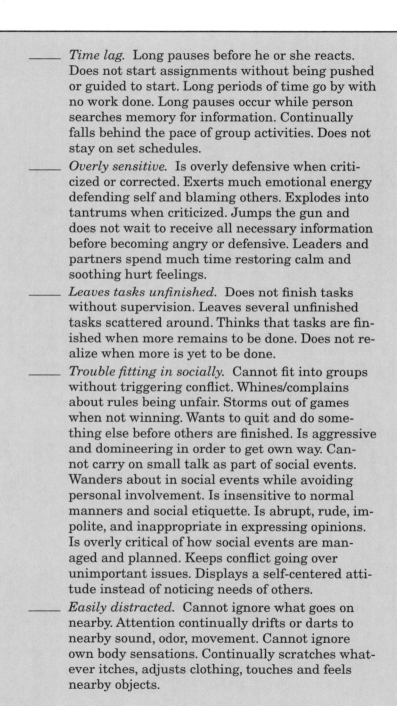

_____ *Time lag.* Long pauses before he or she reacts. Does not start assignments without being pushed or guided to start. Long periods of time go by with no work done. Long pauses occur while person searches memory for information. Continually falls behind the pace of group activities. Does not stay on set schedules.

_____ *Overly sensitive.* Is overly defensive when criticized or corrected. Exerts much emotional energy defending self and blaming others. Explodes into tantrums when criticized. Jumps the gun and does not wait to receive all necessary information before becoming angry or defensive. Leaders and partners spend much time restoring calm and soothing hurt feelings.

_____ *Leaves tasks unfinished.* Does not finish tasks without supervision. Leaves several unfinished tasks scattered around. Thinks that tasks are finished when more remains to be done. Does not realize when more is yet to be done.

_____ *Trouble fitting in socially.* Cannot fit into groups without triggering conflict. Whines/complains about rules being unfair. Storms out of games when not winning. Wants to quit and do something else before others are finished. Is aggressive and domineering in order to get own way. Cannot carry on small talk as part of social events. Wanders about in social events while avoiding personal involvement. Is insensitive to normal manners and social etiquette. Is abrupt, rude, impolite, and inappropriate in expressing opinions. Is overly critical of how social events are managed and planned. Keeps conflict going over unimportant issues. Displays a self-centered attitude instead of noticing needs of others.

_____ *Easily distracted.* Cannot ignore what goes on nearby. Attention continually drifts or darts to nearby sound, odor, movement. Cannot ignore own body sensations. Continually scratches whatever itches, adjusts clothing, touches and feels nearby objects.

_____ *Immaturity.* Behavior is obviously less mature than expected for that age. Behaves like a much younger person. Cannot get along with age-mates. Prefers to play or be with younger persons. Has interests and thought patterns of much younger individuals. Does not make effort to "grow up." Refuses to accept responsibility or to become responsible. Behavior is impulsive/often compulsive. Acts on spur of the moment instead of thinking things through. Refuses long-range goals. Insists on immediate satisfaction of desires and wishes. Blames others for own mistakes. Triggers the displeasure of companions. Often is disliked by others.

_____ *Insatiability.* Desires never are satisfied fully. Clamors for more regardless of how much has been received. Cannot leave others alone. Demands attention. Is bored quickly and wants something different. Complains that others get a larger share. Drains emotions of those who must be involved in this person's life. Triggers desire in others to push this person away. Often is dreaded by others. Becomes target of rejection by others.

_____ *Impulsivity.* Does not plan ahead. Acts on spur of the moment. Does whatever comes to mind. Shows no common sense in making decisions. Does not think of consequences. Demands immediate satisfaction of wishes and desires. Is a "now" person. Cannot put off desires or wishes.

_____ *Disruptiveness.* Is a disruptive influence in a group. Keeps things stirred up. Triggers conflict within a group. Disturbs neighbors during study time. Causes others to complain about how he or she is behaving. Others are relieved when this person is absent.

_____ *Body energy overflow.* Some part of the body is in continual motion. Cannot sit still or be quiet. Can hold body motions under control briefly, but energy overflow soon starts again. Fingers fiddle with things. Feet scrub the floor and bump furniture. Body squirms around. Mouth makes irritating sounds. Cannot stop fiddling with things that make noise.

(continues)

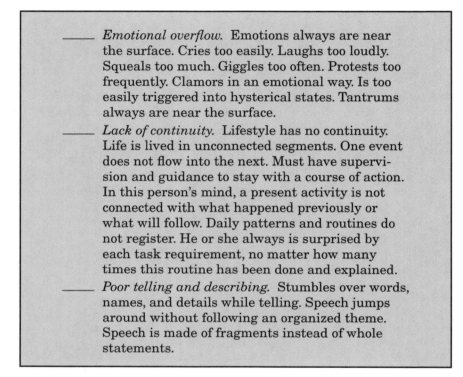

_____ *Emotional overflow.* Emotions always are near the surface. Cries too easily. Laughs too loudly. Squeals too much. Giggles too often. Protests too frequently. Clamors in an emotional way. Is too easily triggered into hysterical states. Tantrums always are near the surface.

_____ *Lack of continuity.* Lifestyle has no continuity. Life is lived in unconnected segments. One event does not flow into the next. Must have supervision and guidance to stay with a course of action. In this person's mind, a present activity is not connected with what happened previously or what will follow. Daily patterns and routines do not register. He or she always is surprised by each task requirement, no matter how many times this routine has been done and explained.

_____ *Poor telling and describing.* Stumbles over words, names, and details while telling. Speech jumps around without following an organized theme. Speech is made of fragments instead of whole statements.

Separating Layers of Learning Difficulty

Later chapters show how to pinpoint dyslexia as individuals read, spell, write, listen, remember, and do arithmetic computation. If overlapping layers of attention deficit (ADHD or ADD), scotopic sensitivity, or central vision disorder are not identified, then special tutoring strategies will not bring success to dyslexic learners. Until these patterns are explained and described, few dyslexic persons are aware that they see differently or attend poorly. Knowing why reading, copying, and listening are difficult opens new doors to self-understanding. The most common reaction when struggling learners learn why they stumble is, "You mean I'm not dumb? I've always thought I was too dumb to do better. You mean I'm not really dumb?" This astonishing self-discovery is the most powerful encouragement that a dyslexic learner can receive.

Overcoming Visual Dyslexia

4

The new dad is doing well a few copeing problems but we made it through. Only be cause Julie is supper mom and haveing her mom here has proven invaulable.

—Note from a tenured university professor who is dyslexic

C hapter 2 presented the concepts that reading is an unnatural invention, and not all individuals have a neurological talent for reading. When early childhood is filled with the nurture of rich language stimulus, rapid neuron pruning occurs in all regions of the brain (see Figure 1.3). Oral language skills develop naturally as neuron pathways within the left temporal lobe become pruned and well connected. Except for individuals with severe neuron deficits within the left temporal lobe, most children are born with neurological talent for oral language that develops naturally without formal training. Not everyone is born with neurological talent for learning to read.

How the Left Brain Learns To Read

Reading Is Unnatural

The human brain is not naturally "wired" for reading, spelling, or handwriting (Lyon, 2000; McGuinness, 1997). The brain does not come prepared to deal with the inventions of alphabet letters, math numerals, or penmanship symbols. However, in four out of five individuals, the brain is remarkably plastic with the capacity to grow specialized neuron pathways in response to the stimulus of learning to read. For a person to learn to read, neurons throughout the left brain must be shaped and "hardwired" through intensive practice at recognizing alphabet symbols, shapes of words, and word clusters. Before talent for reading can emerge, complex neuron connections must be developed through the cultural process of learning to read. With intensive instruction over several years, two out of five persons develop a rich complex of neuron pathways throughout the left brain to become fluent in literacy skills. They are the "stars" of the classroom and workplace in tasks requiring rapid reading with full comprehension. Another two out of five individuals develop enough neural capacity to become average readers with basic literacy skills adequate for necessary reading. The remaining one out of five persons never develops the required neuron connections to become competent at reading no matter how much tutoring they receive. Most of these nonreading individuals are dyslexic (Denckla, 1993; Galaburda, 1983; Geschwind, 1984; Hardman & Rennick, 2000; Irlen, 1991; Jordan, 1996a, 1998, 2000a, 2000b; Orton, 1937; Rawson, 1988; Steeves, 1987; Weisel, 1992, 2001).

The Challenge of Learning To Read

Parents and teachers seldom think of the enormous task children face in learning to read, spell, and write by hand. Changing speech into print or handwriting confronts the brain with awesome challenges that our culture takes for granted. To learn to read, the brain must figure out how to connect oral language to printed symbols. Young children who have only just begun to master the complexities of speech are required to develop fluency in a two-way literacy process. First, they must learn how to decode what they see by translating print into "words we say." Second, they must learn how to encode what they hear and say into "speech written down." With this cognitive challenge in mind, the surprise is not that many fail to learn to read—the surprise is that so many learn to read at all.

Learning the Direction of Reading

Every oral language has a semantic structure that requires learners to memorize which way words should go. This verbal structure determines where a speaker places naming words, action words, and describing words. Some languages place describing words ahead of naming words. Other cultures use naming words first, followed by describers. Verb placement also varies from culture to culture. Outsiders to an oral culture often are bewildered when they hear names, actions, and descriptions used "out of sequence" or in different semantic directions. Much of the excitement of learning a second language comes through discovering differences in the direction that another language takes.

Learning to read requires the brain to develop automatic memory for the direction that written language takes. All cultures that use a printed alphabet establish rules for which direction each symbol must face. Reading can take place only if everyone follows the same directional rules. Languages based on the Roman alphabet, such as English, Spanish, and French, require the reader to decode left to right and top to bottom.

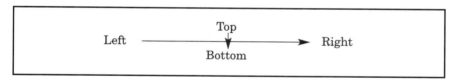

Every alphabet symbol must follow this directional rule so that all readers see the same thing. Otherwise, it would be impossible to have an effective reading culture. To be correct, each letter must face a certain way whether it stands alone, is part of a word, or joins a sea of letters covering a printed page. No letters may flip upside down or backwards, and all letters must be scanned left to right. Furthermore, the brain must develop the capacity to recognize thousands of letter combinations automatically without pausing to figure out which alphabet symbols these are.

How Many Letters Are in the Alphabet?

When asked how many letters are in the alphabet, most English-language speakers think 26. In fact, by the time a child enters fourth grade, he or she is expected to be fluent at encoding and decoding 104 alphabet letters. As a rule, children begin to practice reading and writing with manuscript printed letters. This requires their brains to memorize 26 capital letters and 26 corresponding lowercase letters. Several of these capital/lowercase pairs do not look alike.

A B C D E F G H I J K L M N O P Q R S T U V W X Y Z
a b c d e f g h i j k l m n o p q r s t u v w x y z

These 52 alphabet letters always must face the same way. Adults say "You made a mistake" whenever a learner turns letters backwards or upside down.

For the first 3 years in school (kindergarten through second grade), children spend many hours developing automatic memory for these 52 alphabet symbols. As third grade begins, a surprising thing happens in most classrooms. Students are told that now they must learn another way to read and write alphabet letters. Much of what they have learned about written language symbols since kindergarten no longer will be appropriate. Now they must learn to "write cursive." In third grade most youngsters face a new version of 52 alphabet symbols. Again, many of the lowercase cursive letters do not look like their capital letter companions.

Aa Bb Cc Dd Ee Ff Gg Hh Ii Jj Kk Ll Mm
Nn Oo Pp Qq Rr Ss Tt Uu Vv Ww Xx Yy Zz

By age 9 youngsters are expected to be fluent in reading and writing countless combinations of alphabet letters. This is possible only if the brain has the capacity to develop specialized neural connections for processing this unnatural, invented language.

How the Neurologically Talented Left Brain Reads

During the Decade of the Brain, Sally Shaywitz (1996) at Yale University documented the "hardwired" neuron loop within the left brain that permits individuals to read. Figure 4.1 shows the sequence of left-brain activity that never comes naturally for

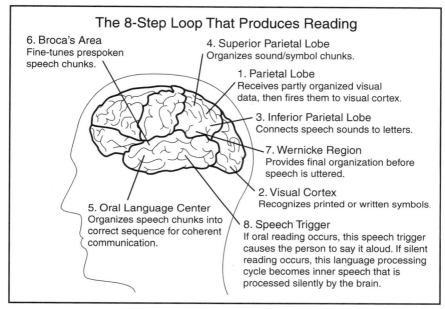

Figure 4.1. Shaywitz (1996) has shown this eight-step loop within the left brain for persons who have neurological talent for reading. Dyslexia interrupts this reading sequence because too many neurons are incompletely developed.

those who are dyslexic. When printed information passes the safety test described in Chapter 1, the geniculate nucleus fires that data up to the left parietal lobe (1) where the visual image is partially organized. The parietal lobe then fires the print-related data to the visual cortex (2) where alphabet symbols are recognized. From there the print images go to the inferior parietal lobe (3) where speech sounds are connected to letters. This sound/symbol information then goes to the superior parietal lobe (4) where the letter/sound chunks are organized. These data then are fired to the oral language center (5) within the temporal lobe where letter/sound chunks are sorted into correct sequence. From there the prereading data pass to the Broca's area (6) where fine-tuning of prespeech segments is done. Then the print-related information is fired to the Wernicke region (7) for final organization, and finally to the speech trigger (8) for vocal utterance. If the person reads silently, this speech information is translated into the brain's "inner voice" instead of being spoken aloud. With enough stimulus from formal reading instruction, four out of five individuals have the neurological capacity to develop this neural loop well enough to acquire adequate literacy skills. Those who are dyslexic do not.

Visual Dyslexia

The subtype of dyslexia that interferes with reading is called *visual dyslexia*. This learning difference is not caused by the eyes. Visual dyslexia occurs within the left visual cortex where printed or written symbols are recognized. Figure 4.2 shows the point in the visual perception sequence where dyslexia first blocks word recognition. If the individual does not have scotopic sensitivity, Aubert–Foerster syndrome, or an uncorrected vision problem, print-related data reach the parietal lobe on schedule (see Figure 4.1). Figure 4.2 shows where visual dyslexia first appears. When images of printed symbols reach the left visual cortex,

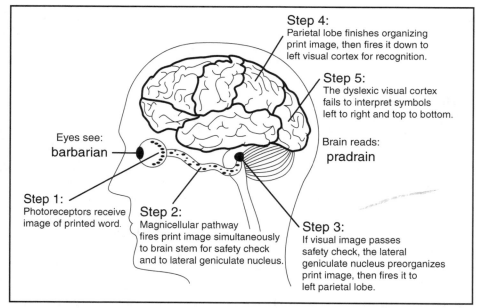

Figure 4.2. Visual dyslexia occurs at step 5 within the left visual cortex. Incomplete development of neurons in this region of the left brain make it impossible for the individual to develop automatic memory for this left-to-right, top-to-bottom orientation of printed symbols. This person does not have neurological talent for reading. (Based on research by Atkinson, 1984; Johnson, 1994; Khan, 1994; Shaywitz, 1996; and van Essen & Gallant, 1994.)

dyslexia prohibits the brain from recognizing some of the printed or written language symbols. Visual dyslexia interferes with memory for which direction alphabet letters should face. The visual cortex fails to follow the sequence of printed language symbols. Mental images of what the person sees are scrambled with some of the individual letters reversed or upside down. As dyslexic individuals try to read, copy, or write from memory, certain letters or numerals often are backwards (*b–d, p–q, 3–E, Z, L, S*). Other symbols often flip upside down (*M–W, N–U, p–b, f–t, 6–9, 7–L*). Visual dyslexia often causes inside portions of words to be read or written backwards (*brid–bird, gril–girl, bran–barn, form–from*). Frequently, whole words or number units are read backwards (*on–no, was–saw, 81–18*). This is called *mirror image.* Individuals with visual dyslexia tend to scramble the sequence of what they see, as when they see 451 but say "five-four-one." In reading words and phrases, dyslexic readers confuse familiar words for something else. For example, a dyslexic man in a restaurant saw a sign:

> Hamburgers
> 3 for $1.00.

He asked a friend, "Why would they be selling hummingbirds in a restaurant?" A dyslexic individual saw the sentence *These items are inedible.* His dyslexic brain read, "The times are indelible." This lifelong tendency to reverse, flip upside down, and scramble the sequence creates constant confusion in reading traffic signs, interpreting newspaper headlines, finding information in directories, and so forth.

The Signature of Visual Dyslexia

Identifying Visual Dyslexia

Chapter 2 presents the Checklist Signature of Dyslexia (pages 55–58), which summarizes the many ways in which dyslexia interferes with classroom learning. The signature of visual dyslexia is discovered by asking struggling learners to do certain things that involve interpreting printed information, copying, writing from dictation, matching words, and matching number groups. An especially useful screening test for visual dyslexia is presented in Appendix C: the Jordan Test for Visual Dyslexia. This test quickly identifies dyslexia. Other widely use tests for dyslexia are the *Slingerland Screening Tests for Identifying Children with Specific Language Disability* (Slingerland, 1984), and Malcomesius's *Specific Language Disability Test* (Malcomesius, 2000). Visual dyslexia occurs when the left brain cannot remember how to interpret language symbols accurately, how to read words left to right, or how to remember language details in sequence. These screening tests are designed to bring these dyslexic patterns to the surface through informal assessments that seldom trigger fear or feelings of danger.

Backward or Upside Down Symbols

The Jordan Test for Visual Dyslexia begins by asking the student to write the alphabet, then the days of the week, and finally the months of the year from memory. These simple tasks quickly reveal dyslexia if it exists. *First seen* is any struggle to remember the alphabet sequence, as well as the sequence of the days and months. *Second seen* is any tendency to turn letters backwards or upside down. *Third seen* is a chronic struggle to write legibly. *Fourth seen* is how soon the person reaches burnout that forces the individual to stop trying to encode and decode language symbols. Figure 4.3 shows the effort of an 11-year-old boy to write the alphabet. He was greatly frustrated because he could not remember which way each letter should face. As he wrote the backwards Z, he put down his pencil and refused to try to write the days or months. "My brain is too tired," he said.

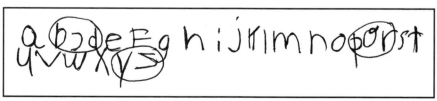

Figure 4.3. This 11-year-old boy scored mental age 13 years, 8 months on an intelligence test, yet he struggles very hard to write the alphabet from memory. After finishing this task, he was too exhausted to attempt to write the days or the months. Rapid "burnout" is a major problem for him in the classroom.

Figures 4.4 and 4.5 show visual dyslexic struggle as two bright students tried to write the alphabet, then the days of the week. Their work shows mixed capital and lowercase letters along with reversed letters, scrambled sequence, and great difficulty spelling correctly. Figure 4.6 shows lack of left-to-right, top-to-bottom orientation. This 15-year-old student always is confused by these language directions. Unless he is reminded or

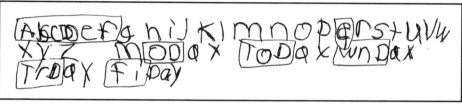

Figure 4.4. This 10-year-old boy has had constant tutoring in reading skills since he was 7 years old. He cannot develop permanent memory for written language data such as the alphabet or days of the week. However, he can recite orally the full alphabet and all the days in correct sequence.

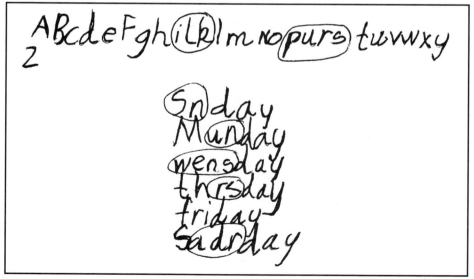

Figure 4.5. The work of this 12-year-old girl shows the dyslexic characteristics of mixing capital and lowercase letters, along with mixing manuscript print with cursive writing style.

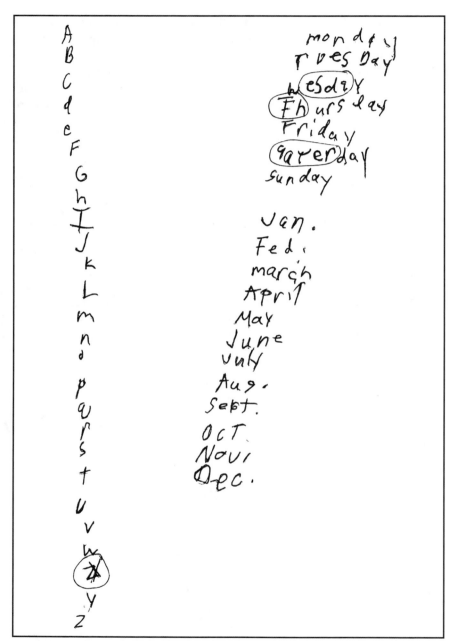

Figure 4.6. This 15-year-old boy never has learned left-to-right, top-to-bottom orientation. His natural spatial orientation is top to bottom. In all of his classroom work he shows confusion when asked to work left to right. He needs continual coaching and reminding to follow a left-to-right sequence.

prompted, he starts downward instead of across. In Figure 4.7 a highly intelligent 12-year-old student wrote the alphabet in cursive style. Each letter was carefully drawn. However, when she began to write words (days of the week), her brain reverted to the manuscript print style she had mastered during her first 3 years in school. Figure 4.8 shows the kind of gleaning that most dyslexic individuals do when their memory fails to deliver the data they need. This 17-year-old student had a wide range of strategies for gleaning clues when his brain failed to make memory connections. Figure 4.9 shows the multiple problems that confront many dyslexic individuals. This 13-year-old girl continually turned letters backwards. She constantly lost the sequence of mental images, and she never was sure which way to turn the pencil in writing. To recall simple data related to reading and writing, she had to be prompted and reminded. Her handwriting mixed capital and lowercase letters, as well as cursive and manuscript styles. Figure 4.10 presents the writing of an adult who had extraordinary right-brain talent for creating

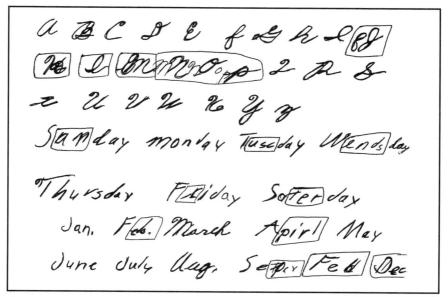

Figure 4.7. This 12-year-old girl has struggled hard to learn to write in cursive style. With great effort she drew each cursive letter separately in writing the alphabet. However, she reverted to manuscript print style as she wrote words. This is characteristic of visual dyslexia.

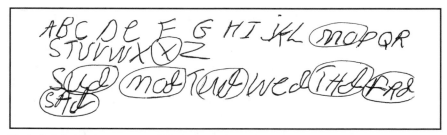

Figure 4.8. This 17-year-old boy wrote the alphabet with confidence, although he did not notice that he skipped *n* and wrote *y* backwards. He could not remember the sequence of the days, so he looked at his digital watch for clues. His struggle to write the days is typical of dyslexia.

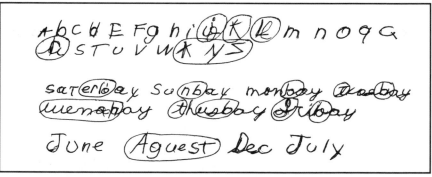

Figure 4.9. The work of this 13-year-old girl shows several signs of visual dyslexia. She has a continual tendency to turn letters backwards. She continually loses the sequence of her thoughts and must start over. Her handwriting is filled with bits and pieces that show where her pencil turned the opposite way to write the next stroke. She cannot remember details in sequence without being prompted or coached. She mixes capital/lowercase letters, and she mixes cursive/manuscript writing styles.

custom furniture. However, he had virtually no neurological talent for reading, spelling, or writing.

Struggle to Match Speech with Print

The *Slingerland Screening Tests for Identifying Children with Specific Language Disability* and Malcomesius's *Specific Language Disability Test* reveal a wide array of dyslexic patterns. Figure 4.11 shows poor ability to focus and refocus the eyes to-

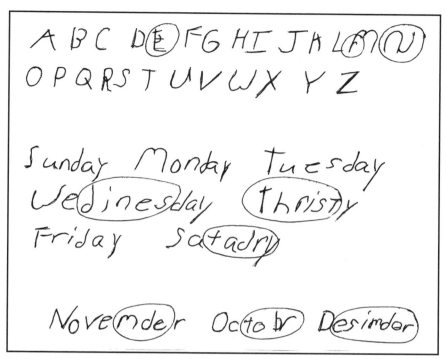

Figure 4.10. This 21-year-old man dropped out of school at age 14 because he was overwhelmed by failure. He had extraordinary talent for woodwork. By age 16 he was earning more than $20,000 per year designing and building custom furniture. By age 21 he owned a successful business with five full-time employees. A patient office manager helped him process paperwork and helped him stay on work schedules.

gether in reading and copying. This student was forced to exert great effort to maintain eye tracking as he focused back and forth while copying from the board or from a projector screen. He could not keep the place as his focus changed to far, then back to near. This kind of poor visual control often overlaps dyslexia. Figure 4.12 shows immediate loss of memory for what this 13-year-old girl saw as she did classroom assignments. She struggled hard in any copy activity. In working math problems, she made inadvertent mistakes that caused adults to think that she did not know math concepts. Figure 4.13 shows constant dyslexic struggle to match words that are alike. This 10-year-old boy taught himself how to eliminate choices that did not

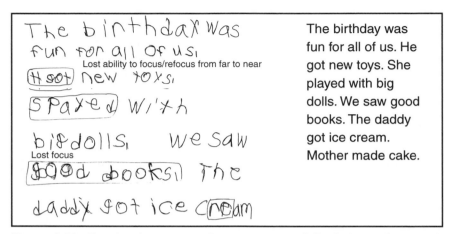

The birthday was
fun for all of us. He
got new toys. She
played with big
dolls. We saw good
books. The daddy
got ice cream.
Mother made cake.

Figure 4.11. Copying from across the room is very difficult for students with visual dyslexia. This 11-year-old boy struggled hard to focus successfully back and forth from far to near. He constantly lost the place and left out chunks of visual data. All copying tasks overwhelm him with failure. He reached "burnout" before finishing this task. *Note.* From *Slingerland Screening Tests for Identifying Children with Specific Language Disability,* Form B, by B. H. Slingerland, 1984, Cambridge, MA: Educators Publishing Service. Copyright 1984 by Educators Publishing Service. Reprinted with permission.

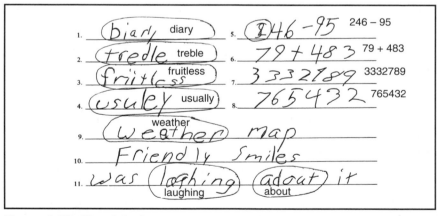

Figure 4.12. Visual dyslexia emerges as students try to write from memory what they have just seen. This 13-year-old girl's short-term memory could not maintain mental images of the word patterns she had just seen on cards. Her memory for number groups was stronger than her memory for alphabet symbols and letter sequences within words. *Note.* From *Slingerland Screening Tests for Identifying Children with Specific Language Disability,* Form C, by B. H. Slingerland, 1984, Cambridge, MA: Educators Publishing Service. Copyright 1984 by Educators Publishing Service. Reprinted with permission.

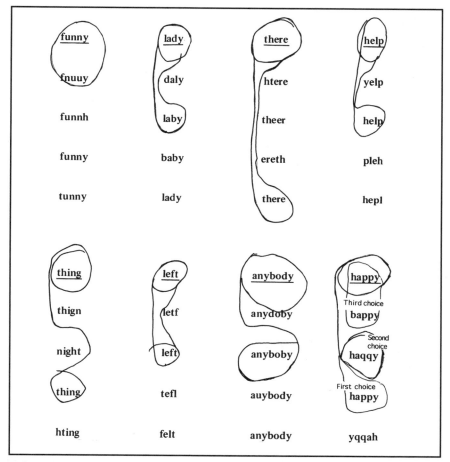

Figure 4.13. Visual dyslexia was a major problem for this 10-year-old boy as he tried to match words. He attempted to control his confusion by linking matching choices with loops to exclude patterns that did not appear to match. *Note.* From *Slingerland Screening Tests for Identifying Children with Specific Language Disability,* Form C, by B. H. Slingerland, 1984, Cambridge, MA: Educators Publishing Service. Copyright 1984 by Educators Publishing Service. Reprinted with permission.

seem correct. By drawing elaborate loops to link his matching choices, he managed to follow a process of elimination without reaching a point of burnout. Figure 4.14 shows the frustration most dyslexic readers face as they try to decode words. This 19-year-old man could not maintain left-to-right, top-to-bottom mental images even for a few seconds. As he did this matching

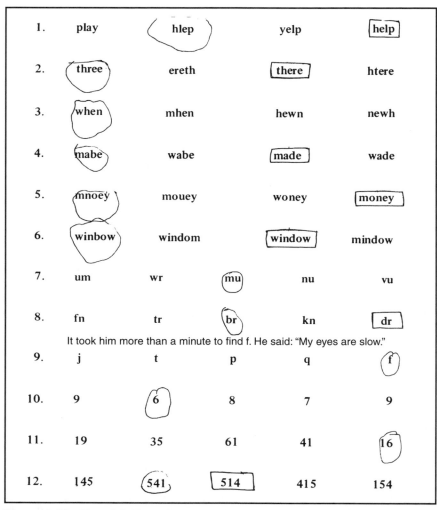

Figure 4.14. Visual dyslexia is a constant problem for this 19-year-old man as he tries to read. He has no control over when letters or numbers reverse, turn upside down, or scramble out of sequence. *Note.* From *Slingerland Screening Tests for Identifying Children with Specific Language Disability,* Form C, by B. H. Slingerland, 1984, Cambridge, MA: Educators Publishing Service. Copyright 1984 by Educators Publishing Service. Reprinted with permission.

activity, he said, "The words keep on changing." Figure 4.15 illustrates how words change as individuals with visual dyslexia try to read. This 23-year-old woman explained that "letters jump around all the time" while she reads. She touched each word with

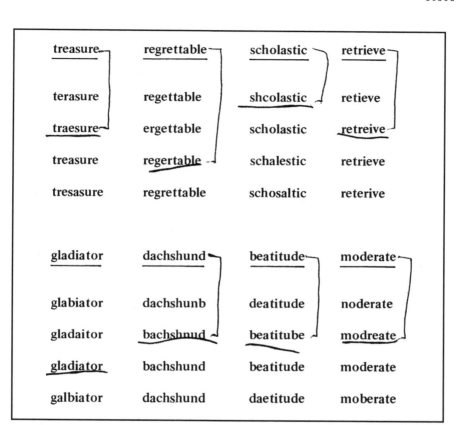

Figure 4.15. This word matching activity shows why reading is almost impossible for this 23-year-old woman. As she looks at printed words, they change. She has the impression that letters "jump around," causing words that change from moment to moment. *Note.* From *Specific Language Disability Test,* by N. Malcomesius, 2000, Cambridge, MA: Educators Publishing Service. Copyright 2000 by Educators Publishing Service. Reprinted with permission.

two fingers to slow down the "letter jumping" effect. Figure 4.16 shows how difficult it can be for a dyslexic person to match what he or she hears with printed words. Even as an individual repeats words accurately, his or her dyslexic brain scrambles letter sequence as the person tries to match speech with print.

Confusion with Time and Sequence

Few individuals with visual dyslexia develop automatic or fluent awareness of time, sequence, or details in a certain order. For

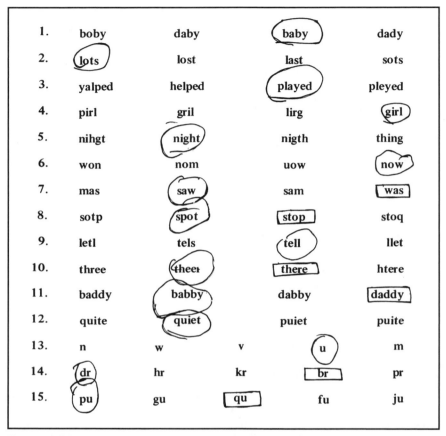

Figure 4.16. Visual dyslexia interferes with matching printed words and spoken words. On this activity, this 14-year-old boy had to listen to a word or sound pattern, then find the correct spelling on each line. These dyslexic patterns also are active when he tries to read. *Note.* From *Slingerland Screening Tests for Identifying Children with Specific Language Disability,* Form C, by B. H. Slingerland, 1984, Cambridge, MA: Educators Publishing Service. Copyright 1984 by Educators Publishing Service. Reprinted with permission.

example, 8-year-old Brian is an intelligent child who struggles with reading, spelling, and writing. On the *Wechsler Intelligence Scale for Children–Third Edition* (WISC–III; Wechsler, 1994b), his verbal IQ is 121, performance IQ is 97, and full-scale IQ is 118. However, instead of recalling an orderly progression of experiences over a period of time, Brian's memory of early childhood is a jumbled collection of events that do not fall into an orderly time sequence. In his perception of time, his broken arm 2 months ago happened right after he badly bruised his elbow when he was 3 years old. Brian's grandmother's death 5 years ago seems like last month to him. Most children have a somewhat confused memory of their early years, but as they mature, those with normal ability to remember sequence learn to connect life experiences within a consistent time frame. In spite of high intelligence, individuals like Brian seldom do. They do not have neurological talent for developing sequential memory of events over time. Because mastery of reading depends on remembering letters in the right sequence, this learning difference (visual dyslexia) is one of the greatest curriculum challenges facing students like Brian.

Brian's confusion with time and sequence always has been a major factor in his difficulty accepting responsibility. Because of his general frustration with order and sequence, he continually is in conflict with adult demands. Brian's parents expect him to carry out the following responsibilities each weekday morning:

1. Make your bed before breakfast.
2. Brush your teeth after breakfast.
3. Feed and water the pets before catching the school bus.
4. Take homework back to school.

They have told him this list over and over, but they never have written it in a visible outline for Brian to see.

After school Brian faces another set of responsibilities that also have been relayed to him verbally but never put into writing:

1. Empty the trash on Monday, Wednesday, and Friday.
2. Feed and water the pets every afternoon.
3. Attend Cub Scouts on Tuesday afternoon.
4. Take a shower by 8:30 p.m. and be ready for bed by 9:00 p.m.

Then there are Brian's weekend chores:

1. Sweep the garage on Saturday.
2. Pick up toys and tools from the yard by Saturday evening.
3. Bathe the dog either Saturday or Sunday afternoon.

Brian never has seen a visible outline of any of these adult expectations. In repeating these routines orally, his parents have assumed that he perceives time and sequence as clearly as they do. The child's dyslexic tendencies to scramble the order of things leave him with an unstructured mass of responsibilities. In spite of his intentions to obey his parents, Brian lives in a state of confusion and frustration. When chores remain undone, adults conclude that he is lazy, stubborn, disobedient, or forgetful. In reality, this dyslexic boy is filled with dread and self-defeat. He has no way to communicate his dilemma to adults who continually are displeased with him. This silent despair generates family friction and constant emotional misery for Brian.

As Chapter 7 explains, continual failure smothers a dyslexic person's self-esteem in a heavy sense of shame that leads many youngsters like Brian into rebellion, depression, or aggressive anger. When confusion with time and sequence goes unrecognized and uncorrected for several years, many dyslexic children do become disobedient and hostile. By the time they enter middle school, these frustrated youngsters are convinced that they are worthless and incapable of success.

Visual Dyslexic Patterns in the Classroom

If teachers do not understand why Brian fails to meet expectations, similar frustration occurs in the classroom. He continually is in conflict with teachers because of his inability to function as adults expect. With many students to care for, Brian's teachers assume that their oral instructions to group A have been clear. As they turn to group B, his teachers are annoyed to see that Brian is not following directions. Again he has failed in his relationship with the adult world. Because he cannot communicate his confusion to his teachers, Brian lives at risk of being judged lazy, careless, or insubordinate. Teachers who make these conclusions about the surface behavior of struggling students unwittingly set the stage for misbehavior and unhappiness. Brian's failure to follow class instructions is due to perceptual difficulty in comprehending time and sequence, not willful disobedience.

Trouble with Sequence

An alert teacher can identify confusion with sequence as students work on tasks involving details in series. For example, learners like Brian usually are fluent in giving oral reports and carrying on conversations. Casual listeners are impressed by their stock of information and the concepts they glean through listening and observation. However, there is a noticeable flaw in this oral performance—difficulty recalling the correct sequence of details when talking.

In spite of high intelligence, many individuals with visual dyslexia cannot remember the day, month, and year of their birth. The teacher can check for this tendency through informal conversation in the classroom. Although Brian may know reams of statistics about his favorite sports team, he stumbles when asked to tell his full birth date.

Learners with visual dyslexia also have trouble naming the days of the week and the months of the year in correct sequence. When asked to write this information, Brian keeps track by tapping his fingers, whispering a rhyme, or humming the alphabet song. He also struggles to learn math information, such as multiplication tables, long division, fractions, or percentages. Dyslexic students have great difficulty dealing with money and measurement. Surprisingly, Brian often does mental arithmetic better than he can write it on paper.

Figures 4.4 through 4.10 show the critical signs of visual dyslexia that appear in Brian's daily classwork. As teachers work with him, they see clearly that his ability to tell information is far ahead of his ability to write the same data. All of Brian's handwritten work shows the same kinds of struggle illustrated by others with dyslexia in Figures 4.4 through 4.10.

Faulty Reading Comprehension

Faulty perception of sequence is a major reason for poor performance on tests of reading comprehension. Brian struggles hard to get the meaning of reading-based information that requires his brain to retain ideas and facts in sequence. Chapter 3 describes several types of poor vision for reading that overlap dyslexia more than half the time. As students like Brian read line after line, several dyslexic patterns begin to interfere with their understanding of what the inner voice is saying about what they see on the page.

Awkward, Jerky Oral Reading

Chapter 3 describes saccadic eye movements that must work smoothly if individuals are to become fluent readers. Most readers with visual dyslexia cannot maintain smooth forward rhythms that team both eyes together along lines of print. Readers like Brian take two steps forward in word recognition, then one step back to correct errors or to find the place again. It is easy to hear this stumbling decoding pattern when Brian reads aloud. He starts to say the next word, stops or pauses, gets stuck trying to say the sounds in sequence, then backs up to try it again. He touches words with a finger, slides a finger below the line, or frames words with two fingers. Forward motion in reading is awkward, jerky, and never certain.

Transposing Words

Individuals with visual dyslexia tend to transpose words as they read. Peripheral vision (described in Chapter 3) causes them to pick up nearby words and insert them in the wrong place. These struggling readers often pull a later word back and insert it earlier in the sentence. As dyslexic individuals read, they tend to scramble the sequence of printed words on the page.

Rapid Burnout

Brian's teachers see how quickly he gives up and stops trying to do assignments. Rapid burnout is a major characteristic of visual dyslexia. Within a short time, Brian's vision becomes over-stressed as his eyes rapidly become too tired to continue focusing clearly. As vision fatigue develops, his mental images begin to fade away. At a certain point of perceptual overload, Brian's thoughts "go blank," forcing him to get away from the act of reading, copying, or writing by hand. Few dyslexic persons have the stamina to continue to read, spell, or write longer than 3 to 5 minutes without taking a break.

Slow Multisensory Compensation

All of these dyslexic factors combine to make it impossible for Brian to hurry. In following instructions, he must repeat to himself over and over what he thinks he was told to do. In all types of classroom work he must touch his work, pause, back up, and try again. In reading he is forced to move slowly from word to word while he touches, whispers, and practices saying words several times. In writing his pencil moves slowly as he "draws" each letter, trying his best to please adults with his penmanship. Many times in any writing task he erases and changes what he wrote the first time. It is impossible for Brian to force his brain to think faster, remember more quickly, or produce work at a quicker pace. Dyslexia produces a work style that is slow, tedious, time-consuming, and labored. If adults press a dyslexic learner to work faster, errors multiply, accuracy deteriorates, and frustration soars. The more Brian is pressed to hurry, the stronger his negative emotions surge. Eventually he reaches the point of burnout, feeling that his emotions are about to erupt in anger against pressure to hurry.

Mind Mapping and Comprehension

An important product of recent brain research is the explanation of how the brain builds mental images. In extremely rapid sequences, regions of the midbrain and higher brain develop complex images of what is happening all around the individual. These constantly changing mental images are called *mind maps* that inform the brain of every event millisecond by millisecond. With incredible speed, these changing mind maps create conscious and unconscious images of every event in one's life. This automatic brain process is much like a camera filming everything in view of the lens. Frame by frame, the brain edits important data that should be saved as long-term memory while discarding irrelevant details (Block, Flanagan, & Guzeldere, 1997; Damasio, 1994, 1999; Dennett, 1991; McGinn, 1991; Penrose, 1994; Schacter, 1996; Searle, 1997).

For example, suppose that a person prepares to drive a vehicle on an hour-long trip. Like countless snapshots taken in sequence, mind maps are formed as the driver closes the door and buckles up before starting the engine. As the eyes look ahead over the steering wheel, mind maps inform the brain of all peripheral details around the edges of the visual field. These mind maps blend details inside and outside of the vehicle. As the driver's eyes move downward, upward, and side to side, mind maps change by deleting things no longer in view while adding new details that come into view. At the same time, the driver's mind maps include impressions of color, shape, size, and spatial relationships of features inside and outside the vehicle. In addition to these visual factors, the driver's mind maps integrate odors, textures, temperature, and body comfort with the emotions and feelings the person is experiencing. These multisensory mind maps change so rapidly that the driver is conscious only of entering and starting the vehicle, then driving away. As the car picks up speed, mind map editing becomes more rapid. As the outside world speeds past the moving vehicle, the driver's mind maps change equally fast so that the person is not confused or disoriented. Mind mapping of the driving trip slows down as the vehicle's speed diminishes. When neuron development is normal, individuals are not bewildered or disoriented by countless changes in mental images during events. When dyslexia exists, lifelong confusion over mind map content keeps dyslexic individuals under emotional stress because they cannot trust their experiences to be accurate.

Mind Mapping and Long-Term Memory

Long-term memory depends on how accurately neurons interpret mind mapping sequences. For example, persons with neurological talent for reading develop accurate memory of language rules that govern literacy skills. Accurate mind mapping of the reading process enables the higher brain to build long-term memory of literacy skills. Neurologically talented individuals with accurate mind mapping become competent, fluent readers with good spelling and writing skills. Dyslexic individuals do not.

Conservation of Form

A critical factor in building accurate long-term memory is the brain's ability to memorize permanent images that stay the same over time. This has been called *conservation of form* (Inhelder & Piaget, 1974). The brain is designed to conserve the form of whatever is learned so that each time a memory is activated, the person recalls the same memory content. When neurons are pruned normally through cultural stimulus, individuals collect a wide variety of memory forms, including memory for faces, shapes, colors, and how objects appear in position-in-space relationships. During one's lifetime, the higher brain accumulates vast knowledge of forms in the environment, symbols of one's culture, and differences in voices and sounds that distinguish each person from all others. Long-term memory requires the brain to conserve countless forms throughout one's lifetime.

Conserving the Form of Reading

The act of reading could be described this way. As readers see visual forms on the printed page, memory systems throughout the left brain are expected to make lasting impressions that will be recalled accurately after the book has been put aside, or after the eyes have moved away from a particular point of focus. Readers with visual dyslexia do not have neurological talent to perform this perceptual act automatically or fluently. Students like Brian do not conserve the form of what they see on the printed page. Once the visual pattern is no longer in view, mind map images fade away or become scrambled in the reader's memory. Individuals like Brian conserve only bits and pieces of the printed patterns they have seen. In addition, they reverse or scramble the sequence of the printed data that contributes to reading.

Transformation

A critical component of long-term memory is the brain's ability to make changes in original forms. A natural skill in maturing and becoming well educated is learning how to see familiar things from new perspectives. Changing a familiar form into a similar yet new configuration is called *transformation*. For example, in changing a written statement into a question, the reader must hold the author's meaning (conserve the original form) well enough to restructure the order of the words. Brian manages to read the sentence: "Four boys played ball in the park." But when his class is asked to change this sentence into a question, the dyslexic boy is confused. What does the teacher mean? How can this sentence be anything else than what it is right now? Transformation also is a problem when dyslexic learners face changes in math structure. After much practice Brian finally understands the vertical structure of number problems:

$$\begin{array}{r} 9 \\ +5 \\ \hline \end{array}$$

When the direction of the problem is transformed from vertical to linear ($9 + 5 = \quad$), he is confused. The task of transforming a familiar pattern into another often overwhelms dyslexic learners with strong emotions and threatening feelings.

Mind Mapping and Language Transformation

Mind mapping plays a key role in the thought process of transformation. Human consciousness depends on the brain's ability to interpret variety as individuals learn new information and add richness to language usage. Transformation of mental images enables children to learn synonyms and other variations in word usage. Becoming a fluent reader or writer requires the brain to create different ways to express important ideas. For example, most learners enjoy playing word games in which they invent as many ways as possible to describe events. Fluent use of synonyms, homonyms, and other word variations depends on instant transformation of mind maps. Interpreting and creating changes in word images requires rapid transformation of mind maps to see how words are alike or different. When visual dyslexia exists, this manipulation of language forms never is fluent or natural.

Mind Mapping and Timed Tests

Achievement tests that require individuals to read paragraphs quickly, then answer questions within a strict time limit, are almost impossible tasks for students who are dyslexic. When Brian must mark bubbles on a separate answer sheet, he gives up in frustration and feels overwhelmed by shame. Again he has failed to satisfy adult expectations. If he is given enough time, often Brian can figure out satisfactory answers through trial and error or by logically eliminating wrong answers (see Figure 4.13). Having to hurry on tests multiplies his mistakes in comprehension and problem solving.

Teachers complain about Brian's tendency to guess on timed tests. However, skipping down the page, marking answers at random, or refusing to check back over his work are perfectly reasonable responses in view of his dyslexia. Brian has experienced several years of failure to comprehend what he reads. Under pressure to hurry, there is little else for him to do but guess. This is especially true when he is told that no allowance will be made for his slow pace, which is the only speed at which his brain can succeed in literacy tasks.

Mind Mapping and Alphabet Processing

Parents and teachers always are concerned when a child cannot cope with the alphabet. The unstructured way in which the alphabet usually is taught to primary pupils is largely to blame for unnecessary visual dyslexic struggle. For the past half century, alphabet sequence seldom has been taught to beginner pupils. Young learners who are curious about letters always have discovered alphabet sequence displayed on wall charts in most classrooms. Grandparents and other relatives often try to teach the alphabet sequence to children before they start to school. However, it is rare to find classroom teachers presenting the alphabet sequence in an organized, systematic way to beginner learners. This unstructured approach fails to generate mind maps of the alphabet letters in sequence.

For children with natural talent for reading, this unstructured approach has posed no long-term problems. However, children who are predisposed to being dyslexic must have clearly structured, systematic, and repeated exposure to mind maps of the alphabet letters in sequence. The foundational challenge of visual dyslexia is faulty perception of sequence. Having little or no mind mapping experience with alphabet sequence provides no structure for youngsters like Brian. Had he been well grounded in the alphabet sequence at the beginning of his school experience, he could have learned to handle beginning reading tasks more successfully. Starting formal education with well-repeated mind mapping of reading structure helps struggling readers to learn conservation of form with reading symbols.

Figures 4.3 through 4.10 show the simple technique for determining a student's perception of the alphabet. In the classroom, teachers watch as students write the alphabet on ruled paper. Any dyslexic tendencies quickly emerge. Individuals with no dyslexic tendencies soon develop confidence in writing the alphabet sequence. Those with visual dyslexia do not.

When Brian is asked to write the alphabet, he hesitates and asks whether he should "print or write cursy." When told that it does not matter, he may want to know if he should use "big or little letters." Students with dyslexia seldom remember the terms *capital* and *lowercase.*

Next, Brian may ask whether he should go across or down the page. The instructor explains that it does not matter. "Write it the way that is most comfortable for you," the teacher advises. When he finally starts to write, Brian soon reaches a stalling point, often at the letter *M.* Whenever he bogs down, he goes back to *A* and whispers the letters one by one, trying to remember the whole sequence. Occasionally he hums or sings the alphabet song to remind himself of the alphabet sequence. When Brian gets stuck, he touches each letter with his finger or pencil as he goes back to *A* and reviews what he has written. An observer can easily note the dyslexic problem of sychronizing speech with writing. As Brian touches the letters while saying them, his voice usually is ahead of his eyes or finger. Consequently, reviewing while saying his written work does not help him find his mistakes.

Brian is very slow as he writes or prints the alphabet. The letters *m, n, p, u,* and *v* often are in scrambled positions. In addition to this sequence problem, Brian often confuses similar-looking letters, such as *b–d–p–q, h–u–n, h–y, t–f–j, M–W, N–Z, r–s, v–w–k–y–x,* and *o–e–c.* As he writes, Brian makes circular letters with backward pencil motions. He frequently writes the circular parts of letters with a clockwise motion that leaves a small tail or hook at the top of the letter. He makes several letters with a bottom-to-top stroke (*t, f, p, g, b, d*). Unless adults carefully observe his pencil at work, they might not be aware of this backward motion, which is a signal of dyslexia.

Individuals with visual dyslexia often mix capital and lowercase letters when writing the alphabet and also mix manuscript and cursive styles. Brian's reasons for this inconsistent writing actually are quite practical. Because he has not been taught the alphabet sequence, he has never encountered the letters in left-to-right sequential relation to each other. The best he can, Brian has devised his own mind map system for remembering or recognizing certain letters. The forms of *B* and *D* are conserved in his long-term memory, although they may be written backwards. Brian's memory recalls that *B* has two loops while *D* has only one loop. The single loop on *b* is too easily confused with the single loop on *d, p,* or *q.* So long as Brian continues to deal with isolated letters in manuscript style, there is no dependable left-to-right form in his mind maps to which he can anchor his perceptions of the alphabet. It is unfortunate that well-meaning adults often misinterpret this handicapped work as a sign of limited intelligence or laziness. Students like Brian struggle very hard to produce the quality of work shown in Figures 4.3 through 4.10.

Reversing Written Symbols

A reliable signal of visual dyslexia is the student's confusion about which direction certain symbols should face. This faulty conservation of form causes dyslexic individuals to write or read symbols backwards, upside down, or partially turned over (see the writing examples in Figures 4.3 through 4.10). Students like Brian generally write *B* and *D* instead of writing their lowercase transformations. The two loops on *B* help Brian remember which way to turn that letter. It is easier for him to remember which way *B* and *D* face than it is to recall the correct direction of *b* and *d.*

Visual Dyslexia in Oral Reading

The tendency to reverse or transpose symbols is a handicap in reading. Persons with visual dyslexia often read whole words backwards (*was* for *saw, but* for *tub*). Sometimes only certain kinds of syllables are reversed within words (*bran* for *barn, form* for *from, sliver* for *silver*). Beginning letters, especially *b, d, p, q, h, r, m, w,* and *u,* are frequently perceived upside down or backwards. This causes the dyslexic reader to misperceive similar words (*daddy* for *baby, dark* or *park* for *bark*). This results in nonsense, forcing the reader to go back over the context of the sentence to figure out what is wrong. Dyslexic students like Brian usually can learn how to correct these reversal errors when their backward patterns are pointed out over time. Repeating correct mind maps strengthens long-term memory for correct letter orientation and position.

Adults can detect visual dyslexic reversal tendencies by listening as students read aloud. Within a few minutes, the listener hears reversal habits. As struggling readers like Brian read aloud, adults can make rapid notes of dyslexic errors. The following oral reading errors often indicate visual dyslexia:

1. Reversal of beginning letters: *dark* or *park* for *bark, dump* or *pump* for *bump*

2 Transposing blends and digraphs: *preform* for *perform, there* for *three, star* for *stream, porfit* for *profit, frame* for *farmer*

3. Substituting one letter for another: *sleep* for *sheep, come* for *came, some* for *same*

4. Transposing letters within words: *vigener* for *vinegar, magilant* for *malignant, macilous* for *malicious*

5. Reversal of whole words: *no* for *on, saw* for *was, but* for *tub*

6. Failure to see small details (including habitual failure to see punctuation marks): *house* for *horse, with* for *wish, butter* for *better, hungry* for *hunger*

7. Omission of endings: *ever* for *every, her* for *here, happen* for *happening*

8. Telescoping: *standarize* for *standardized, consently* for *consequently, sudly* for *suddenly*

9. Perseveration: *hopenen* for *hope, farmerer* for *farmer, sudendely* for *suddenly*

Dyslexia is suspected only when several of these symptoms exist in the individual's oral reading. Adults must be careful to distinguish between dyslexia and the word blind or off-center foveal patterns described in Chapter 3.

Errors in Copying

Figure 4.11 shows how hard it is for dyslexic students like Brian to copy from the chalkboard or from a projection screen. Success at copying (also called *vision-to-motor transfer*) involves a high-level talent for conservation of form. To copy successfully, mind maps must remain intact as eyes refocus near to far, then back again. Successful copying requires at least six complex steps that must be done in a given sequence:

1. See the forms clearly.

2. Hold these mental images intact (conserve the form).

3. Refocus to the writing space without getting lost.

4. Transform mental images into handwriting (fine motor coordination).

5. Space the symbols properly on the writing paper (figure-ground control).

6. End up with a legible resemblance to what was on the chalkboard, projection screen, or in the textbook.

Adults who write well often forget what a complex task copying is. It is a monumental challenge for dyslexic individuals like Brian who cannot conserve form without enormous concentration and effort. Figure 4.17 shows how well a higly motivated 14-year-old dyslexic boy can compensate for dyslexia when he is

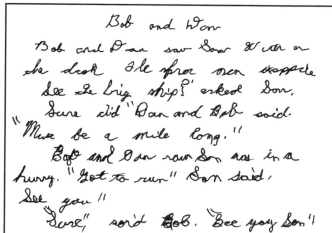

Bob and Dan
Bob and Dan saw Sam Watts on the dock. The three men stopped. "See the big Ship?" asked Sam.
      "Sure did," Dan and Bob said. "Must be a mile long."
      Bob and Dan saw Sam was in a hurry. "Got to run," Sam said. "See you.":
      "Sure," said Bob and Dan. "See you, Sam."

Figure 4.17. This 14-year-old boy needed 37 minutes to copy this story from the Jordan Test for Visual Dyslexia (see Appendix C). As a highly motivated person, he asked for enough time to finish this task. Rarely do teachers give him this much extra time for copying or writing. His classroom work seldom reflects how well he can compensate for dyslexia when he has enough time.

given all the time he needs. The use of projection screens increases the pressure on many dyslexic students if they are required take notes or copy data while a teacher lectures. Chronic confusion with symbols forces individuals like Brian to work slowly. If he tries to hurry, he quickly becomes too frustrated to keep details in correct sequence. When he cannot touch the text, he becomes too lost to keep on trying to copy.

It is easy for instructors to identify students who have problems with copying. When individuals like Brian are asked to copy a paragraph from the chalkboard or from a projection screen, the teacher should watch for the following tendencies:

_____ Loses the place on the board or screen.

_____ Erases frequently.

_____ Overprints or overwrites to correct writing mistakes.

_____ Misspells words as they are copied.

_____ Fails to observe or copy capital letters.

_____ Fails to observe or copy punctuation marks.

_____ Fails to space handwriting properly.

_____ Reverses letters or syllables.

_____ Reverses whole words.

_____ Works unusually slowly.

_____ Whispers over and over while copying.

_____ Squints both eyes to see clearly.

_____ Shades eyes to read from a whiteboard or projection screen.

_____ Closes one eye to read from the board or screen.

_____ Points toward the board or screen to aim the eyes together to the right place.

_____ Bogs down and has to start over to find the place.

_____ Erupts into strong emotions by sighing heavily, muttering complaints, or thrashing around with noisy body motions.

_____ Skips words or leaves out phrases or whole lines.

_____ Writing is too messy to be legible.

_____ Uses heavy hand pressure that produces smeared writing.

As with oral reading, observers must be careful not to mistake word blindness or off-center foveal vision for dyslexia.

Errors in Spelling

A unique pattern of spelling errors distinguishes visual dyslexia from auditory dyslexia (described in Chapter 5). The primary disability in visual dyslexia is failure to process details in sequence. Individuals like Brian who have visual dyslexia cannot recall a clear mental image of whole words. They can hear and identify most of the individual speech sounds within common words. In fact, Brian often can spell words correctly orally, but as he writes, letters inadvertently jump out of sequence. Brian made the following errors on a dictated spelling test of 15 words for which he had spent many hours preparing. The night before the test he correctly spelled each word orally with his mother. He came to school next day confident that this time he would make a good grade on the weekly spelling test. When his paper was returned with red marks showing the following errors, once more he was devastated by the shame of failure.

Word in Brian's Mind	His Written Response
rode	roed
goes	gose
play	paly
suddenly	sundedly
railroad	railraod
brother	borther
mailbox	mialbox
friend	frenid

Activities for Overcoming Visual Dyslexia

As Brian's parents and teachers seek ways to help him overcome visual dyslexia, they must look for strategies that provide practice in building vivid mind maps of details in sequence. Each strategy must stimulate Brian's brain to integrate several senses at the same time. He must combine seeing it, saying it, hearing it, and touching it at the same time. Multimodality practice is the only way he can build correct long-term memory to help him overcome visual dyslexia. Even though he is 10 years old, Brian's teachers and parents must not assume that he has mastered essential cultural information that requires sequence.

Frequently he must go back to basic sequential information to reinforce long-term memory.

Learning Time Sequence

Chapter 2 presented the severity scale used to show how much difficulty a dyslexic individual faces in classroom learning (see page 38). At age 10 Brian is at level 7 on this severity scale. Everything related to reading, spelling, writing, and recall of sequence is difficult for him. Because he is talented in oral language, away from school he hides much of his dyslexia through good conversation and lively storytelling. However, listeners notice how often he stumbles over time sequence. Brian does not have fluent recall of the sequence of events. He stumbles over days of the week and months of the year. As he tells stories of movies he has seen or things he has done, he shows confusion about when things occur. Adults notice how often elements of his oral stories are out of sequence. It is important for Brian's teachers and parents to help him practice with accurate mind maps of time sequence.

Calendars as Visible Reminders of Time

Brian must be surrounded by visible reminders of time sequence. He must see time represented on a variety of calendars that stimulate mind maps of how days make a week, how weeks make a month, and how months make a year. Several times each day Brian must be reminded to look at calendars to practice time sequences. All of his activities should be written on calendars that remind him of such time sequences as *yesterday / today / tomorrow, last week / this week / next week, last month / this month / next month, how long until Thanksgiving* (November), *how long until Hanukkah or Christmas* (December), and so forth. Part of Brian's education must be to learn how life flows forward through the units we call minutes, hours, days, weeks, months, and years. Also, he must learn how to look back in time for accurate memory of when events took place. As adults guide this practice with time sequence, Brian will develop concepts of chronological order, when birthdays occur, when important events happened in the family, and when future events will take place. Adults must guide him in rehearsing knowledge of time sequence the way they tutor him in reading and arithmetic skills.

Personal Pocket Reminder

Brian must develop the lifestyle of keeping track of time by carrying his own calendar in a pocket, in a notebook, or in an electronic organizer. He must be tutored in how to write every event on his calendar so he can look at it several times each day. It does not matter if he makes dyslexic mistakes as he jots down information on his calendar. So long as he can read his own writing, he must gain the sense that this is his personal guidebook for staying on schedule and meeting appointments on time. Every event he is expected to attend should become a note on his private calendar: sports events, private lessons, when grandparents are coming to visit, when assignments are due, when tests are scheduled, when he will see the dentist for a checkup, when his next scout meeting will occur, and so forth. Adults in his life must guide Brian in developing brain maps of which day of the week this is and what the coming days will require him to do. Over time, this kind of tutoring with time sequence will teach him how to compensate for dyslexia well enough to build a successful lifestyle based on knowledge of time. If he does not receive this training in time awareness, Brian will become a time-handicapped adolescent and adult. For his future, having a functional command of time sequence will be as important as knowing how to read.

Learning Alphabet Sequence

For half a century, U.S. education has concealed the alphabet sequence until after children have learned to read. For most youngsters, this has done no harm, largely because inquisitive children with a talent for reading figure out the alphabet sequence from what they see displayed in the classroom. Youngsters like Brian who have dyslexia do not absorb the alphabet because they do not comprehend sequence that is presented indirectly. Dyslexic learners are stymied when called on to alphabetize words, find entries in the dictionary or phonebook, or locate information in reference books. When the alphabet letters are doled out in random order, there is no left-to-right point of reference by which dyslexic youngsters can visualize where letters are positioned within the alphabet sequence. Not having quick recall of alphabet sequence poses serious classroom problems when students like Brian must respond to alphabetic information in upper grades.

Multisensory Practice

Because of differences in how their brains perceive, students with dyslexia must memorize cultural and literacy-based landmarks through seeing/saying/hearing/touching activities. If the alphabet sequence is to be mastered, it must be done through memory drill that produces multisensory mind maps. Students like Brian must have consistent practice that teaches them alphabet forms. This foundational experience prepares long-term memory for future success with transformation of the alphabet sequence. From their earliest classroom experiences, children should begin learning the alphabet by handling cutout, three-dimensional letter forms. This hands-on multisensory practice is especially important for youngsters who show signs of not being ready to learn to read. Adults must provide all kinds of tactile experience by making alphabet letters out of clay, pipe cleaners, or cutout forms that have enough texture to let fingers feel differences in shapes and sizes.

One Concept at a Time

Individuals who are dyslexic must learn only one major concept at a time. Youngsters like Brian must not be overwhelmed by experiences that introduce phonic principles at the same time that letter shapes are being memorized. Brian should begin his literacy training by associating names of letters with their shapes. He should not begin by connecting phonic sounds to letter shapes. For example, Brian should match the letter shape *A* with its name "aye." He should call the letter shape *B* "bee," and so forth. Phonic sounds should not be introduced until his brain is sure of each capital and lowercase alphabet symbol. For dyslexic learners, phonic sounds for letters should come after the brain has mastered the letter shapes, their names, and their sequence in the alphabet.

Steps in Learning the Alphabet Sequence

Alert teachers and parents can tell when a child is ready for a more advanced level of handling alphabet sequence. The following learning sequence shows the kinds of multisensory activities a child like Brian should do:

Step 1: Master the alphabet sequence with movable letter forms. Practice over and over seeing/saying/hearing/touching each capital/lowercase pair of letters until the child's brain knows them all in sequence.

Step 2: Trace over the alphabet sequence on a chalkboard. Then practice typing the alphabet sequence on a keyboard.

Step 3: Trace over the alphabet sequence on paper or on plastic wipe-off sheets. Practice typing the alphabet sequence.

Step 4: Copy the alphabet sequence at the chalkboard as the student looks at model cards or the teacher's model. Copy alphabet sequence on a keyboard by looking at a printed alphabet sequence chart.

Step 5: Copy the alphabet sequence on lined paper as the student looks at an alphabet card or the teacher's printed model. Practice copying the alphabet sequence on a keyboard.

Step 6: Practice writing and typing the alphabet sequence with a model nearby so the student can see it if he or she forgets.

Step 7: Write and type the alphabet sequence from memory with no reversals, upside down letters, or letters out of sequence.

Adults have made the mistake of rushing students like Brian too rapidly through this developmental sequence. Today's kindergarten programs often introduce steps 1 through 3 with randomly presented alphabet letters that are not in sequence. Adults assume that youngsters have mastered all seven steps of this learning sequence by the the time they enter second grade. This assumption is correct only for those four out of five children who have neurological talent for learning to read. Youngsters like Brian quickly fall behind in classroom literacy expectations. For many years, one in five children who do not have natural talent for reading have fallen through the cracks to become nonreading adolescents and adults who flood the workplace. The most urgent literacy need for dyslexic individuals is to master the alphabet sequence, no matter how old they are when their reading deficit is discovered. It is irrelevant for students like Brian to struggle and fail with book reports and writing themes if they have not yet developed correct memory for the alphabet sequence.

Comprehending Instructions

As dyslexic students like Brian try to cope with classroom expectations, one of their most frustrating experiences is trouble understanding the mind maps that emerge as they listen to oral information. Brian almost never escapes criticism from adults who give him oral instructions. No matter how carefully he tries to listen, he cannot transform new mind maps into accurate memory quickly enough to remember all of what he hears. When the speaker stops talking, Brian retains only bits and pieces of mental images that seldom follow the same sequence that the speaker said. This inability to comprehend oral instructions brings Brian into frequent conflict with classmates who understand fully, instructors who are irritated by his failure to comprehend, and family members who think he should do better.

Because of his difficulty with reading, Brian also struggles to comprehend written instructions. His left brain does not remember the sequence of steps that each task requires. He does not automatically think in terms of sequence such as *first / next / last* or *first, second, third.* In both listening and reading, Brian falls through the cracks of comprehending fully what he is expected to do.

Written Outlines

Helping dyslexic students pay attention to sequential steps in carrying out instructions actually is rather simple. Instead of forcing Brian to depend on memory, adults should give him simple written outlines of whatever is expected. Dyslexic students who have achieved dependable basic reading skills can use written outlines that list each step or responsibility. This technique is especially suitable for routine work such as daily chores or work schedules that stay the same from day to day.

When clearly written instructions are given in textbooks or workbooks, teachers have a ready-made visual aid for teaching students like Brian how to follow sequence interpreting instructions. Otherwise, instructors must make new daily lists and outlines for him to see. Teachers in kindergarten and primary grades often solve this problem by creating right-brain picture codes, such as animal pictures, colored shapes, or other nonreading markers to remind pupils of what they are to do next. Children who easily lose track of sequence can refer back to the outline or chart to see what comes next.

Listening to Instructions

As students like Brian grow older, they continue to need help keeping track of sequence. As he listens to a series of directions, Brian starts to lose the sequence of what is expected. The mind maps of listening do not transform into permanent memory without visual help. Most adults are unaware of how complicated their oral directions can be. For example, in getting her math class under way, Brian's fourth-grade teacher usually makes 20 or more short statements. Most children are adept at "tuning in" and "tuning out" as adults deliver a stream of speech. Children seldom pay attention to everything adults say. In fact, one of the signs of maturing brain processing is when youngsters begin to filter and do mental editing of what they hear.

For example, Brian's teacher delivers oral instructions something like this:

> Now class, it's time for math. Put away your social studies books and get out your math books. Tom, please sit down. Yes, Mary? No, you don't need two pencils. Now, class, be sure you have your pencils ready. Open your workbooks to today's lesson. Yes, Joe? No, I didn't say get them out, but you know I meant for you to. Now, children, open your books to page 25. What, Sue? Yes you may get a drink for your hiccups, but hurry. Now, on page 25 we are ready to review short division. . . .

This steady flow of speech is supplemented by the teacher's paralanguage that includes gestures, facial expressions, variations in tone of voice, and other nonverbal actions that support effective communication. Most children become skilled at editing running speech as adults give instructions. As they hear the teacher's voice, most students tune in only when the adult or a fellow student says something important that must be remembered. Most of Brian's classmates monitor the teacher's instructions as follows:

> . . . It's time for math. . . . Put away social studies books. . . . Get out math books. . . . Don't need two pencils. . . . Open workbooks to today's lesson. . . . Open books to page 25. . . . Review short division. . . .

Because of dyslexia, Brian cannot do this kind of editing. He cannot separate essential data from nonessential parts of the oral message. Brian's left brain does not filter the content of mind maps that must be condensed so that long-term memory can form. Without a visual outline to guide language filtering, Brian is lost. If his teacher provides a written list for him to see later, then he has a chance to be successful in following instructions as he works at his own pace. Brian's classroom success increased dramatically when his teachers learned of his special need for visual points of reference. For each assignment, he receives a simple outline on the chalkboard or a stick-on note placed at the top of his work area:

Today's Math
1. Have one pencil ready.
2. Open math book to page 25.
3. Open workbook to page 97.
4. For tomorrow, 15 problems on workbook page 97.

Tape-Recorded Instructions

Many teachers have learned to help dyslexic students by making tape recordings of daily instructions in addition to simple outlines. After the class has begun to work, those who did not understand the instructions put on headphones and listen to the assignment again in private. Brian can listen to the instructions as many times as he needs to be sure he is doing what the outline shows. If a written outline with the tape recording is still not enough, students may go individually to the teacher. When this kind of face-saving safety net is provided for students who are dyslexic, the class is spared arguments that are triggered when the same few students disrupt the learning atmosphere by clamoring for repeated explanations.

Failure to comprehend the sequence of instructions is the main cause for confusion with arithmetic story problems, science experiments, and chronological order in social studies. Learning how to create brief outlines that show details in sequence is a critical skill for Brian to learn as early as possible in his school experience. The first step in learning how to outline important data is to understand the purpose of outlining. An outline is a "word picture" that shows the most important parts of what we read or say. Before they are held accountable for making their own outlines, students like Brian must be taught to think in sequence. They must have guided practice in spotting what comes first, then next, and finally last as they read story problems and paragraphs in books. This practice should start with using a colored marker to highlight data that will become part of the written outline.

For example, Brian's math book presents the following story problem:

> On Monday morning, Maria's mother gave her $10.00. That afternoon Maria bought a can of soda for 60 cents. On Tuesday she bought a candy bar for 70 cents. On Wednesday she bought a bag of chips for 95 cents. How much money did she have left on Thursday morning?

If Brian is required to read this story problem by himself, this is what dyslexia causes him to see the first time he reads the passage:

> No Monbay ming, Mar's mom give her $10.00. The afnon Mari ??? can soba of 60 sent. No Thrsbayshe ??? canbar from 70 sent. On ???? she bite same chip for 59 sent. Who must wony bid she has felt no Thurbay?

As usual, Brian's independent reading makes no sense. After struggling for several minutes to read the math problem, his mind maps are so cluttered by dyslexic "glitches" that he gives up in frustration. Again he has experienced the shame of failure to do what most of his classmates do easily and quickly.

Before he can succeed with narrative information, Brian must have one-on-one help to read the text correctly. As he hears his voice say the words correctly, his intelligence makes sense of the printed information. Once he has practiced reading each word correctly, he is ready to talk through the problem with his study partner. Together they decide the sequence of the story. What did Maria do on Monday, then Tuesday, then Wednesday, and finally on Thursday? Brian highlights these story facts with a blue marker. Next, he and his study partner find the math information for each of those days: $10.00 on Monday, then 60 cents on Monday, 70 cents on Tuesday, then 95 cents on Wednesday. Finally on Thursday, how much money is left from the $10.00? This math data are highlighted with a yellow marker.

After Brian has done this preliminary filtering and organizing, he is ready to create the written steps of the math problem. First he decides whether he should add or subtract. Does Maria add more money to the $10.00, or does she take money away? At this step in problem solving, all guessing must be removed from the computation process. Brian is guided to understand the sequence of the problem. First, Maria adds to find out how much she spent. Next, she subtracts to find out how much is left on Thursday. Once he knows these transformations, Brian constructs two vertical addition problems:

$0.60 Monday	$10.00 Monday morning
0.70 Tuesday	−2.25 Spent by Wednesday
0.95 Wednesday	$ 7.75 Left on Thursday
$2.25 How much Maria spent	

Brian talks his way through this process as he sees/says/hears/touches at the same time. His study partner guides this process to make sure that he follows the correct sequence of the story data. Over time with this kind of visually based practice, Brian's brain develops enough permanent memory of math processes to let him succeed with basic math computation. As Chapter 6 describes, he likely never will become talented with math computation without using a calculator.

If Brian is to grow in reading comprehension, outlining textbook information must follow a similar procedure. Until his word recognition and phonic skills are strong enough to let him read alone, he must do reading tasks one on one with a study partner. Brian must develop habits of color-highlighting facts, ideas, and other essential information. Then he must transform these filtered data into written outlines that show him the sequence of what the author presented. Most of this outlining can be done through keyboard writing to save time and give Brian a stronger sense of success.

Correcting Reversals and Rotations

Teaching dyslexic students like Brian not to turn things upside down or backwards is not always possible in a mainstream classrom setting. This dyslexic pattern often requires one-on-one tutoring that few teachers can provide during the school day. However, teachers can take certain steps within a mainstream classroom to help Brian deal more successfully with letter reversals and rotations.

Begin with Openness

Remediation of learning differences must begin with openness. Often it is uncomfortable or difficult for adults to deal openly with situations involving a specific learning disability. However, if students like Brian are to find relief from shame of failure and constant frustration, conflicting patterns must be acknowledged and dealt with openly. Obviously, adults must never shame or embarrass struggling learners through critical remarks made in front of the class. The approach to successful remediation requires adults to start with Brian privately as they talk about the kinds of differences that show up in his writing and reading. Once he knows what must be done again in his writing, spelling, copying, reading, and math, Brian and his teachers can work out reminder systems to help him spot his differences more quickly.

For example, in a quiet conference away from the prying eyes and ears of classmates, the teacher explains how Brian's work has been analyzed for certain things that should be done differently. This might include showing him a checklist of visual dyslexia patterns (see pages 55–58 in Chapter 2). The tone of this conference is positive and encouraging. The teacher tells Brian how proud he or she is of his effort and how much he or she enjoys the boy's ideas. But in order for him to learn how to show all that he knows, he must practice spotting things that are backward, upside down, or out of sequence. The teacher explains carefully that these differences have nothing to do with intelligence. The use of words like "dumb" or "stupid" never are condoned or implied when struggling learners compare themselves with classmates who work more rapidly without making mistakes. The teacher emphasizes the concept of individual difference and explains why there is nothing wrong with being different. For example, the teacher explains that the goal now is for Brian to learn to be an editor, a specialist who looks for things that are different and that cause incorrect answers or misspelled words. The teacher assures Brian that he can learn to be an editor to spot most of his own differences and correct them.

Adults sometimes recoil from this sort of frankness on the grounds that it is cruel and risky to expose a child to such self-knowledge. In fact, it is cruel not to explain to a bright student like Brian exactly what things in his work produce conflict. It would, of course, be foolish to tell an overly fearful or less mature child that he or she has dyslexia. But if the student is mature enough to wonder what the problem is, he or she should be told. Half of the success of remediating these tendencies depends on the person's full cooperation. It is impossible to enlist Brian's full cooperation if he never is fully informed of the nature of the differences he is expected to correct.

Adults might understand more readily the need for openness by recalling how they feel when physicians withhold information about a patient's illness. Adults instantly become anxious when an examining doctor mutters "Hmmmm!" or "Aha!" but does not explain those vocal reactions. If teachers and parents can realize that children have the same need to know what is happening and why, then remedial work becomes much more effective.

Quietly, unemotionally, and openly, the teacher draws Brian's attention to examples of dyslexic difference in his daily classwork. The teacher explains that these differences are the reasons for low grades and criticism. He or she points out examples where Brian wrote *beb* for *bed, mnst* for *must, gril* for *girl,* or *on* for *no.* Brian and his teacher look at some math papers on which *51* was flipped to *15, 5* and *3* were written backwards, and he accidentally added when the sign told him to subtract. Brian and his teacher discuss how this caused his math work to appear incorrect. During this conference they look at examples of Brian's copying in which he switched the position of letters (*abel* for *able, paly* for *play*). In this conversation the teacher does not criticize or sound judgmental. The tone of this conference is matter of fact and un-emotional. "Brian, would you like to learn how to be an editor so you can change these differences when they happen?"

It may be hard for adults to understand how this kind of frank, simple, factual explanation brings relief to Brian's emotions and feelings. After all, he has known for a long time that something has not been right. At last someone is explaining it in simple language. His first response likely will be, "You mean I'm not dumb? I thought I must be dumb or stupid. You mean I can't help getting things backwards or upside down? I thought it was because I'm dumb!"

As this kind of open discussion occurs, the teacher asks Brian to suggest ways to correct his writing accidents. Once he under-stands that actually he is bright, Brian is ready to help his teacher plan how he can learn to become an editor. The teacher makes clear what he or she expects from Brian. This often is done by making a simple contract that outlines the daily dyslexic patterns (backward letters, transposed syllables, reversed num-bers) and what Brian promises to do each day to overcome them. The teacher makes it clear how much one-on-one time he or she can provide during the school day. If the teacher can manage three 5-minute periods during recess, the lunch hour, or class work periods, this must be specified. The important thing is that Brian knows how much individual attention he can expect.

Study Partners

It usually is possible to pair Brian with a classmate who is ma-ture enough to help him practice editing skills. Students with dyslexia need immediate personal feedback that comes from working with a partner. The "study buddy" does not teach new skills but rather walks through familiar tasks with Brian. They talk about how and where he gets stuck. Together they practice using editing skills until Brian feels sure of himself in spotting reversals and other kinds of dyslexic differences. The study buddy becomes a reading partner when Brian must read a story or textbook assignment. His study partner helps him edit his writing so that most of the dyslexic differences are corrected be-fore the work is given to the teacher.

Older Students as Study Partners. A promising source of one-on-one help during the school day is older students who can fit into

Brian's routine without disrupting classroom procedures. Older students are especially effective as tutors, provided there is no clash between them and the dyslexic learner. A small amount of personal attention from an older student goes a long way in building self-confidence and replacing shame with pride, especially if the older student has overcome similar learning differences. Two or three 30-minute sessions during the school week often are enough to unlock perceptual blocks, allowing younger students to make significant progress in overcoming specific challenges.

Finger Touching and Marking

Chapter 3 describes several central vision problems often seen in individuals who are dyslexic. Figures 3.2 through 3.5 show the distortion patterns many dyslexic readers see when they look at black print on white paper (scotopic sensitivity syndrome). Figures 3.6 and 3.7 explain what happens during reading when an individual has off-center foveal vision, or Aubert–Foerster syndrome. When these or other types of poor central vision exist, the person has no choice but to touch everything seen in print along with using some kind of marking system.

Dyslexic students like Brian must do something physical to transform visual mind maps into usable knowledge. If they try to read silently without touching the page, they have no visual boundaries to help both eyes focus on the same spot. Without visual boundaries, Brian cannot develop complete mental images just by looking at new information. He must see/say/hear/touch at the same time to stimulate neural pathways enough to make good connections. This means that Brian cannot succeed with passive, silent reading or with silent math processing. He must incorporate vision, speech, hearing, and touch to override loose neural connections. He must be encouraged to figure out the best way of touching his work. One finger sliding beneath the line might be enough tactile stimulus. Or Brian might need to touch each word with a finger while the other hand lies just above the line. At times he might need to frame words between two fingers to keep his eyes focused on that spot. Or he should hold a card marker beneath each line to mask the print just below his point of focus. Figure 3.8 in Chapter 3 shows the kind of slotted marker that enables some struggling readers to eliminate visual distraction on the page.

Reading Orally

Reading orally is essential for correcting Brian's reversals and rotations. As he reads slowly from printed information, his study partner monitors by following the same text. As dyslexic glitches occur, the study partner quietly says, "Look at that word again, Brian. How is it spelled? Spell it to me and touch each letter with your finger." This sort of cuing is low-key and does not embarrass Brian by labeling dyslexic stumbling as mistakes. By immediately pinpointing dyslexic differences, the study partner reinforces accurate symbol perception. Brian soon begins to catch his own errors by integrating what he sees, says, hears, and touches as he reads.

Keyboard Writing

Most students who are dyslexic can develop satisfactory writing skills through a keyboard system that has self-correcting spelling and grammar features. The positive benefits of keyboard writing for dyslexic individuals were first demonstrated by Joyce Steeves (1987) at Johns Hopkins School of Education. Steeves recruited a group of boys with dyslexia for training with keyboard writing skills. Each boy had his own computer to use as often as he wished. Steeves taught the boys a simplified touch typing technique developed by Diana King (1985). The King method of typing teaches only the left-hand keys first. Students learn a rhyming chant that is vocalized as they practice finger movements on the keyboard. This multisensory process rapidly creates permanent memory for which fingers touch which keys. Soon this say/hear/see/touch strategy enables dyslexic students to type several left-hand words without mistakes. Then the right-hand keys are learned in the same multisensory way. Within 2 or 3 days with this keyboard practice, students like Brian are ready to produce accurate keyboard writing with the left hand, right hand, and both hands together. Steeve's research demonstrated that learning multisensory keyboard writing techniques permits dyslexic individuals to develop 15 times better written language skills than they can achieve through penmanship.

Recent brain research has explained how brain regions team together to produce such positive results with students who are dyslexic (Barnard & Brazelton, 1990; Dechesne, 1992; Goodale &

Milner, 1992; Gottfried, 1990; Johnson, 1990; Khan, 1994; Killackey, 1995; Muller & Homberg, 1992; Romand, 1992; Ungerleider & Haxby, 1994; van Essen & Gallant, 1994). Figure 4.18 shows the few regions of Brian's brain that are activated if he only looks at print. Passively viewing print does not evoke enough mind maps to let his brain process printed information. Figure 4.19 shows what happens when Brian writes by hand. Again, too few mind maps emerge to help him compensate for left-brain dyslexic patterns that interfere with penmanship. Figure 4.20 shows what occurs throughout Brian's brain when he does multisensory language processing through keyboard writing. When he sees, says, hears, and touches at the same

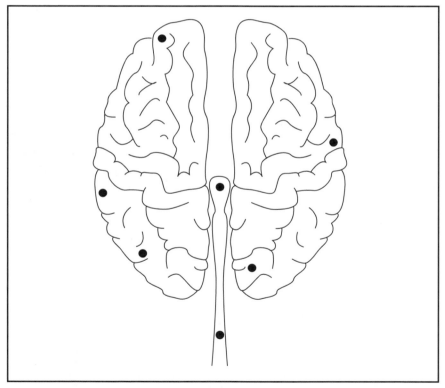

Figure 4.18. These regions of the left brain, midbrain, and right brain participate in the passive act of looking at print on a page. When dyslexia exists, too little stimulus occurs to create effective neuron communication. (Based on research by Johnson, 1990; Khan, 1994; Shaywitz, 1996; Steeves, 1987; and van Essen & Gallant, 1994.)

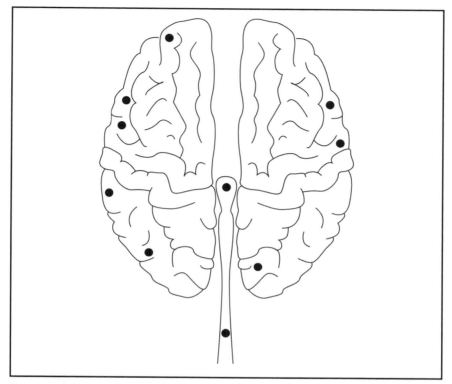

Figure 4.19. During the act of handwriting, these regions of the left brain, midbrain, and right brain are activated. When dyslexia exists, not enough stimulus occurs to trigger effective neuron connections to carry out accurate handwriting tasks. (Based on research by Atkinson, 1984; Johnson, 1990; Khan, 1994; Shaywitz, 1996; Steeves, 1987; and van Essen & Gallant, 1994.)

time, multiple mind maps are stimulated to create whole brain activity. As these many brain regions team together in thinking and acting, Brian can encode a great deal more creative ideas and information than is possible through handwriting alone.

Personal Portable Computer

Rapid development of computer technology has created a wide variety of personal computer systems, including "laptop" models that Brian can bring into the classroom, then carry home after school. His personal computer is as portable as books in a backpack. Having a compact personal computer in the classroom permits him to take adequate notes, produce much better written

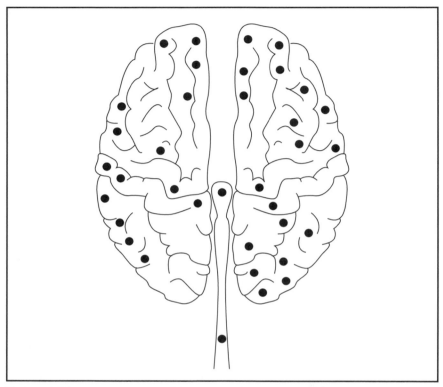

Figure 4.20. During the multisensory act of keyboard writing at a computer, these regions of the left brain, midbrain, and right brain are activated. Combining the sense of sight with tactile senses in the right-brain and left-brain sensorimotor cortex stimulates enough neuron connections to generate whole brain involvement in written language. (Based on research by Atkinson, 1984; Johnson, 1990; Khan, 1994; Shaywitz, 1996; Steeves, 1987; and van Essen & Gallant, 1994.)

work during the school day, and store unfinished tasks on the computer hard drive to be finished at home. Keyboard writing has helped countless dyslexic students transform shame of failure into self-confidence by allowing them to compete successfully with everyone else in the classroom. Computer-based writing sets Brian free to put his thoughts and knowledge onto paper without losing mental images. As Steeves (1987) has demonstrated, keyboard writing sets students with dyslexia free to learn how to express creative ideas and complex information. When adults accept keyboard writing as a legitimate alternative way of doing schoolwork, much of the conflict over dyslexic writing disappears. Brian's study partner continues to help him edit for mistakes, and keyboard writing allows him to become skilled with encoding far beyond the level he can achieve with pencil or pen.

Matching Word Forms

Daily practice activities that require the brain to notice likenesses and differences in words can be devised by parents, teachers, and study partners to increase Brian's word discrimination skills. For example, Figure 4.21 shows a word matching activity from the *Jordan Dyslexia Assessment / Reading Program* (Jordan, 2000a). Line by line, Brian studies a word on a card. He has all

---

Practice with Matching Words

Mark the word just like the word you saw on the card.

1.	bran	pran	puar	bnar	narb	uarp	barn
2.	spot	tobs	tops	stop	stob	sbot	tods
3.	sliver	silver	vilser	revils	revlis	selvir	verlis
4.	trad	brat	rapt	part	prat	bart	trap
5.	tums	tsum	smut	swnt	tsuw	must	wnst
6.	severe	esrever	reverse	eversen	servere	neverse	nervese
7.	sheeb	speeh	sheed	sdeey	sheep	speey	peehs
8.	tarsh	shraf	farsh	shart	trash	frash	sharf

Figure 4.21. This kind of word matching practice can be done with many words seen and spoken each day. The same worksheet can be used several times if different words are shown on cards. *Note.* From the *Jordan Dyslexia Assessment / Reading Program* (2nd ed., p. 91), by D. R. Jordan, 2000, Austin, TX: PRO-ED. Copyright 2000 by PRO-ED. Reprinted with permission.

the time he needs to read this word. He is encouraged to say it, hear it, and touch it to increase his visual perception. When he is ready, he finds the matching word from memory. Over time this kind of multisensory practice teaches his left brain to transform mind maps into reliable memory for letters and words.

Keeping Track of Progress

Parents, teachers, and study partners who help students like Brian overcome dyslexia must keep track of progress. This should be a simple procedure that requires a small amount of bookkeeping. As they mature, dyslexic students can be taught to record their own progress, as they do in other individualized study programs.

Figure 4.22 shows the type of individualized record that the teacher and Brian can develop together. As they talk about the writing and spelling differences that he must learn to edit, they prepare his progress chart, which outlines all of the dyslexic differences that appear in his work. This progress chart can be entered on Brian's personal computer to give him immediate access wherever he is. When he no longer needs help to spot and correct a dyslexic difference, he enters that date on his progress chart. The goal is for him to develop editing skill at spotting and changing most of his dyslexic patterns before turning in papers as finished assignments.

The progress chart offers two advantages for editing practice at home and in the classroom. First, Brian's goals are straightforward, once the specific differences are identified on his checklist. His teachers and tutors help him to build consistent work habits that include finding and changing his dyslexic differences before turning in assignments. Until specific items on the progress chart have a "Learned To Edit" date, those points of conflict will not be labeled mistakes that lower his grades. Second, at all times Brian knows exactly how much remains to be overcome in his schoolwork. With this contract frankly understood by adults and students, most of the typical conflict over dyslexic differences can be avoided.

The most reliable index of how successful Brian's editing is will be the level of his frustration. Chapter 7 reviews the wide range of negative emotions and feelings that disrupt learning for all dyslexic individuals whose needs are not met. So long as

---

Brian's Progress Chart

Differences To Be Edited

Date of Contract _____   Date When Brian Learned
                                            To Edit

_____ Letters turned backwards: *b d p q*   _____

_____ Letter turned upside down: *n u m w*   _____

_____ Numbers turned backwards: *3 5 7*   _____

_____ Numbers turned upside down: *6 9*   _____

_____ Parts of words spelled backwards   _____

_____ Punctuation marks left out   _____

_____ Capital letters left out   _____

_____ Forgot to check it again   _____

_____ Forgot to bring homework to school   _____

_____ Forgot to listen or read instructions _____
      again

Figure 4.22. This kind of simple checklist can be prepared for every student who must overcome dyslexic patterns. Working together, teachers and students develop a contract that shows exactly what kinds of differences the student must learn to edit. When that self-editing skill has been learned, a date is written to show that step of progress.

adults observe tension, frustration, anxiety, dread, avoidance tactics, or disruptive behavior, they know that Brian has not overcome the dyslexic stumbling blocks that trigger strong emotion. Regardless of the student's age or the lateness of the school year, it is useless and unwise to push overly frustrated learners further and further through the curriculum when clearly they are too overwhelmed to succeed. Instructors will know when editing skills and perceptual maturity have been gained. As he overcomes specific dyslexic tendencies, Brian exhibits longer stamina without becoming upset, compared with his former quick frustration during study activities. When he can work calmly for half an hour with tasks that used to trigger emotional outbursts within a few minutes, teachers and parents know that his brain pathways are ready for next steps in classroom tasks.

Teaching Individuals with Visual Dyslexia To Read

This chapter has emphasized multisensory learning strategies that help the left brain, right brain, and midbrain build permanent memory. It is impossible for most dyslexic individuals to learn through passive, silent strategies. To learn to read, those who are dyslexic must be involved in multisensory reading instruction that stimulates the whole brain to incorporate vision, hearing, and touch along with positive emotions and feelings.

For example, one of the most successful reading instruction methods of the 20th century has been the Lindamood program. During the 1960s, Charles Lindamood, a specialist in linguistics, and Pat Lindamood, a specialist in speech and hearing therapy, designed a multisensory reading program they called *Auditory Discrimination in Depth* (ADD). The ADD reading program organizes lessons around the speech sounds (phonemes) of the English language. Beginner pupils start by learning each of the 44 English-language phonemes and how they are produced by the throat, mouth, tongue, and lips. This instruction follows the alphabet sequence so that pupils practice alphabetic order while connecting sounds to letters. Instructors of the ADD method are certified through extensive hands-on training at one of the Lindamood–Bell clinics. The ADD program is based on each teacher's intuition, imagination, and ability to "read" body and facial signals from each student. Students in this program use a mirror to learn how their lips, tongue, mouth, and throat form speech sounds. Every lesson is based on vigorous physical and vocal activities that engage sight, hearing, speech, touch, and positive emotions and feelings. Every moment of success is praised by the teacher. Students follow imaginative verbal cues that remind them of how speech sounds are produced. As time goes by, permanent memory emerges for how we speak, how we listen, and how we connect sounds to printed letters (Lindamood, Bell, & Lindamood, 1992; McGuinness, 1997).

The ADD reading program has proved highly effective for teaching literacy skills to persons with visual dyslexia. As Chapter 5 explains, this intensely verbal language training program is not always successful with individuals who have auditory dyslexia that keeps them from "hearing" how soft/slow speech chunks are alike or different. The Lindamood–Bell ADD reading program is excellent for "late bloomer" youngsters who are behind normal developmental schedule. It also is effective for persons who are learning English as a second language. ADD and other Lindamood–Bell language training methods are available only at one of the Lindamood–Bell private clinics or at schools whose teachers are certified to present the ADD method. The high cost of private ADD instruction and the limited number of classrooms where ADD is taught mean that only a few dyslexic individuals can receive the benefits of this excellent reading program.

Making Referrals

Three out of five dyslexic individuals can respond well enough to the techniques suggested in this chapter to cope or thrive in mainstream class activities. Two in five dyslexic students must have specialized help away from a mainstream environment. When youngsters like Brian reach the end of their tolerance in the classroom, teachers and parents should seek special help that mainstream instructors cannot always provide. When daily classwork continually triggers disruptive emotions and feelings, it is time for special intervention to take place. A rule of thumb for referral to learning specialists might be this:

> So long as the student is making some progress without too much emotional upset, I will keep up my efforts to meet his or her special needs. When behavior becomes too disruptive, or when the student becomes so frustrated he or she cannot continue to learn in this situation, then I will refer that individual to someone who can provide special help.

Diagnosing Dyslexia Is Controversial

One of the great ironies of U.S. education is the reluctance of most educators to use the label *dyslexia*. Chapter 2 summarizes scientific research that has defined the nature and causes of this specific learning disability. At a national symposium on dyslexia where 100 years of research was reviewed, Drake Duane (1985) from the Mayo Clinic declared, "Dyslexia now is the most thoroughly researched type of learning disability."An enormous body of scientific literature has been devoted to the study of dyslexia, yet most educators continue to avoid using this label when bright students struggle to read, spell, and write. Instead of openly acknowledging this brain-based learning difference, examiners who evaluate students for learning difficulty universally say "LD" (learning disability). When asked by anxious parents and teachers if a child might have dyslexia, few licensed educational examiners acknowledge or discuss this issue. Instead, they talk about LD without explaining which type of learning difficulty is indicated by diagnostic tests results.

Until 1984, struggling learners like Brian were given special help on the basis of test scores combined with the observations of teachers, parents, tutors, coaches, and others who knew the child. Adults on those assessment teams used checklists and anecdotal information to decide which students were eligible for special help. Before 1984, the term *dyslexia* was used freely by adults who recognized it and were familiar with dyslexic patterns.

In 1984, a national standard was proposed by the American Psychological Association (APA) for evaluating students for learning disability. This diagnostic model became known as the score-disprepancy model for identifying specific learning disabilities. Beginning in 1984, most schools and governmental agencies have adhered to the score-discrepancy model from the APA. This so-called scientific method for identifying learning disability requires certain score profiles from standard tests before an individual can be labeled LD. This diagnostic model mandates that a standard intelligence test be administered to establish a baseline IQ score. Then the student is given a standard academic achievement test that yields standard scores for reading, language usage, and math. Finally, the standard scores for reading, language usage, and math are subtracted from the IQ score. For a person to be labeled LD by this method, he or she must show an arbitrary discrepancy between IQ and classroom achievement. However, no national standard has been established for how much discrepancy a student must show to be eligible for special educational help because of LD. Each state is free to set its own score-discrepancy standard. Within many states, individual school districts may set their own standards, which might differ from other schools in the same state.

For example, students who struggle to read, spell, write, and do math may not be eligible for special educational help. To qualify for special help at his school, Brian's standard achievement test scores in reading, language usage, and math must be an arbitrary number of points lower than his IQ score. Suppose that he lives in Oklahoma when his parents seek special educational help because of Brian's constant struggle with dyslexia. That year Oklahoma might require a 20-point discrepancy between Brian's IQ score and his standard scores in reading, language usage, and math. Suppose that his IQ score is 110. To be eligible for special help in the Resource Room or another special class, his standard achievement scores must be below 90 (20-point discrepancy or greater). Brian's score profile from standard tests is as follows:

IQ	110
Reading	91
Language usage	89
Math	87

That year in Oklahoma he would be designated as LD because his standard scores met the score-discrepancy criteria (20 points below IQ). According to the score-discrepancy method, schools are permitted to make exceptions when score discrepancy is borderline, as when Brian's reading score of 91 is 19 points below his IQ of 110.

Suppose that Brian's family moved to North Carolina during a year when 25 points of discrepancy were required before a child is eligible for special help. Brian, who was legally LD in Oklahoma, suddenly would not be LD in his new home because his score discrepancy pattern failed to meet the 25-point criteria. This frustrating dilemma in determining who is eligible for special educational help remains unresolved as our culture enters the new millennium.

Rebellion Against Score Discrepancy

Many teachers and parents never have accepted the APA score-discrepancy method as being the best way to determine which struggling learners may receive special help with literacy skills and math. Groups of parents, educators, and other professionals have protested strongly that standard scores alone cannot analyze the special learning needs of students like Brian. Two parent/professional organizations, the Learning Disabilities Association (LDA) and the International Dyslexia Association (formerly the Orton Dyslexia Society), have led the movement toward less rigid assessment of special learning needs. These and other organizations have supported federal legislation to make sure that regardless of test score profiles, every struggling learner receives the special help he or she needs. In 1975 Congress enacted the Education for All Handicapped Children Act that became known as Public Law 94-142. That law required that each child be provided the "least restrictive environment" with the most appropriate educational opportunities. In 1990 that legislation was revised as the Individuals with Disabilities Education Act (IDEA). These federal laws stipulate that dyslexia is a type of specific learning disability that requires help within the school curriculum. In 1986, the Texas state legislature amended the Texas Education Code with Section 38.003 to establish a new category of special education called dyslexia. This legislation mandated that every child within the Texas public schools be evaluated for dyslexia. In 1995, subsequent legislation through Act 1995 established the following definitions:

> (1) "Dyslexia" means a disorder of constitutional origin manifested by a difficulty in learning to read, write, or spell, despite conventional instruction, adequate intelligence, and sociocultural opportunity.
> (2) "Related disorders" includes disorders similar to or related to dyslexia, such as developmental auditory imperception, dysphasia, specific developmental dyslexia, developmental dysgraphia, and developmental spelling disability. (Moses, 1998, p. 4)

The Texas model for treating dyslexia combines formal diagnosis by licensed examiners, informal assessment by valid checklists, and score profiles from achievement tests. The Texas model goes beyond test scores to determine who is eligible for special educational help. Data about student needs are gathered by using such informal assessment tools as the *Jordan Dyslexia Assessment / Reading Program* (Jordan, 2000a), the *Slingerland Screening Tests for Identifying Children with Specific Language Disability* (Slingerland, 1984), and the *Learning Disabilities Diagnostic Inventory* (Hammill & Bryant, 2000).

What Is Required To Overcome Dyslexia?

No book can include all of the useful techniques for overcoming dyslexia. Parents, tutors, and teachers must tailor corrective strategies to fit the specific needs of each student. Figure 4.22 shows how a simple checklist of dyslexic differences can become a teaching/learning guide into which a wide variety of techniques can be incorporated. Regardless of what remedial strategies are used, some fundamental principles must be observed in working with dyslexic students like Brian.

Principle 1: Providing Accommodations for Dyslexia Is Fair

Chapter 2 begins with the assertion that reading is not a natural process for the human brain. Two out of five individuals are born with the neural capacity to develop excellent skills for reading. Another two out of five persons can acquire enough literacy skills to become adequate readers. One out of five individuals cannot become competent readers, no matter how hard they try. Of those who struggle to read, many are dyslexic because of genetic predisposition or physical mishaps that inhibit neural functions within the left brain. When an individual is dyslexic, he or she faces lifelong frustration in any situation that requires fluency in literacy skills.

Perhaps the most difficult challenge for teachers and parents who read well is to understand that being dyslexic is not a choice. Being dyslexic is beyond the control of the individual. Struggling to read, write, and spell is a brain-based difference that cannot be remedied through trying harder. For half a century the American culture has worked toward erasing social and workplace barriers for individuals who have disabilities. Our society has decided that it is fair for every public place to provide equal access so that every person has equal opportunity to enjoy the benefits of living in the United States. Often it is difficult for educators to understand that it is fair to provide accommodations in classroom learning for those who do not have natural talent for literacy skills required by the curriculum.

What is fair in teaching those who are dyslexic? When educators truly believe that every person is entitled to an education according to his or her abilities and special needs, then relaxing pressure to hurry is fair. Giving dyslexic learners enough time to do their best is fair. Adjusting academic goals to fit the neurological abilities of dyslexic students is fair. Providing accommodations so that dyslexic learners have equal opportunity to become all they are capable of being is fair.

Principle 2: Positive Self-Fulfilling Prophecy

Chapter 1 presents the concept of the proto-self that develops very early in an infant's life (see page 27). How each person thinks of self plays a powerful role in how individuals approach or avoid formal learning. Among the most powerful factors in classroom success or failure are the attitudes that teachers and parents display. Chapter 7 discusses the critical role of emotions and feelings in dyslexic students like Brian. A vital principle can be stated as follows: *Learners tend to behave the way that teachers and parents expect them to behave.* In other words, students tend to return the feelings and attitudes they sense in their leaders. If the adults in Brian's life believe that he can succeed with their help, he will do his best to live up to their expectations. If, however, Brian senses that adults do not believe in him or do not expect him to succeed, his self-image (proto-self) will be negative and turned toward failure. Positive teachers who respect their students are respected in return. Negative teachers who regard students like Brian as failures who will not succeed witness the fulfilling of that negative prophecy. If his teachers believe that he will fail, Brian responds in negative, disrespectful ways that defy adult authority and disrupt the class. What dyslexic learners achieve is closely tied to adult attitudes and expectations.

The attitude of the classroom leader is a critical factor for students who are dyslexic. Some adults are not suited temperamentally for working with struggling learners. Such adults are put off by repeated failure when students do not have talent for reading, spelling, writing, or math. If working with these individuals is uncomfortable or offensive for an educator, it will be impossible to establish a warm, accepting relationship. Students who learn differently do not respond positively to leaders who are critical and aloof. More harm than good comes from forced associations between educators who dread dealing with such students and learners whose teachers feel that way. It is essential that instructors have positive expectations and affection for individuals who struggle with literacy skills for which they have little talent.

Principle 3: Work on What the Learner Needs

Unless teaching strategies actually meet the learner's needs, valuable time and energy are wasted while no educational growth occurs. This principle can be expressed in a practical three-point guide:

1. What does the student need?
2. What would be nice for the student to know?
3. What is beside the point at this time?

Answers to these questions are important in overcoming dyslexia. Earlier, this chapter explained why it is critical to identify the student's literacy needs. If Brian does not know the alphabet, then learning the alphabet is his most important need. It would be nice for him to read 10 books this year, but that goal is not yet feasible or possible. It is beside the point for him to try to write book reports. In other words, if a building's foundation never has been laid, it would be foolish to try to build upper floors. If Brian needs the foundation skill of knowing the alphabet, then that is where his literacy instruction must begin.

Principle 4: Relax the Pressure

Students who are dyslexic face two mortal educational enemies: (1) *a work rate that goes too fast* and (2) *pressure to produce more quantity than limited skills make possible.* Students like Brian must work slowly as they read, write, and spell because they cannot make left-brain language centers process symbols faster. Chapter 7 describes lifelong emotions and feelings that quickly surge into panic when dyslexic persons are forced to hurry. Time-limited tests are especially threatening for individuals who are dyslexic. The click of a stopwatch or the relentless tick of a timing clock triggers intense fear of failure. Time penalties for dyslexic learners are as cruel as being forced to run a track meet would be for a person with an injured leg. Adults who are unaware of time-triggered emotions can inflict deep anguish in students whose thought patterns are slow in processing symbols.

Pressure to produce quantities of handwritten work is equally devastating for students like Brian. When confronted by demands to produce quantities of handwriting quickly, he panics and gives up. However, if Brian is encouraged to use his personal computer for writing, he can meet most of the written language goals his class faces.

Principle 5: Keep Assignments Simple

There is nothing simple about today's classroom curriculum. Talented adults who delight in manipulating complex theory have designed a wide range of advanced programs for children. Each new texbook adoption startles parents and teachers who see advanced abstract concepts introduced into kindergarten and primary education. All kinds of pressures are exerted by special interest groups to cram more and more into the already complex curricula of most children. This escalation of high expectations is overwhelming for dyslexic students who are easily confused when bombarded by new information at every turn. Even fun time often is so overorganized that sensitive children dread recess.

Dyslexia involves the inability to sort out sensory impressions rapidly enough to stay on group schedules. Classroom success is not a matter of learning how to react appropriately to the flow of new data. Instead, academic achievement comes through learning how not to react to the overload of irrelevant stimuli that bombards students from every side. Those who have dyslexia cannot tune out irrelevant information well enough to keep up with the flow of what is essential to remember. They cannot edit their environment quickly enough to identify what is relevant. The result is a mass of inaccurate, overly cluttered, or incomplete mind maps that leave the student unable to cope.

Dyslexia can be overcome only when outside stimulus is carefully controlled. Teaching students like Brian requires clearly stated step-by-step routines that expose them only to the amount of stimulus they can handle at a given time. For example, Figure 4.23 shows a math lesson that includes several concepts on the same work page. When he sees this assignment, Brian is overwhelmed by too many visual cues at the same time. Figure 4.24

LESSON 24

ᔓ ᔓ ᔓ ᔓ ᔓ ᔓ ᔓ ᔓ ᔓ ᔓ ᔓ ᔓ ᔓ

- **See how quickly you can work the following problems**

$6.41	$11.51	$4.73	$10.10	$9.95	$3.44
+ .39	− 4.20	−1.13	− 3.14	+ .42	−1.22

* * * * * * * * * * * * * * * *

Try to work these problems without using a pencil.

1. Juan sold half of his baseball cards for $2.00. Then he traded 12 cards for new ones. How much money did Juan make with his cards? _____

2. Marie spent 3 hours in the store shopping for new shoes. Then she spent 1 hour eating lunch. Before she went home, she spent 2 hours at a movie. How many hours did Marie spend at the mall? _____

~ ~

// Circle the problems that have mistakes.

$14.12	$5.19	$61.20	$11.45	$15.77	$9.11
+ 2.27	− .18	− 1.44	+ 3.20	+ 2.99	−4.10
$12.29	$5.01	$62.64	$ 8.65	$18.76	$4.11

Figure 4.23. This kind of busy, overcrowded work page is impossible for students with visual dyslexia. Teachers cannot tell whether the student does not know math or whether he or she cannot interpret the page format.

shows the kind of simple work page he must have to avoid perceptual overload. When work pages are too busy with too many details, teachers cannot tell whether Brian does not know how to do the task or whether his brain is overly confused by the page format.

Principle 6: Keep It Structured

Chapter 2 presented the concept of neurological talent that explains the variety of skills and abilities that teachers find in every classroom. Persons who are dyslexic often have outstanding

LESSON 24

$6.41
+ .39

$11.51
− 4.20

$4.73
+1.13

$10.10
− 3.14

$9.59
+ .42

$3.44
−1.22

Figure 4.24. This kind of simple, open format is ideal for students with visual dyslexia. There are no extra visual details to interfere with the purpose of the task.

right-brain talent for intuitive problem solving and creative thinking when they are not involved with literacy-based instruction. However, when classroom information is centered on reading and writing, dyslexic learners become overwhelmed by too much variety along with too little structure. A prominent concept in today's curriculum is that good teaching guides learners to discover essential information rather than being told about it. The ability to discover within the context of reading and writing is a specialized talent not shared by everyone. In every classroom, some students are talented discoverers. Others are not. Classroom teachers often are confronted by curriculum goals based on the premise that all students can and should discover fundamental concepts if they have enough experience through exploring. In fact, millions of students of all ages have not acquired basic skills in reading, spelling, grammar, math, or science in spite of attractive materials designed to let them explore and discover for themselves.

A cardinal truth regarding dyslexia is that learning new reading-based skills must be highly structured. This principle does not contradict theories of self-discovery. Individuals who are dyslexic cannot cope with loosely structured situations. For them, discovery learning is impossible if they do have enough structured practice and drill to develop competence in foundation skills. Without structure, Brian cannot assemble mind maps into coherent memory unless he is given clearly defined models to show him how. Abstract reasoning without visible structure often is a major stumbling block for dyslexic learners.

Parents and teachers must provide clearly structured, familiar routines on which students with dyslexia can depend. This rules out certain kinds of multiple-stimulus activities that often are prescribed in teachers' manuals and guidebooks. Words with multiple meanings, variant spellings of vowel or consonant sounds, open-ended grammar or punctuation rules, and indefinite elements of math, science, and social studies are threatening to students who cannot function when things change too much from lesson to lesson.

Figure 4.25 shows what happens when students like Brian are expected to filter and organize several perceptual tasks on the same page. Brian's teacher decided to make a phonics work page more interesting by showing each picture task inside a basket. Brian's task was to write the name of each picture inside each basket. A problem called *perceptual crossover* occurred as he tried to cope with this unstructured task. His brain was expected to remember that the basket was only the frame for the picture. Brian was expected to focus attention on the picture inside the basket, figure out how to spell the object in the picture, then write that word below the basket. This multilayered task triggered many overlapping mind maps that Brian's dyslexic left brain could not organize. What he saw (visual perception) crossed over into what he heard and said (auditory perception). Then he had to translate vision and speech into writing. In each instance, he correctly wrote the first letter/sound for each picture. But the predominant hard consonant cluster /sk/ in *basket* crowded out his perception of the rest of the word. When Brian looked at the visual image of a basket, he could no longer concentrate on the auditory image of the object name. Instructors must not pile perceptual tasks on top of each other as they create work pages for students with dyslexia.

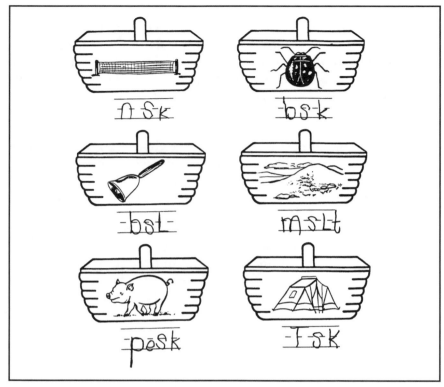

Figure 4.25. The instructions were: "Write the word for each picture." Brian saw two pictures. His mental images crossed over and produced mixed images. Every time he wrote the first letter of the *inside picture,* his mental image finished the *outside picture* (basket).

Principle 7: Individuals with Dyslexia Must Accept Supervision

The most critical skill that individuals with dyslexia must develop is knowing how to maintain structure in their lives. It is the nature of dyslexia that details are continually out of order or sequence. Having dyslexia means not holding onto clear mental images of how parts go together to produce a functional whole. Every moment of every day, persons with dyslexia must cope with mixed images, such as partial memory of details, confused sense of passing time, incomplete awareness of direction, and inability to recall where things are located. Dyslexic individuals never are sure of when it is time for the next important activity, how much money already has been spent, or how much money is left to pay bills before the next payday. Dyslexia makes it hard for individuals to remember how many steps are yet to be done before tasks are completed.

Individuals with mild dyslexia can learn how to stay organized if, during early childhood, they are coached in noticing cues and reminders. They learn to mask their scrambled thinking well enough so that others rarely suspect that these uncertain moments exist. Persons with moderate dyslexia cannot hide their trouble staying organized. If they receive enough coaching during childhood and early adolescence, moderately dyslexic individuals manage to get by with frequent help from certain ones they trust. However, friendly coaching does not erase the likelihood that they will be labeled "forgetful" or "scatterbrained." When dyslexic symptoms are severe, having continual supervision is not an option. To function successfully in the classroom, the workplace, or within personal relationships, those with severe dyslexia must have help all of their lives to stay organized and on schedule.

Perhaps the greatest problem adults face in working with children who are dyslexic is their habit of resisting supervision. Yet, these vulnerable youngsters cannot cope with the stress of being dyslexic without help from a supervisor. This universal reluctance to accept supervision is due partly to the fact that individuals with dyslexia view the world differently. They do not see the same panorama of events, nor do they scan their world with the same degree of insight. They come away from experiences with incomplete impressions, causing them to recall events from a different perspective. They do not judge time, dimension, distance, space, or reality the same way as do others who are not dyslexic. Individuals with dyslexia do not react to stimuli with a whole, fully integrated response. They continually leave out important ingredients that alter how they should have reacted, and they tend to respond more slowly than others, causing their understanding to be delayed.

They "freeze" in unexpected situations, which appears to be balking or stubborn refusal to cooperate. Often they do not know what to do in situations where others know automatically or quickly figure out the right response. Having dyslexia in today's fast-paced culture is like standing in the middle of a busy free-way. If dyslexic individuals are left alone to decide for themselves at their slower rate of processing, they are out of step, in conflict, at cross-purposes, and at emotional risk from all sides. A cluster of differences places these individuals in need of help: slow re-action time, faulty interpretation, incomplete recall, misunder-stood signals, scrambled impressions, cluttered mental images, and uncertain body-in-space orientation. To cope successfully, these individuals require the help of gentle supervisors who re-mind them patiently again and again.

Supervisors Reduce the Level of Fear

Parents of children with dyslexia face the never-ending task of keeping the youngster's life structured to reduce the number of loose ends the child faces each day. Without supervision, it is impossible for these children to be on time for meals, gather up necessary things for school, get dressed on schedule, remember strings of oral instructions, finish a series of tasks, keep every-thing picked up in their rooms, bring all outside things into the garage at night, take care of pets, and so forth.

Because their memory cannot cope with the hundreds of facts and sequences that are part of normal living, dyslexic persons of all ages must have friendly supervision that is kind, nonaggres-sive, helpful, and not overly critical. The supervisor must be pa-tient, must stay calm, and must not yell or lash out at the con-fused reactions of the individual who is dyslexic. Whoever is the supervisor must walk as a guide by the person's side, not push from the back as a prodder. Those who are dyslexic need super-vision because they cannot see the next few steps clearly, much like someone peering into a dark corridor while wondering what is just ahead. Anyone would naturally pause before starting down a dark, unknown passageway. Individuals with dyslexia pause hundreds of times each day because the next moment is not clear. Those who supervise must be aware of this fact.

If the supervisor takes time to shed enough light on these dark "unknowns," the apprehensive individual will feel safe enough to move forward in confidence. If, however, the supervi-sor impatiently shoves the indecisive person forward, the dyslexic individual is overwhelmed by panic and the ghost of im-pending failure. These individuals with faulty memory and incomplete perception respond best to a guiding hand that reassures them all is well. Those who supervise must not forget that individuals with dyslexia will freeze, panic, or rebel the moment that stress is felt too keenly. Regardless of age, fear is a constant shadow over the lives of those who are dyslexic—fear of failure, of being incompetent, of being rejected, of being criticized or belittled, of being humiliated or embarrassed, of being impotent at tasks that others do well, of losing loved ones or cherished relationships, of dying, of being "dumb," and of not living up to the expectations of special persons in their lives. Such fears would cause anyone to freeze. These chronic fears are invisible lifelong campanions of those who are dyslexic.

The underlying aura of fear colors every decision that dyslexic individuals make. The emotional aftertaste of fear alters one's feelings the way a bad odor fills a room. Haunting memories of other failures trigger faster heartbeat and physical constrictions that cause the chest to tighten, breathing to quicken, and blood pressure to soar. Momentarily frightened individuals are on guard, overly defensive, and on the verge of running away from the unknown. These emotionally vulnerable persons want to hide or escape from unknown situations that rise before them at every turn. From their point of view, it is less painful to be scolded again for forgetting homework or failing to pay a bill on time than to go through the agony of making more mistakes. It is easier to endure reprimand for being lazy than it is to do one's best and still be criticized.

Adults who have dyslexia often are criticized for "not taking that good job." They are subjected to such comments as, "Why did you quit your job? That's four jobs you've quit already this year!" What the critic does not realize is that invisible pain within the fearful worker finally became too acute to be endured. Those who have dyslexia never are fully free from uncertainty. If the right kind of supervision is provided early enough, most dyslexic youngsters learn to control this innate fear and develop coping strategies for stress.

Kinds of Supervisors

Supervision can come in a variety of ways. Individuals with moderate or severe dyslexia need a key person who is the main source of their supervision. For children, this usually is a parent, typically the mother. In single-parent families, the parent cannot always be available to supervise and keep the child on schedule. Then the child must have a "substitute parent" to provide reminding and help. It is natural for anyone who is dyslexic to bond with someone who offers safe, reassuring companionship. Adults often complain about the kinds of friends whom dyslexic youngsters prefer. It is natural for fearful, apprehensive, or insecure young people to seek out companions who do not judge, criticize, or scold. Individuals who have dyslexia usually become attached to others who also are dyslexic because no one else is patient enough to be safe. When two or three dyslexic individuals form a group, they are developing their own community or substitute family where they feel welcome and free from the stress of judgment. Why should they want to associate with people who continually nag, criticize, judge, scold, or otherwise make them feel like failures? Bonding with a group of companions who accept their differences as being normal is part of the process of finding a source of help that gives without always taking away. Occasionally, someone with dyslexia finds supervisory companionship in an older brother or sister. Sometimes a grandparent, an uncle, or an aunt can fill this important role. Often the supervisor is a scout leader, a coach, a religious leader, a teacher, a school custodian, or a neighbor.

Strategies for Supervisors

Visible Reminders. The most important type of supervisory strategy is something the dyslexic individual can see. Few persons with dyslexia can develop full mental images just by listening or doing abstract thinking. They must see some kind of outline, sketch, graph, chart, Post-it sticker, or diagram before most concepts make sense. Even those who have natural talent for learning through listening need some kind of visible pattern that helps the higher brain build permanent memory. Most individuals who are dyslexic must combine several senses by seeing/touching/saying/ hearing at the same time.

Written Lists and Outlines. As soon as children can read simple words, the supervisor starts making written lists and outlines. Each task to be done is written or printed on a list with each step clearly numbered. The child learns where the list always will be. Once the child is told where the list will be, that place stays the same. When the supervisor says, "Jai, go look at your list," Jai does not have to wonder where it is. Written lists help to remove nagging from the relationship between supervisor and child. When adults try to supervise orally, they inevitably end up in shouting matches with the forgetful child. "Jai, I told you to feed the dog." "No, you didn't!" "Yes, I did! You never listen to a word I say!" This kind of verbal argument could have been avoided by posting a simple list:

1. Feed the dog.
2. Water the dog.
3. Wash your hands.

Supervisors of children whose lives are disorganized must be prepared to split hairs. Most adults make the mistake of under-estimating the intelligence of dyslexic youngsters who are loose and poorly organized. As noted previously, individuals with dyslexia often are much brighter than average. They do not score well on standard tests, yet they are quite intelligent. With those who are dyslexic, usable intelligence often is loose, poorly orga-nized, and beyond their reach at those moments when rapid or-ganized thinking is required. This underlying intelligence fos-ters a lot of splitting. Supervisors of individuals with dyslexia often become intensely frustrated by the tendency to quibble and argue. Most dyslexic youngsters spend much of their mental en-ergy splitting hairs over what adults say. This frequently occurs because the supervisor assumes that the child will use common sense when interpreting what was said. A simple statement like "Feed the dog" includes a lot of assumed material that the su-pervisor did not think was necessary to say.

The following dialogue is typical of the splitting that occurs when supervisors take shortcuts:

SUPERVISOR: Jai, don't forget to feed the dog this evening.

JAI: OK.

When the supervisor comes home from work at 5:30 p.m., the dog has not been fed.

SUPERVISOR: Jai! I told you to feed the dog when you got home from school! You don't ever do anything I say!

JAI: No, you didn't.

> SUPERVISOR: I certainly did! This morning I told you to feed the dog when you got home from school! Don't tell me I didn't tell you!
>
> JAI: That's not what you said. You said to feed the dog this evening. It's not evening yet. Evening starts when the sun goes down.

This illustrates the hazard of giving oral instructions. Obviously, the best way to reduce or eliminate the problem is to make a specific, detailed, in-sequence list:

1. Feed the dog when you come home after school.
2. Check the dog's water.
3. Close the garage door so the dog can't get out.

The supervisor need only ask, "Jai, did you do everything on your list?" This places the responsibility back on Jai and avoids nagging and yelling over what was said that morning. If Jai has chosen not to look at the list, then he is reponsible for the consequences. He cannot squirm out of responsibility by splitting hairs over what was or was not said.

Calendars and Daily Logs. As children move upward through school grades, they must learn to handle a multitude of memory tasks. Each new year introduces still more things to be remembered. Homework materials must arrive at home. Finished homework must be returned to each teacher to receive a grade. Long-term assignments such as book reports, science projects, and research papers must be done on a schedule. Many youngsters do not go directly home from school. From kindergarten upward, life becomes increasingly complex for today's children and families. It is imperative that children who lack natural talent for organization be taught how to keep their duties and obligations in order.

A major symptom of dyslexia is a poor sense of time and chronology. Individuals who are dyslexic have no internal awareness of events in sequence or of how one event relates to a series of others. They must *see* time in order to deal with it successfully. Dyslexia requires early use of a personal calendar. As soon as children become involved with day-to-day activities, they must begin seeing the days, weeks, and months represented on a calendar. Before they can read the names of days and months, they need right-brain symbols. For example, each day could be a certain color. On the blue day, they take lunch money to school. On the red day, they have a special lesson after school. On the green day, they ride in the carpool to soccer practice. On the yellow day, they have gymnastics lessons, and so forth. As soon as children begin to work with letters, words, and numbers, these are added to the calendar. The supervisor takes a few minutes each day to go over the week's calendar with the child. This continual, consistent repetition begins to build a foundation for helping him or her think in terms of time and how events are related. The youngster begins to see how one event comes first, another comes next, another occurs later, and so on. By the time the child has seen his or her life represented in this calendar form for several years, a lifelong organizational skill has been established.

Teaching children with dyslexia how to keep a daily school list also is an important part of learning how to stay organized. Each evening, the supervisor guides the student in making a simple list of everything that must go back to school next day. Everything means everything—nothing is assumed. Together, the child and supervisor check the list: pencils, tablets, art supplies, erasers, or whatever the student needs to do his or her work properly. Does Joy need some new supplies? Have her teachers announced that certain things will be required for upcoming assignments or projects? Are all of her homework assignments finished? Together, the supervisor and Joy go over the list before bedtime. Next morning the supervisor gives reminders: "Joy, go over your list again. Don't forget anything that needs to go back to school." If Joy protests that she does not have time, the supervisor reminds her that she is responsible. Joy is not to call from school saying that she left something important at home. Again, the list becomes the source of pressure. If Joy chooses to take shortcuts, then she must face the consequences. If it was on the list, then the list becomes the final authority.

Electronic Organizers. As dyslexic youngsters become skilled with computers, they can form lifelong habits of using electronic organizers that fit into a pocket, bookbag, or purse. As the new millennium unfolds, most individuals will become skilled in using electronic devices for communication, record keeping, and accessing information. Earlier, this chapter pointed out that right-brain keyboarding skills are natural for most of those who are dyslexic. By the time Brian, Jai, and Joy enter middle school, they should be skilled at using their personal electronic organizers to order their lives and reduce the stress that comes from being too poorly organized.

Overcoming Auditory Dyslexia

5

"mr. jorgen, Donna don't nede to
go see the nirs. She alredy
had her nesary shouts"
—Note from a mother with auditory dyslexia to Mr. Jordan, her child's teacher

Chapter 4 explained what causes visual dyslexia: Regions of the left brain cannot learn which direction written symbols must face or the sequence those symbols must maintain. Visual dyslexia has little to do with vision. Most individuals with visual dyslexia see quite well, but they do not have natural talent for learning to read. Historically, nonreaders were called "word blind." Chapter 4 presented illustrations of how the dyslexic brain turns symbols backwards, flips them upside down, and scrambles details out of correct sequence.

Another type of dyslexia arises when the brain cannot "hear" individual sounds of speech. Historically, the inability to perceive soft/slow speech sounds (vowels and soft consonants) has been called "tone deafness." Today this inability to distinguish sounds of speech is called *auditory dyslexia*. Specialists who evaluate speech and hearing often use the label *central auditory processing disorder*. Auditory dyslexia has nothing to do with ability to hear. Most tone-deaf individuals have normal hearing for non-speech sounds. Yet when it comes to interpreting speech, they cannot identify the individual sound chunks that fit together to create spoken words. Figure 5.1 shows the neurological loop that enables the human brain to translate oral language into mind maps of what others say. Most individuals are born with brain structures ready to respond accurately to oral language. Those who cannot do so usually are dyslexic.

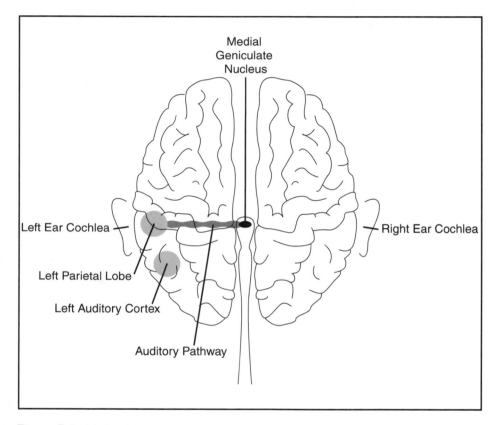

Figure 5.1. The cochlea in each middle ear gathers speech sounds that are changed into electrical codes. These speech codes are sent to the medial geniculate nucleus within the midbrain. The medial geniculate nucleus organizes soft/slow and hard/fast speech chunks into word patterns, then fires that data to the left parietal lobe, which sends it on to the auditory cortex within the left temporal lobe. The auditory pathway between the midbrain and parietal lobe contains two types of cells that work together as a team. Larger cells along the auditory pathway process soft/slow speech sounds (vowels and soft consonants). Small cells process hard/fast speech sounds (hard consonants). Auditory dyslexia occurs when underdeveloped larger cells fail to transfer soft/slow speech sounds in the correct sequence. The auditory cortex receives and interprets only part of the original oral language flow. (Based on research by Bredburg, 1985; Eliot, 1999; Hepper & Shahidullah, 1994; Lous, 1995; Peck, 1995; Pujol, 1990; and Tallal, Miller, & Fitch, 1993.)

During their research since 1980, Paula Tallal, Steven Miller, and Robert Fitch discovered the neurological cause for auditory dyslexia. Their research identified a double deficit in neuron formations within the medial geniculate nucleus and along the auditory pathway (see Figure 5.1). The primary function of the medial geniculate nucleus is to separate and organize the hard/fast and soft/slow speech chunks that are received from both ears as individuals listen to oral language. Then these speech data are fired down the auditory pathway to left-brain regions that assemble speech chunks into recognizable language. When auditory dyslexia exists, neurons within the medial geniculate nucleus are incompletely developed (Tallal et al., 1993). This deficit in cell structure makes it impossible for the medial geniculate nucleus to separate speech chunks correctly or to organize them adequately. These incomplete speech units then encounter further problems in their journey to the auditory cortex. Within the auditory pathway that links the medial geniculate nucleus with the left-brain language center are two types of cells that work together as a team. One set of smaller cells rapidly carries hard/fast speech sounds to the parietal lobe, where these speech chunks wait. At a slower pace, the second set of larger cells transfers soft/slow speech sounds to the parietal lobe. Auditory dyslexia occurs when the larger cells fail to deliver soft/slow speech sounds to the waiting hard/fast chunks. This difference in neural structure makes it impossible for the left brain to build adequate mind maps of what dyslexic individuals hear others say.

Phonemes

All human speech is built from chunks of sound called *phonemes*. All languages incorporate chains of fast/slow/fast/slow phoneme chunks to create speech. Infants and toddlers whose brain pathways are developing on schedule soon begin to mimic and repeat the language chunks they hear. As youngsters mature, four out of five become increasingly skilled at repeating the phoneme patterns of whatever language they hear at home and in the community. One out of five do not. Neurons within the medial geniculate nucleus and along the auditory pathway fail to mature on schedule. These tone-deaf youngsters do not hear phoneme chunks accurately. They cannot mimic or accurately reproduce their oral culture fluently (Jordan, 1998, 2000a, 2000b; Nagarajan et al., 1999; Tallal et al., 1993).

For example, the word *cat* is made of three sound chunks: hard /k/–soft /a/–hard /t/. Persons with normally developed neurons within the medial geniculate nucleus and along the auditory pathway instantly process these three sound chunks in correct sequence. Tone-deaf individuals do not. For example, Julia entered school without her auditory dyslexia being recognized. All her life she has been bewildered when teachers say, "Listen as I say *cat* . . . *cat*. Julia, tell me the sound of the vowel in *cat*." Julia, who is tone deaf to soft/slow speech sounds, is confused. She does not hear the soft /a/ vowel inside the word *cat*. What is the teacher talking about? She hears the hard /k/ at the beginning of *cat*. She hears the hard /t/ at the end of *cat*. But she has no idea that there is a soft /a/ sound in the middle of *cat*.

Julia faces growing auditory perception problems when she is required to listen to complete sentences. For example, her teacher says, "Get out your blue notebook." This simple oral sentence is made from a chain of hard/fast and slow/soft sound chunks:

▶ **/g/e/t/ou/t/yuh/oo/r/b/l/oo/n/o/t/b/oo/k/**

Julia's tone deafness fails to hear several of the slower, softer sound chunks. She hears only part of this string of speech sounds:

▶ **/g/-/t/-/oo/r-/b/l/-/b//-/k/**

Julia's brain heard the teacher say, "Go tour blow book." This makes no sense. Her first impulse is to blurt out "Huh? What? What do you mean?" But being scolded for interrupting and not trying to listen has taught Julia not to ask these listening questions. The teacher notices that she has not responded to the instructions. "Didn't you hear what I said, Julia?" the teacher asks impatiently. "I said get out your blue notebook." Still the oral message is not clear. Quickly Julia glances around to see what her classmates are doing. She gets through the school day by gleaning clues from her neighbors more than from understanding what her teacher says.

Students who have auditory dyslexia struggle with the consequences of not hearing all the chunks of oral language. They cannot rhyme words successfully, nor do they understand words in songs. They cannot hear rhyming words in poetry, they misunderstand conversations, and they misinterpret what is said on the radio and television. All their lives they have great difficulty connecting sounds to letters from memory. This makes it impossible for persons with auditory dyslexia to become talented at spelling or word sounding. Children like Julia are forever in conflict with adults because they do not interpret oral instructions correctly. We can understand the mystery of auditory dyslexia more clearly if we think of individuals who are tone deaf to differences in musical tones. Music is processed by nonlanguage regions of the left and right temporal lobes the same way that oral language is processed by the midbrain and left brain. One of the most painful experiences for music teachers and vocal coaches is to work with a monotone student who cannot carry a tune. No matter how much musical drill this person receives, he or she never learns vocal music skills. Persons like Julia are tone deaf to sounds of speech the way that others cannot hear notes and tones of music.

Recognizing Auditory Dyslexia

Appendix D presents the Jordan Auditory Dyslexia Test, which produces an inventory of the points in language processing where students like Julia bog down. By identifying specific stumbling blocks in language processing, teachers and tutors can develop remedial strategies that are designed to overcome auditory dyslexia. The following descriptions also pinpoint the patterns of auditory dyslexia in the classroom.

Print Does Not Match Speech

It is not difficult to identify tone-deaf persons who struggle to convert oral language into writing. When trying to create original sentences or paragraphs, Julia cannot think of what to put on her paper. Even when she says good sentences orally, she does not realize that she can encode those same words to make written sentences. When trying to read, Julia does not recognize that written words stand for oral words she uses in daily speech. Even though she has fluent speaking skills, Julia often cannot make the connection between what she or others say and what she sees in print. An observer will notice that dyslexic individuals struggle to connect what they see on the page with their own oral language. For them, reading and writing are foreign languages even though the words are pronounced the same. Auditory dyslexia is like a bridge that is out between written words and what those words mean in speech.

Tone Deafness to Phoneme Chunks

A red flag characteristic of auditory dyslexia is the inability to hear variations of vowel sounds. Most reading programs emphasize the long and short sounds of five vowels: *a, e, i, o, u*. Although *w* and *y* also are vowels (called *semivowels*), teachers do not always teach specific sounds for *w* and *y*. Educators have assumed that students who have clear speech should have no trouble telling the differences between long vowel and short vowel sounds. This is not true for students with auditory dyslexia. They have great difficulty distinguishing such close-sounding words as *big* and *beg* or *cat* and *cut*. For them, subtle distinctions in speech sounds do not exist.

A similar problem exists when tone-deaf students encounter consonant clusters (also called blends and digraphs). Few students with auditory dyslexia can hear separate consonant sounds in such clusters as *st, sp, gr,* or *pl*. For example, Julia usually can hear the first consonant letter sound in familiar words. Yet it frequently is impossible for her to hear the second or third sound in clusters such as *str, spl,* or *shr*.

Auditory dyslexia often remains undetected during the primary grades, particularly when formal phonics and spelling instruction are postponed until late second grade or early third grade. Most beginner pupils stumble in their first encounters with organized reading and writing instruction. These unnatural inventions challenge young brains to learn how to decode and encode a written alphabet. When the whole word (sight memory) approach or whole language method is used in primary grades, teachers often remain unaware that certain pupils are not hearing speech sounds accurately.

Confusion with Words: Alike or Different?

A major symptom of auditory dyslexia is the student's inability to tell whether words are the same or different. Julia is typical of an individual who struggles with auditory dyslexia. Her teacher has begun to suspect that she does not hear sounds accurately. Classroom teachers can screen students informally for tone deafness by using portions of the *Slingerland Screening Tests for Identifying Children with Specific Language Disability* (Slingerland, 1984) or the *Jordan Dyslexia Assessment / Reading Program* (Jordan, 2000a). These structured listening activities identify the accuracy of Julia's auditory perception of the phoneme chunks of oral language. The following is a sample of her performance on a simple listening activity:

Julia, listen carefully as I say two words. Tell me "same" if they are exactly the same. Tell me "different" if the words are not exactly the same.

Pronounced by Teacher	Julia's Responses
"bed–dead"	Different
"dime–time"	Same
"back–pack"	Same
"look–look"	Same
"tam–dam"	Same
"pane–bane"	Same
"dill–bill"	Different
"say–say"	Same
"fat–vat"	Same
"no–no"	Same
"not–what"	Same
"vetch–fetch"	Same
"mile–Nile"	Different
"where–hare"	Same
"got–got"	Same

It is difficult for dyslexic students to follow instructions well enough to give the standard answers adults expect. For example, the teacher may instruct Julia to say "alike" or "different." In her effort to concentrate and do her best, Julia's oral responses may range over several ways of expressing her decisions. She might say "same" instead of "alike." Then she may shift to "yes," meaning that the words are alike. Then she may shift again to responding "no" or "not the same" instead of saying "different." Such responses must not be regarded as incorrect. The point is to find out whether Julia hears sound patterns accurately, not whether she can parrot back stereotyped answers. Much of the conflict in the classroom between teachers and dyslexic students is triggered when adults fail to interpret correctly the student's confusion with signals.

This kind of informal listening evaluation reveals some significant deficits in Julia's auditory perception of speech sounds. From the activity shown above, her teacher has discovered several important differences that can respond to corrective tutoring. Julia's tone deafness keeps her from hearing differences with four sets of similar sound chunks: /d/ and /t/, /b/ and /p/, /f/ and /v/, /h/ and /hw/. The teacher now will be alert for other areas of faulty auditory perception as she guides Julia's reading and spelling practice. A peculiar pattern sometimes is seen as tone-deaf learners do these kinds of alike/different activities. Sometimes they make a perfect score when they deal only with single words or pairs of words. When they return to processing phonemes within phrases or sentences, they cannot cope with differences in speech sounds.

Mishearing Words

Mishearing words creates continual problems for dyslexic individuals as they respond to what goes on around them. For example, Julia's teacher kept a record of word misunderstandings that occurred in the girl's listening during one school day.

Teacher Said	Julia Heard
leopard	leprosy
pity	picky
Thermos	furnace
curiosity	cures
grief	grease
compare	repair
rose	roll
gulf stream	gull stream (later, golf stream)
difference	defends

This kind of record of a student's auditory misperception helps adults to understand much of the conflict that flares in Julia's relationships with others. Every time she misunderstands what her parents or teachers say, an argument follows. Because she is bright, Julia wants to tell what she knows. Her intelligent thinking often is masked by incorrect word usage because she does not hear differences between familiar words everyone in her life uses each day.

Verbal Rabbit Trails

Individuals with this type of faulty auditory perception are forever wandering off on verbal rabbit trails. Because she has misheard *grief* as *grease,* Julia's thoughts shift to thinking about an experience involving grease, while everyone else is thinking about the issue of grief. In the middle of the class discussion of what grief means, Julia blurts out a statement that her grandmother was burned by hot grease. Again, group discussion has been interrupted by an irrelevant comment that makes no sense. Julia's teacher and classmates react with irritation that sends the message "Oh, be quiet! There you go again!" It is hard for adults and classmates to realize that Julia is not just being stubborn or difficult when she gives this kind of response to what she hears. The tendency for her brain to wonder off on verbal rabbit trails sets her apart in social relationships.

Individuals with this oral language difficulty tend to become misfits in group situations. Often they are rejected by peers as being "weird." Chapter 7 describes the strong emotions and feelings that color the lives of individuals who are dyslexic. Oral language deficits triggered by auditory dyslexia bring much unhappiness and conflict into Julia's life. She cannot understand why she is unpopular with friends and has so much trouble getting along with adults.

Confusion with Spelling

Auditory dyslexia is a major cause for poor spelling. Because Julia does not hear separate speech sounds accurately, there is no way for her to remember how to spell. Traditional spelling instruction fills dyslexic children with frustration. When an arbitrary list of unrelated words is assigned on Monday to be memorized for Friday's dictation test, Julia faces a frustrating predicament that is intensified by fear of failure. Creative students often devise their own memory systems for remembering spelling patterns ("when" is *h-e-n* with *w* in front. "Mother" is *t-h-e* with *mo* in front and *r* at the end). Today's curriculum involving thousands of words presented at an ever faster pace soon produces impossible demands for students who are dyslexic. Few of them have the language talent required to figure out memory devices for all the words they must write.

Frequent Erasing

A major symptom of auditory dyslexia is chronic erasing, crossing out, and marking over to correct written mistakes. A careful observer soon understands why dyslexic students struggle through writing activities so nervously. They usually "think out loud" as they work, whispering over and over, trying it several ways, erasing, then writing another combination of letters. They never are sure that they have spelled a word correctly. Handwriting is an unusually threatening challenge for anyone who is dyslexic. Every word committed to paper exposes the insecure speller to probable failure. These students erase again and again, trying to "luck out" with the correct combinations of letters, hoping to please critics but not really expecting to succeed. Many students with dyslexia try to hide their work as they write, a further indication of their deep dread of failure.

Spelling Mistake Patterns

Certain mistake patterns are seen in the spelling efforts of individuals with auditory dyslexia. As Julia copies, writes from memory, or writes from dictation, four basic error patterns repeat over and over in her work. Sometimes she catches a spelling or writing mistake and does her best to correct it. Usually, however, her brain does not notice these dyslexic differences. Figure 5.2 shows the spelling struggle of a tone-deaf 19-year-old man with extraordinary talent for mechanical engineering. When he must deal with written language, he is at a serious disadvantage. Figure 5.3 shows the careful, time-consuming work of an 11-year-old boy who often figures out correct spellings if he has plenty of

word	response	word	response
rope	*roonla*	snake	*snonk*
	butter	family	*faimy*
bird	*birt*	getting	*geting*
pot	*pocty*	aid	*Rist Ade*
star	*stare*	blame	*Blende*
dress	*dresse*	crowd	*crecw*
even	*ening*	address	*Addredresse*
making	*menun makeing*	leaving	*lesseing*
every	*evetng*	parade	*prade*
moving	*moveing*	evening	*enrdeng*
plan	*plane / Plane*	single	*sneiny*
found	*fanihg*		*talking*
taken	*takiing*	listen	*lesing*
paint	*plang*	homesick	*homeself*
cast	*Cartsing*	delay	*den puh*
hardly	*horing / bite*	true	*tasgu*
		o'clock	*ockea*
		cabin	*capeng*
		careful	*king em*
		wear	*wripe*

Figure 5.2. This 19-year-old man is severely tone deaf when he tries to identify separate sounds within words. Occasionally he recalls a correct spelling pattern, but usually he is helpless to process the hard/fast, soft/slow speech chunks in correct sequence. He continually misunderstands conversations, oral instructions, phone messages, and what he hears on radio and television programs. However, he is a talented mechanical engineer with unusual skills in working with machinery.

time with freedom to whisper to himself. Figure 5.4 shows the best that a 21-year-old dyslexic man could do when asked to write 39 familiar words from dictation. Figure 5.5 shows how difficult these 39 words are for a severely tone-deaf 13-year-old girl

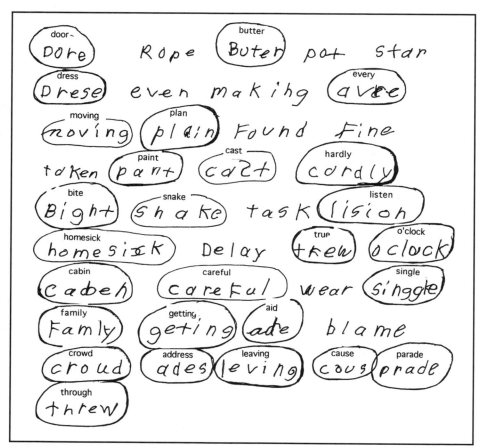

Figure 5.3. This 11-year-old boy is moderately tone deaf to hard/fast, soft/slow speech sounds. When he has all the time he needs to whisper to himself over and over, he often figures out correct spellings. He needed 35 minutes to do this dictated spelling activity that most students his age finish in 10 minutes.

to write. Figure 5.6 illustrates the value of asking a student to write the alphabet, days of the week, and months of the year as a screening test for auditory dyslexia. The problem of uncertain mind maps is shown in Figure 5.7. Many individuals with auditory dyslexia cannot maintain steady mental images long enough to finish thinking through a writing task. Figures 5.8 and 5.9 show how difficult it is for dyslexic students to write phrases or sentences from dictation.

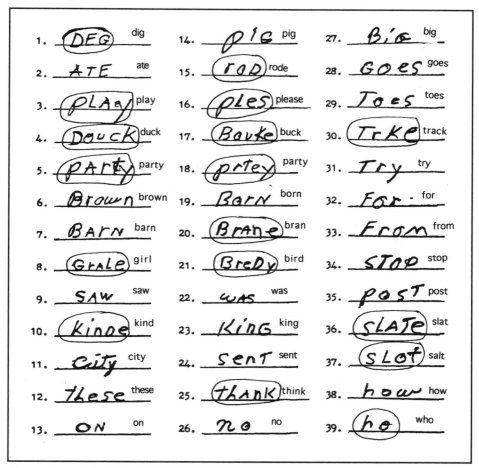

Figure 5.4. This 21-year-old man is moderately tone deaf in spelling. With enough time to whisper to himself, he often can figure out the sequence of speech sounds within words. This dictated spelling activity is from the Jordan Auditory Dyslexia Test (see Appendix D).

Transposed Consonants and Vowels

In trying to spell, Julia habitually turns consonant/vowel patterns backwards. *Barn* becomes *bran, play* becomes *paly, girl* becomes *gril.* Students with auditory dyslexia seldom recognize these transpositions because of their underlying difficulty connecting sounds to letters in the right sequence.

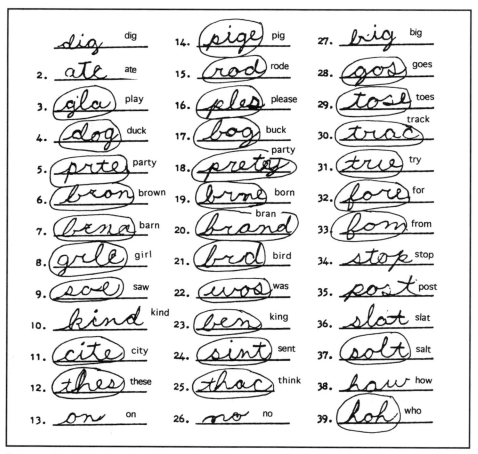

Figure 5.5. This 13-year-old girl is severely tone deaf to hard/fast, soft/slow speech chunks in sequence. It is almost impossible for her to build long-term memory for how to spell familiar words she speaks and hears every day. This dictated spelling activity is from the Jordan Auditory Dyslexia Test (see Appendix D).

Phonetic Spelling

It is almost impossible for Julia to apply phonics rules to spelling. As she tries to write what she hears, her brain creates literal translations that do not follow memorized phonics rules. Julia writes words the way they sound to her. Teachers can analyze this tendency if the student's writing is read phonetically. In her effort to write familiar words, Julia may write *reefews* for *refuse* or *gard* for *guard*. The old cliche that some children can't

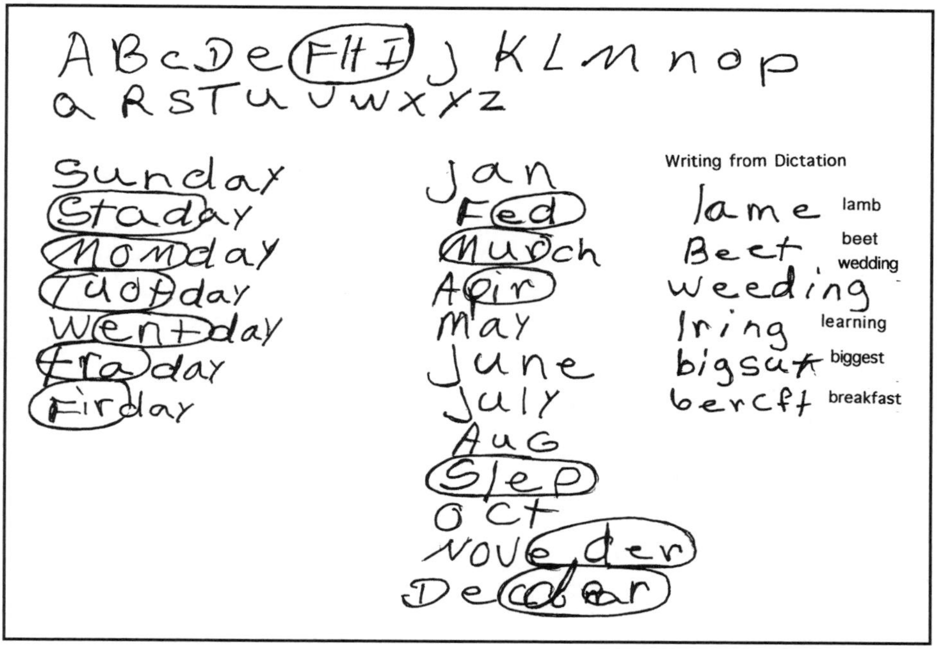

Figure 5.6. Severe auditory dyslexia rapidly emerges in this 10-year-old boy's effort to write familiar words from memory or from dictation. He quickly is overwhelmed by classroom tasks that require him to write from memory, copy, or write from dictation.

spell *cat* sometimes is true. Persons with severe dyslexia often write *kat* for *cat* and *cind* for *kind*.

Sound Chunks Omitted

One of the most significant spelling indicators of auditory dyslexia is the habit of leaving sound chunks out of longer words. This is called *telescoping*. The following examples illustrate this red flag signature of tone deafness:

Dictated by Teacher	Julia's Written Response
remember	rember
November	noveder
suddenly	sundly
candidacy	candasy
indefinitely	indefly

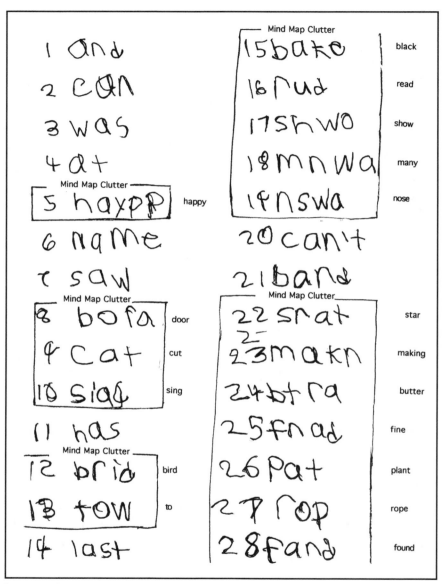

Figure 5.7. This 9-year-old girl cannot maintain clearly focused mind maps as she does classwork. At times her mental images are clear and correct. Then without warning her mind maps "clutter," causing her to become confused and inaccurate. Being tone deaf and having frequent cycles of loose mind maps overwhelms this student with frustration.

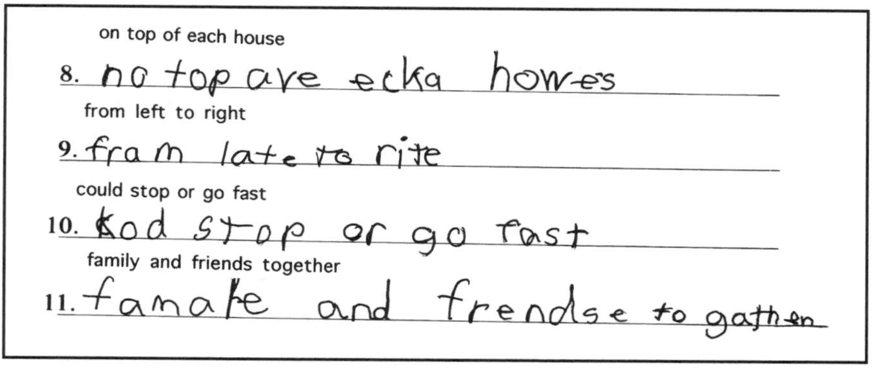

on top of each house

8. no top ave ecka howes

from left to right

9. fram late to rite

could stop or go fast

10. kod stop or go fast

family and friends together

11. famake and frendse to gathen

Figure 5.8. Writing from dictation is almost impossible for this 9-year-old girl who has severe auditory dyslexia. She cannot connect what she hears and says with what she should write. For her, written words are a different language that have little to do with the oral language of her culture. *Note:* From *Slingerland Screening Tests for Identifying Children with Specific Language Disability,* Form C, by B. H. Slingerland, 1984, Cambridge, MA: Educators Publishing Service. Copyright 1984 by Educators Publishing Service. Reprinted with permission.

on top of

13. On top azp

by the old house

14. bie the old howe

from our big yard

15. fram an bie yord

day and night

16. bay and mte

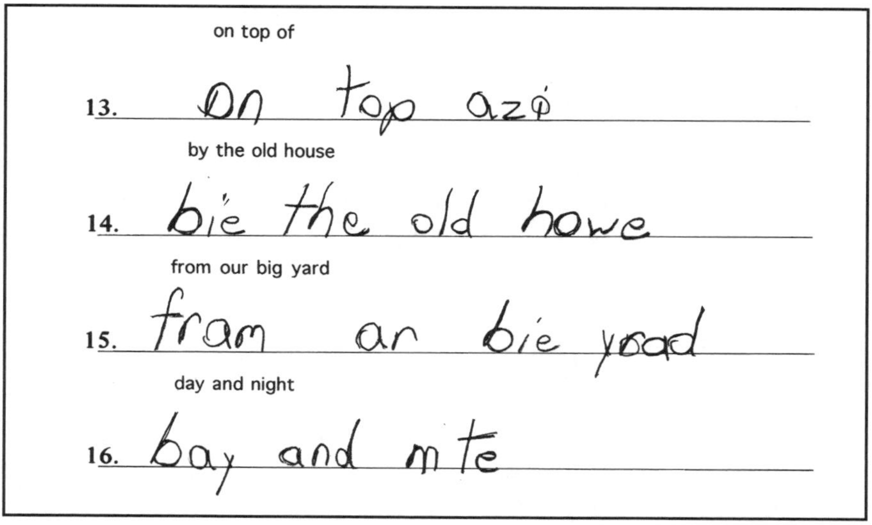

Figure 5.9. Signs of tone deafness emerge as soon as a child is expected to write from dictation. This intelligent boy in second grade is unusually gifted in oral language expression. He has no difficulty remembering details of what he hears. However, when he must write, the underlying auditory dyslexia patterns emerge rapidly. *Note:* From *Slingerland Screening Tests for Identifying Children with Specific Language Disability,* Form B, by B. H. Slingerland, 1984, Cambridge, MA: Educators Publishing Service. Copyright 1984 by Educators Publishing Service. Reprinted with permission.

Sound Chunks Added

A further red flag signature of auditory dyslexia is the tendency to add extra sound chunks when writing or copying. This is called *perseveration*. This tendency is illustrated below:

Dictated by Teacher	Julia's Written Response
party	parteny
duck	duckeny
successful	susisifully
immediate	imediantly
single	singulully
homesick	homsikully
address	addredresse
making	makenening

Writing Problems

Auditory dyslexia is a major handicap when Julia must write essay answers or produce original stories or paragraphs. Dyslexic spelling frequently is associated with dysgraphia, which is discussed in Chapter 6. It is not difficult to see the symptoms of auditory dyslexia in Julia's written work if her teachers study carefully what she writes. No one knows how many intelligent, creative students have been labeled as academic failures because instructors have not known how to identify dyslexic writing or how to recognize intelligent language usage hidden beneath poor penmanship.

For example, Figure 5.10 shows a creative writing assignment by a third-grade student. She was asked to write a story about something interesting she had done. Her illegible work was brushed aside by a school counselor as the work of a child with "borderline mental retardation" because she could not learn to read, write, or spell adequately. As part of a seminar on dyslexia, the girl's special education teacher translated this dyslexic writing and discovered good intelligence hidden beneath the surface of auditory dyslexia. Alongside the handwriting is a typed translation that reveals this 8-year-old child's dyslexic differences more clearly.

Figure 5.11 shows the dyslexic copying of a 9-year-old girl who developed school phobia within a highly structured class-

The Two sisters who went on a trip

Once upon a time there was two girls and their names were Kailey and Subren and they went to Disney World and they saw brown squirrels and they saw dinosaurs and then they got restless to go on the roller coaster and they threw up like any one would do but they had to run then they went to go eat at the eating place and they saw mickey

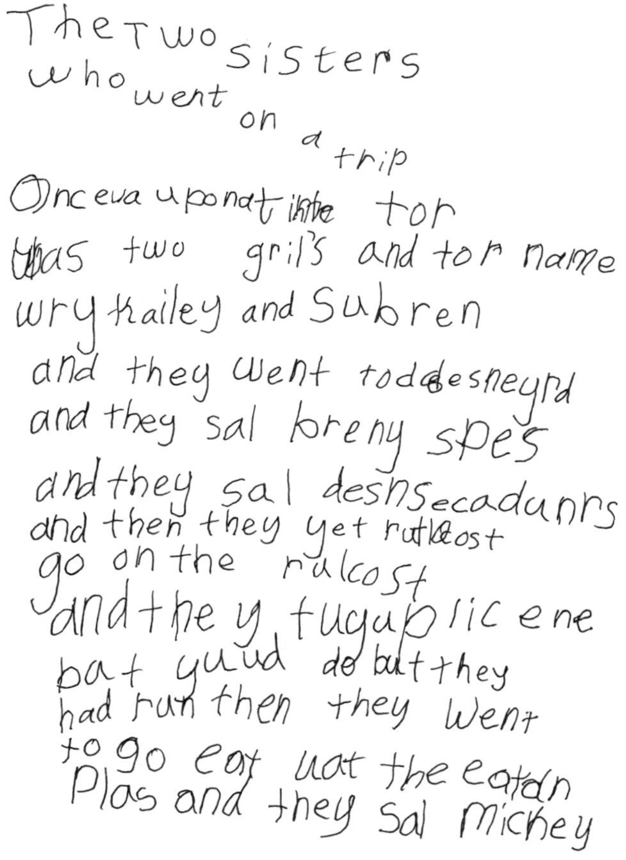

Once eva upon at inte top thas two gril's and top name wry kailey and Subren and they went toddesneyrd and they sal breny spes and they sal deshsecadunrs and then they yet rutleost go on the rulcost and they fuqublicene bat yuud do but they had run then they went to go eat uat the eatdn Plas and they sal mickey

Figure 5.10. This bright 8-year-old girl was placed in a special education class for "trainable" children because she could not learn to read, write, or spell. An intuitive teacher who had learned about dyslexia asked her to read this story to her class. The translation on the left reveals the girl's potential for language skill development.

room where students were required to copy from textbooks as part of their handwriting training. Daily criticism and constant failure overwhelmed this intelligent child who never could meet adult expectations. Copying language assignments, then filling in the blanks, was meaningless and overly threatening because of her lack of talent for reading, handwriting, and spelling.

No one knows how many intelligent, creative students have been written off as academic failures because instructors have not known how to identify dyslexia. Figure 5.12 shows the work of a 9-year-old girl who had been labeled "borderline mentally retarded" when she could not develop adequate skills for reading, spelling, and writing. After attending a seminar to learn about dyslexia, her special education teacher asked the girl to read her story aloud to the class. Beneath the layers of auditory dyslexia and dysgraphia (see Chapter 6) was hidden the good potential for language that is seen in the typed translation of her writing.

Figure 5.13 shows the work of a frustrated 20-year-old college student who was determined to become a special education

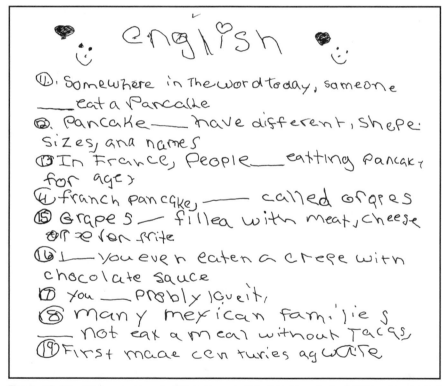

Figure 5.11. This creative dyslexic 9-year-old girl attended a highly structured fourth-grade class where students were required to copy activities from textbooks as part of their handwriting training. Day after day she received criticism for "not trying harder to write neatly." She continually received failing grades for misspelling words as she copied. To cope with fear of failure, she frequently drifted off into daydreams that caused her to doodle fanciful images on her worksheets. Her teacher continually fussed at her for spoiling assignments by drawing "silly pictures."

I was born in califarna (California) S (I) in (am) ten year old my brothers are six and four my dog is three years old my parents are 34 and 33 years old I like my parents wery (very) much my dad is in watnam (Vietnam) he will come home in about 3 months we have a geny (Guinea) pig it is three years old and I got a turdle (turtle) it is aloud (about) a week old S (I) like my turdle he doesn't (doesn't) lite (bite) some times the geny pig lites (bites) but mot (not) very much. my dog doesn't bite ever unless it's a rolber (robber). one tine (time) vhen (when) I was in south american a ruller (robber) tried to get in the door my dog barked and scared the rillers (robbers) away and Im (I'm) glad to be in the united states, my brothers names are robert and Mike may (my) dogs (dog's) name is Oueen (Queen) mygene pig is sweat peat (Sweet Pete) and I don't know (know) what to call the turdle

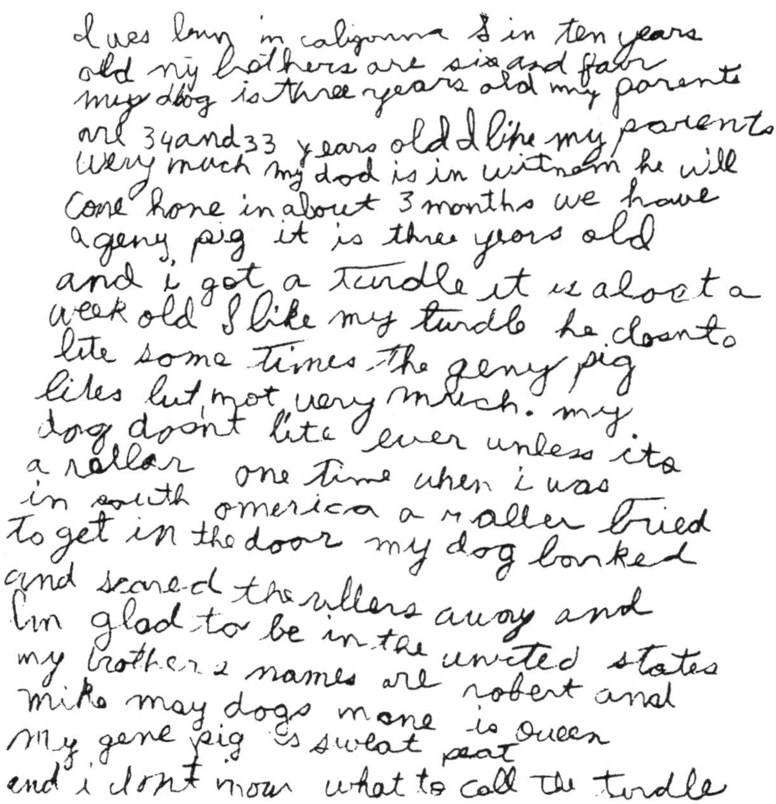

Figure 5.12. The 9-year-old girl who wrote this was labeled "borderline mentally retarded" when adults could not read her penmanship. This translation shows her intelligence that was hidden beneath layers of dyslexic spelling and dysgraphia (poor handwriting).

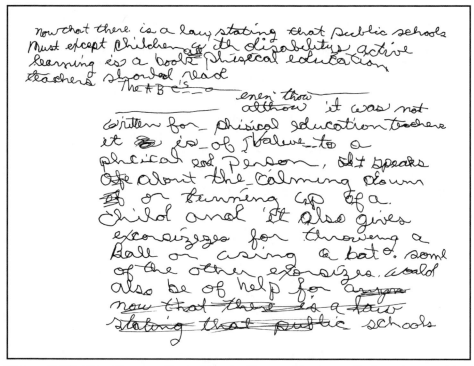

Figure 5.13. This 20-year-old student finally earned a special education teaching certificate and became a talented teacher of youngsters with learning disabilities. Learning to do keyboard writing unlocked her ability to express her ideas without being penalized for poor handwriting and dyslexic spelling.

teacher. A discerning professor spotted dyslexic patterns within this student's tangled penmanship. After a few weeks of training in keyboard writing skills, she began to produce intelligent, well-constructed essays that led to her certification as a special education teacher. Later she became a talented instructor for struggling learners.

Confusion with Rhyming

An easily detected characteristic of auditory dyslexia is difficulty with rhyme. As a standard practice in literacy instruction, teachers often dwell on rhyming words to reinforce pupil awareness of sounds in words. Students handicapped by auditory dyslexia have great difficulty hearing likenesses and differences in words.

Awkwardness in hearing or saying rhymes is a major symptom of tone deafness, or auditory dyslexia.

Educators probably make too great an issue of faulty rhyming ability. Aside from providing a covenient way to practice for phonics skills, rhyming ability actually is of little practical importance in overall reading skill. Rhyming practice helps some individuals build long-term memory for spelling. It is unfortunate that persons without talent for rhyming often are penalized when they cannot hear rhyming patterns or recognize them in print. If it is important for dyslexic students to do rhyming activities, teachers can present simple strategies that do not overwhelm tone-deaf individuals with complex rhyming situations.

For example, Julia's teacher asks her to name all the words she can think of that rhyme with *car*. A person who is not dyslexic immediately thinks of a string of words that rhyme with *car: jar, far, star, bar*. Because she is dyslexic, Julia must have enough time to ponder each word before saying it. Her lack of talent for rhyming is a challenge. When she hears *car*, her brain produces a string of nonsense words that rhyme but are not given credit in this task: *dar, sar, nar, har, zar*. It is easy for Julia to name words that start with the same hard/fast consonant sound /k/ in *car: care, core, cute, can*. However, her left brain struggles to process the soft/slow vowel patterns that follow /k/ at the beginning of *car*. When teachers discover this tone-deaf pattern in rhyming, they can be reasonably sure that auditory dyslexia exists.

Speaker Must Repeat

Instructors often are irritated by Julia's habit of asking to hear something again. Tone-deaf students are very insecure in all situations that require them to comprehend what they hear the first time it is spoken. Individuals with auditory dyslexia cannot cope with a flow of oral instructions or group discussion. In any listening situation, Julia comprehends only bits and pieces instead of the complete flow of speech. Because of their extremely slow rate in changing speech into mind maps, dyslexic listeners lose the sequence of what they hear. This constant uncertainty in listening gives them no choice but to ask the speaker to say it again.

This lifelong habit produces friction in classroom situations. As students like Julia fall behind the group, they tend to become disruptive through restlessness, repeated requests to hear it again, and continually saying "Huh?" or "What?" or "What do you mean?" Less mature students with auditory dyslexia begin to make noise by fiddling with things, shifting around in their seats, and creating foot noises on the floor. It is not unusual for classmates to complain about Julia's behavior. Many tone-deaf students are shunned by classmates who think that these poor listeners are "weird." What begins as a dyslexic difference often leads to social problems and public embarrassment. In reality, little of this disruptive behavior is deliberate.

Vocalizing During Silent Study Time

Many adults remember classroom teachers who snapped their fingers and said "Shhhh!" when students were not silent during study time. A common standard for learning is that students should be quiet. Silent learning is a major challenge for dyslexic students who must vocalize if they are to succeed in matching written words with speech or with mind maps. Because of the underlying problem in connecting sounds to letters, dyslexic readers must use several brain pathways to verify their impressions. This need to reinforce seeing with saying while touching words with a finger should not upset teachers. It is not difficult to let students like Julia use unorthodox ways if the instructor is aware of why these individuals learn differently. Those who are dyslexic have no choice but to respond to reading, spelling, and writing in a variety of ways to check their impressions for accuracy. This need to reinforce seeing with voice and touch is a universal need for those who are dyslexic. They cannot cope with the challenges of literacy if they are not free to combine as many body senses as possible to produce clear, complete mental images.

Struggle To Blend Word Chunks into Whole Words

The heart of the reading handicap for dyslexic students is faulty blending of sound chunks into recognizable words and phrases. For Julia, reading and spelling are filled with dread and the certain feeling that she will fail. The process of "sounding out" words is an emotional experience that threatens to overwhelm dyslexic individuals with feelings of shame. When phonics skills are taught in traditional ways, students must divide words into chunks to discover the speech segments that make up each word, then blend those segments together to create whole words. This two-way word analysis process often is impossible for those who have auditory dyslexia. When Julia is pressed to sound out words, she has difficulty with blending. For example, a familiar word like *bug* can become a major hurdle. With great effort Julia breaks *bug* apart: "buh-uh-guh." As this struggle illustrates, she never has learned how to sound the soft consonants *b* and *g*. Her tone-deaf brain cannot give the quick sound /b/ or /g/ to these letters. Auditory dyslexia triggers a type of perseveration that causes the voice to draw out sounds longer than necessary. Thus /b/ becomes *buh* while /g/ becomes *guh*. Being dyslexic makes it risky and embarrassing for Julia to practice the phonics skill of word sounding.

Traditional instruction in phonics, which emphasizes blending, usually is beyond the comprehension of individuals with auditory dyslexia. Sometimes it is possible for tone-deaf persons to memorize simple techniques for blending and word sounding. Sometimes students like Julia can saturate their left-brain language centers with enough stimulus to gain basic skills in word sounding. However, individuals with auditory dyslexia face lifelong limitations in how accurately they can blend or do word sounding. When these literacy skills take shape, dyslexic persons always must work very slowly while touching each word.

Garbled Pronunciation

Closely linked to difficulty with blending is a socially embarrassing problem of garbled pronunciation. Tone-deaf individuals become the objects of laughter and teasing because of scrambled speech called *tongue twisting* or *echolalia*. Parents and teachers can identify this dyslexic pattern by listening as students repeat words and phrases.

Normal Pronunciation	Julia's Dyslexic Response
aluminum animals	alunimum aminals
olives in vinegar	ollies in vigenar
baskets of spaghetti	baksets of pasghetti

Reading aloud is painfully embarrassing for Julia who cannot control her tongue twists as she pronounces words. Chapter 7 describes the often strong emotions and feelings that overwhelm dyslexic individuals when their differences are exposed to others who laugh or make fun. Adults must be cautious about asking those who read poorly to do so aloud. Countless dyslexic adults refuse to attend events where they might be called on to read aloud. These tongue-twisting patterns can be the most painful part of dyslexia for sensitive individuals who have been teased all their lives for speaking awkwardly.

Confusion with Dictionary Symbols

Auditory dyslexia makes traditional dictionary usage quite difficult. It is unrealistic to expect tone-deaf students to interpret phonetic respellings, accent markings, and pronunciation guides. Highly motivated individuals with dyslexia often manage to cope with the various codes found in reference materials. However, most students who are dyslexic cannot comprehend the variety of symbol systems found in current dictionaries and reference materials. With enough careful training in word analysis skills, persons with moderate auditory dyslexia can benefit from studies in word origins, multiple meanings, and syllable division. Arriving at correct word pronunciation from dictionary keys frequently is impossible and should not be expected when auditory dyslexia has been identified.

Checklist Signature of Auditory Dyslexia

Auditory dyslexia is easily observed by using the following checklist to pinpoint what the student does and says over a period of time. Appendix D presents a comprehensive assessment technique in the Jordan Auditory Dyslexia Test.

_____ Cannot hear vowel or soft consonant sounds in words.

_____ Cannot distinguish between similar speech sounds.

_____ Continually misunderstands what others say.

_____ Mishears familiar words, thinking of something different from what the speaker said.

_____ Cannot understand rules of phonics.

_____ Cannot spell correctly, no matter how much he or she practices.

_____ Cannot sound out words correctly in reading.

_____ Speech includes frequent "tongue twister" errors in saying words.

_____ Cannot hear or repeat rhymes.

_____ Must hear again several times before being sure of what others say.

_____ Continually says "Huh?" or "What?" or "What do you mean?"

_____ Continually asks to hear it again.

_____ Misunderstands conversations, telephone messages, what is heard on radio or television.

_____ Cannot remember oral instructions without being reminded.

_____ Argues that "You didn't tell me that" or "I didn't hear you say that."

_____ Is confused quickly while listening against background noise.

_____ Spells words as they sound, not according to rules of spelling.

Learning Activities for Persons with Auditory Dyslexia

If students like Julia are to be successful in the classroom, they must be surrounded by visible structure that lets them see clues to remind them of what is expected. Emphasis must be on seeing information, not hearing it. Oral information must be supported by visual clues that enable mind maps to merge into memory.

Teach Multisensory Letter–Sound Connections

At the beginning of this chapter, Figure 5.1 explained why over-coming auditory dyslexia requires a multisensory approach that brings all of the senses together in the learning process. Neuron deficits within the midbrain and left brain make it impossible for the person to hear soft/slow speech sounds accurately or to assemble speech sounds in correct sequence. If several sensory pathways are stimulated at the same time, dyslexic individuals can develop accurate mind maps of what reading, spelling, writing, and arithmetic are all about. The four most important sensory learning channels are *sight, sound, speech,* and *touch.* As Chapter 7 explains, positive emotions and feelings also must be involved through praise and encouragement.

Chapter 4 described the Lindamood–Bell ADD method, which is highly effective for teaching students with visual dys-lexia to read. This and other multisensory learning methods are active and stimulating with rapid verbal exchanges between in-structor and pupils. Unless the instructor slows the pace and simplifies the verbal flow, students with auditory dyslexia often are overwhelmed by too much oral information at one time. Stu-dents like Julia quickly feel lost within vigorous listening/speak-ing activities. To be effective with tone-deaf students, multisen-sory learning methods must be like playing tennis. Each player needs immediate, well-focused feedback from a partner. If the learning situation resembles a busy doubles match with several players in motion at the same time, individuals with auditory dyslexia quickly become too confused to make sense of the learn-ing process. If no specialized program is available to provide well-structured oral and visual feedback, students like Julia can learn to simulate a feedback process by talking to themselves, listening to themselves say it, touching with fingers to focus full attention on each word, and making body motions to tie together loose ends in their mental images. An effective multisensory mode of language processing is a slow way to learn, and it can-not be hurried or silenced.

Identify Sound Chunks in Spoken Words

Not all multisensory phonics programs are successful with tone-deaf learners whose brain structure does not hear soft/slow speech sounds. When reference is made to phonics, most adults think only of consonants and vowels. However, these building blocks of reading and spelling are not the beginning points for teaching those who have auditory dyslexia. Because of the neural deficits shown in Figure 5.1, it is virtually impossible for students like Julia to identify the hard/soft/hard/soft sound sequences that make up oral language. This is why instructors should not start with traditional phonics instruction that asks the learner to hear soft consonants and vowels. Tone-deaf individuals do not know that these phonemes exist because their auditory pathways cannot hear subtle speech differences. Instead of pressing Julia to hear and repeat soft consonants and vowels, instructors must begin by teaching her how to see syllable chunks within words. If sight, sound, speech, and touch can be brought together in this experience, it is possible for Julia to bypass her tone deafness well enough to develop most of the basic phonics skills for reading.

Many activities for teaching phonics skills are available wherever reading and spelling materials are sold. The common theme in most of these programs is the same: "Listen to the vowel inside this word. . . . What sound do you hear the vowel make?" Because Julia does not hear vowel sounds, a different approach must be used. First, she must be taught to see softer sound chunks instead of trying to hear them. A system of *visual phonics* must be presented. Second, Julia must learn how to link together several sensory pathways. To learn much about phonics, she must see it, say it, and feel it in an emotionally safe way that does not trigger dread or fear of failure. With enough multisensory practice, she may begin to "hear" some of the softer chunks in spoken language.

Visual Phonics

Individuals with dyslexia seldom have trouble learning which letters are vowels and which are consonants. Chapter 2 explained the importance of mastering alphabet sequence before students like Brian and Julia move on to more advanced word analysis. In learning the alphabet sequence, dyslexic learners usually remember that *Aa, Ee, Ii, Oo,* and *Uu* are called vowels. As they practice with alphabet sequence, Brian and Julia may learn that *Ww* and *Yy* also can be vowels. It is simple for Julia and Brian to learn that all the other letters are consonants. This knowledge of how alphabet letters are classified lays the foundation for learning to see sound chunks when a tone-deaf student cannot hear them.

Many programs that teach reading and spelling present a method of marking vowels to show their sounds. The following procedures for teaching visual phonics to tone-deaf learners can be modified in creative ways. The important fact is that this type of structure teaches students like Julia first to see vowel patterns, then to connect sounds to what they see.

1. *Seeing vowels inside words.* The instructor begins by showing the student how to locate vowels inside words by seeing vowel letters, then marking them with a pencil. The words are arranged so that the vowel letters follow alphabetical sequence. The teacher says, "Julia, let's look for vowels inside some words you've seen in reading."

▶ **cat   bed   did   stop   up**

"Look for the vowel in each word. Underline each vowel you see. Now tell me the name of each vowel you underlined." Julia's task is to say the vowel *names (aye, eee, eye, oh, you)*. At this point, no other sound should be associated with these vowel letters. The teacher then says, "Now, Julia, I'm going to show you some words that have two vowels."

▶ **date   meet   ride   rope   cute**
　　1 2

"Let's count the vowels in each word. What is the first vowel in *date*? Put a small 1 under it. What is the second vowel in *date*? Put a small 2 under it. What is the name of the number 1 vowel? What is the name of the number 2 vowel? Now let's do the rest of the words this same way."

2. *Sounding vowels inside words.* When Julia is fluent in seeing and naming each vowel letter, she is ready to take her first step in sounding the vowels she sees in short words. Her first experience with phonics will be the *short name* of single vowels that come in short words. The teacher says, "Julia, I'm going to show you some short words that have just one vowel. Let's learn a rule: *When I see one vowel by itself in a short word, the vowel*

usually says its short name. Now I will help you learn to say this rule." The instructor guides Julia in saying this rule until she can repeat it rather well by herself. Then the instructor says, "Let's look at some words where the vowel says its short name."

▶ **băg   let   it   mop   up**

"Now, Julia. Let's find the vowel in the first word. This time I'll show you a new way to mark this vowel." Above the *a* the instructor draws the half-moon mark (˘, called *breve*), which stands for the sound of short *a*. "Julia, when one vowel comes in a short word, the vowel usually says its short name. This mark reminds you to make the vowel say its short name." This rule is practiced again and again until Julia is confident in marking the vowel letter in a short word to *see* that it says its short name.

When the instructor feels confident that Julia knows how to apply this short vowel rule, it is time to take the next step. The teacher says, "Julia, let's learn a new rule: *When I see two vowels in a short word, the first vowel usually says its long name. The second vowel doesn't say anything.* Now I'll help you learn this rule." The instructor guides Julia in saying this rule several times until she can repeat it rather well by herself. Then the instructor says, "Let's look at some words and make the first vowel say its long name."

▶ **dātȩ   eat   hide   bone   rude**
   1 2

"Now, Julia, let's practice our new rule. How many vowels do you see in the first word? Put a small number under each vowel you see. Let's say our new rule: *When I see two vowels in a short word, the first vowel usually says its long name. The second vowel doesn't say anything.* Now I'll show you a special mark that tells the vowel to say its long name." The instructor makes the long mark (¯, called *macron*) above the *a*. "Now we see what sound the *a* makes. Let me show you the mark that tells the second vowel not to say anything." The teacher makes a slash mark (/) through the second vowel.

As simple as these beginning rules appear, they open the door for independent reading for Julia. Several dozen familiar short vowel and long vowel words follow these two rules in beginning reading practice. Julia and her instructor can write their own practice reading activities by choosing words that follow these beginning vowel-sounding rules. Again, the instructor and any adults assisting Julia must remember why she cannot benefit from traditional methods for teaching phonics: She cannot hear the soft chunks when she is asked to listen for them. She must start with a method that teaches her to see vowel chunks. Then she can work out vowel sounds by using the multisensory strategy demonstrated here.

3. *Finding word chunks.* Students with dyslexia often are confused by the task of locating syllables. Instructors must remember that syllable division in the dictionary does not always match the oral syllables of speech. Dividing words into dictionary syllables requires a rather high-level talent for word processing. Students with limited talent for reading and spelling do not benefit from traditional practice of dividing words into dictionary syllables. What they see in print often is different from what they say in word usage.

Both Brian and Julia need a different method for locating the breaks between sound chunks as they move to higher levels in sounding out words. After they have mastered the simple phonics rules for seeing short vowels and long vowels in short words, they are ready to move up to finding chunks in longer words. Again, the most effective strategy is one that engages sight, speech, and touch at a slow enough pace to allow the student to keep all of the mind maps organized.

Brian and Julia need to learn an old-fashioned word chunking technique called *chin bumping,* which was taught when children attended only a few years of formal schooling. Chin bumping is a multisensory way to feel, hear, and say the chunks of speech that appear in familiar spoken words. In reading, Julia and Brian must learn how to translate what they see on the page into inner speech that fills the brain as mind maps are interpreted. They must learn learn how to turn printed words into a mental voice that tells them what their eyes are seeing. In chin bumping, the learner holds two or three fingers below the chin to feel what happens as the mouth says longer words. The chin will bob (bump) downward slightly every time the mouth reaches the end of a chunk. When the chin dips downward, the reader marks that place as a dividing point in the printed word. This process does not always match syllable divisions in the dictionary, but beginning readers are not concerned with what the dictionary says is correct word division. Beginning readers need only know how to break words into chunks to reinforce the word-sounding process.

The instructor shows Julia and Brian some familiar longer words: *saddle, yellow, little, Monday, summer.* Together they practice chin bumping these words:

▶ **sad/dle   yel/low   lit/tle   Mon/day   sum/mer**

Now would be a good time for the instructor to show Brian and Julia another piece to the puzzle of word sounding. Each of these longer words starts with a "short word" that contains one vowel. What sound does this vowel say? What mark do we make to show the sound for one vowel in a short word? A complete visual phonics system designed for dyslexic students is provided in the *Jordan Dyslexia Assessment/Reading Program* (Jordan, 2000a).

Use a Keyboard and a Tape Recorder

Chapter 4 summarized the pioneering research by Joyce Steeves (1987) that documented the benefit of keyboard writing for dyslexic students (see pages 127–129). Using a keyboard for spelling and writing is a simple technique for students like Brian and Julia. In fact, the ideal situation would be for each dyslexic learner to have his or her personal portable computer to use in the classroom each day, then carry home to do finish assignments or do special projects.

It is simple to establish keyboard/tape recorder strategies to give important multisensory practice in spelling and sentence writing. Practice words can be taken from the student's personal vocabulary. The teacher or study partner prints practice words on cards. Then Brian and Julia practice this seeing/hearing/saying/touching routine at home or during private time at school.

Step 1.   Read a word aloud into the tape recorder.
Step 2.   Spell that word aloud into the tape recorder.
Step 3.   Type that word immediately from memory.
Step 4.   Read into the recorder the spelling that appeared on the screen.

Then they select the next card and repeat this four-step process. After spelling five words, they rewind the tape to the starting position and review what they spoke into the recorder and typed on the keyboard. They continue this routine, five words in each work segment, until all the words on the cards have been done.

This multisensory procedure produces immediate results. As Brian and Julia feel their fingers tap the keys, they become aware of the sequence of letters within the practice words. Any letter reversals, transpositions, or rotations become apparent. Anyone nearby may overhear Brian or Julia mutter as they work out correct letter sequence: "Where's the *b*? Uh, oh! I got it backwards again. Now where's *o*? a-b-o-v-e. Above! OK. I got it right. Now where's *t*?" This stream of chatter is a vocal mirror of the thought patterns a student with dyslexia experiences with every school assignment. Listening to Brian or Julia work through keyboard/tape recorder exercises reveals much about their dyslexic confusion with sounds and symbols.

Can the Brain Structure of Auditory Dyslexia Be Changed?

Chapter 1 described how the 20th century ended with a surge of research into how the brain develops, how the brain learns, and the role that stimulus plays in pruning neurons into specialized clusters that carry out lifelong tasks. As research progressed into the nature of dyslexia, neuroscientists began to ask: Is it possible to stimulate neurons within the left brain so that dyslexia decreases or disappears? During the 1970s Paula Tallal at Rutgers University began to study brain functions in children with delayed speech development and severe speech problems. Her research focused on how well those children heard individual speech sounds as they progressed from infancy through early childhood (Tallal & Piercy, 1974). Tallal and her colleagues developed specialized computer technology that simulated speech through a voice synthesizer. This technology enabled them to control the precise timing of consonant–vowel combinations that her subjects heard every day. Tallal's research revealed that children who fail to develop normal speech cannot hear rapid variations of speech patterns. These children cannot hear subtle differences between soft consonants (/b/–/d/, /p/–/b/, /m/–/n/) at the normal speech rate of 40 milliseconds per phoneme utterance. The children in those research efforts were tone deaf to many of the building blocks of speech when oral language flowed too quickly (Tallal & Stark, 1981). During the 1980s, Tallal and her colleagues invented what was called "stretched speech" that slowed oral language flow to 20 milliseconds. At that half-speed rate, each sound chunk was clearly heard by tone-deaf children (Tallal, Stark, & Mellitis, 1985).

This information led the Tallal team to investigate neural structures within the left-brain auditory cortex and medial geniculate nucleus (see Figure 5.1). During the Decade of the Brain, Tallal and her colleagues discovered that tone-deaf individuals have deficits in neural wiring within the medial geniculate nucleus and the auditory pathway that carries speech information to the auditory cortex (Tallal et al., 1993).

During the late 1980s a fascinating insight into the auditory benefits of neuron stimulus was reported by Michael Merzenich at the University of California in San Francisco. In researching the plasticity of the brains of monkeys, Merzenich discovered a type of "learning disability" in some adult monkeys who could not process streams of rapid sounds presented at 40-millisecond intervals, which is similar to human speech. Those monkeys displayed the "tone-deaf" symptoms of auditory dyslexia. Brain studies of those monkeys revealed "neural wiring" deficits within the auditory cortex and medial geniculate nucleus (see Figure 5.1). On a hunch, Merzenich developed a brain stimulus technique that slowed sound patterns to half the normal speed. To his surprise, the tone-deaf monkeys clearly heard this altered presentation of hard/fast, soft/slow patterns. Over a period of several weeks, Merzenich had the tone-deaf monkeys practice listening and responding to the half-speed sound patterns. Then he examined neuron formations within the auditory cortex and medial geniculate nucleus. He discovered that the original flaws in neural wiring had changed. The stimulus of listening to altered sound had "rewired" enough of the neurons to produce almost normal auditory perception in the monkeys (Merzenich, cited in Travis, 1996).

Because of the similarities of their research, Merzenich teamed with Tallal and her colleagues to develop a "stretched speech" auditory training program called *Fast ForWord*. This computerized training game slows down consonant-related speech sounds to half normal speed. Tone-deaf individuals listen to stories that to the normal ear sound as if they had been recorded underwater or behind a waterfall. However, these altered speech events are heard clearly by listeners who have auditory dyslexia. Under the supervision of the Scientific Learning Corporation in Berkeley, California, field trials of *Fast ForWord* were conducted at 35 sites throughout the United States and Canada. Following the prescribed number of training sessions with *Fast ForWord,* more than half of the struggling readers in the field trials gained 1 to 2 years in auditory processing speed, speech discrimination, awareness of speech sounds (phonemes), improved spelling, and overall growth in receptive and expressive language skills (Merzenich, Jenkins, Miller, Schreiner, & Tallal, 1996).

Does Fast ForWord Training Change Brain Structure?

Chapter 1 discussed the critical role that sensory stimulus plays in pruning dendrites to help neurons become specialized for doing specific tasks. The intriguing benefits of *Fast ForWord* auditory training suggest that it is possible to improve neural wiring, perhaps even to create new neuron pathways by stimulating regions of the brain. One of the richest benefits of brain training programs like *Fast ForWord* is the hope that this kind of treatment of auditory dyslexia will become available to all who struggle to hear and comprehend oral language. As more is discovered about how brain regions function in classroom learning, it will become possible to design individualized remedial techniques to fit the needs of each person who is dyslexic.

Overcoming Dysgraphia and Dyscalculia

The first discussion of chronic poor handwriting appeared in 1869 when the English neurologist Henry Charlton Bastian published his studies of written language deficits in adults who had suffered aphasia. As he worked with victims of aphasia, Bastian became intrigued by handwriting difficulties many of his aphasic patients developed after suffering brain injury from accident, stroke, or seizure. Figure 6.1 shows the left-brain language regions where aphasia occurs. If brain injury happens within Broca's area, a speech loss called *Broca's aphasia* emerges. The person understands the meaning of words (receptive language), but he or she has great difficulty saying words. Speech becomes forced and slow, requiring enormous effort. An individual with Broca's aphasia might respond as follows:

QUESTION: Did Mrs. Jordan visit you today?

ANSWER: Yu - yu - yu - s. Sh - sh - sh - d-d-d-damn c-c-c-ame af - af - t lun - lun - lun - sh.

Persons with Broca's aphasia know what they want to say, and patient listeners can follow the meaning of this labored speech. These victims of aphasia become intensely frustrated when they cannot speak their thoughts clearly. A common habit in this type of aphasia is to insert expletives that come from an overly frustrated intelligent brain that cannot communicate adequately. Relatives of these individuals often are startled or embarrassed to

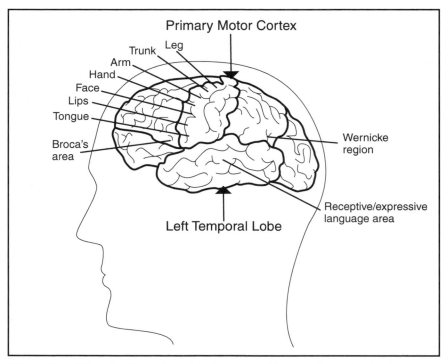

Figure 6.1. When brain regions develop normally, neurological talents emerge in an orderly developmental sequence. Within the primary motor cortex, muscle control emerges in the sequence shown above, beginning with tongue movement during early infancy and ending with coordination of leg movements during early childhood. At the same time, specialized regions of the left frontal lobe (Broca's area) and left temporal lobe (Wernicke region) learn to process receptive and expressive oral language. When neural wiring fails to develop within the hand/arm control regions of the motor cortex, a handwriting disability called dysgraphia makes it impossible for the individual to become competent with penmanship.

hear pious older persons use "cuss words," something they never did before the brain injury.

If damage occurs to neural wiring within the Wernicke region, a different type of aphasia emerges. Persons with Wernicke's aphasia often speak fluently, but their words have no meaning. Sentences are uttered in garbled strings of correctly pronounced words that make no sense. Neurologists often call this meaningless speech "word salad." Someone with Wernicke's aphasia might speak as follows:

QUESTION: Did Mrs. Jordan visit you today?

ANSWER: Where? Oh, dog blue my bags datatata hurt or plunk plink gooobies here.

As Bastian (1869) worked with aphasic patients, he became intrigued by extremely poor handwriting that often accompanied Broca's aphasia. He referred to this illegible penmanship as *dysgraphia*. Others refer to writing disability as *agraphia*. Bastian speculated that some kind of brain damage causes handwriting to be as illegible as speech becomes with aphasia. It was not until the 1980s that the cause for dysgraphia was discovered. As brain imaging science emerged, it became possible to pinpoint the specific regions of the brain that govern handwriting. Approximately 97% of all persons are right-handed. This means that the left motor cortex signals the right arm, hand, and fingers to make handwriting movements. Handwriting in the 3% of individuals who are left-handed is governed by the motor cortex in the right brain.

Illegible handwriting can result from brain injury to the motor cortex. However, dysgraphia that is linked to dyslexia is not the result of brain damage. Dysgraphia usually is part of the genetic predisposition for dyslexia. It is passed down genetic lines along with visual dyslexia and auditory dyslexia.

Regardless of which brain hemisphere controls hand preference, a specific region of the primary motor cortex learns, or fails to learn, how to do legible handwriting. Figure 6.1 shows the regions of the primary motor cortex that control major body functions. When infants and toddlers reach developmental milestones on normal schedule, neural pathways become "hardwired" to perform lifelong tasks. Figure 6.1 shows the developmental sequence that starts with tongue control as sucking reflex and ends with leg control for elaborate motor activities, such as hopping, skipping, running, climbing, leaping, and racing. In most individuals, neural maturity within the motor cortex prepares the fingers, hands, and arms for the fine motor coordination required for handwriting. When dysgraphia exists, this developmental milestone within the motor cortex fails to emerge.

Chapters 2 and 4 present the concept that reading, spelling, and writing are unnatural inventions that not all human brains are capable of learning. When dysgraphia exists, individuals cannot master the fine motor coordination skills required for fluent penmanship. Chapter 4 describes the challenge of learning to read and write 104 alphabet symbols that must be mastered if individuals are to become fully literate (see page 84). Visual dyslexia occurs when regions of the left brain do not have the neurological talent to learn which direction alphabet symbols must face and the sequence in which they must appear. All their lives, persons with visual dyslexia stumble over the task of decoding written symbols that represent oral language. Auditory dyslexia occurs when neuron pathways within the midbrain and left brain fail to develop fully. Dysgraphia occurs when neuron clusters within the primary motor cortex do not develop the ability to encode oral language into written words. Handwriting and reading are opposite brain functions. To write, the brain must translate spoken language into written symbols. To read, the brain must translate written symbols into spoken words. Dyslexia and dysgraphia are brain-based neural differences that prevent each of these language talents from developing adequately.

In most instances, dysgraphia is a subtype of dyslexia (Jordan, 1972, 1989a, 1989b, 1996a, 1996b, 2000a, 2000b). Often dysgraphia is one of several layers of learning difficulty. Most individuals who have visual dyslexia or auditory dyslexia also have dysgraphia. Many dyslexic persons who stumble over reading or spelling learn penmanship rather well. However, dysgraphic individuals may read well or spell adequately, but they cannot write legibly by hand.

Dysgraphia rises from faulty control of muscle systems required to write letters and words accurately. Learners with dysgraphia usually have a clear mental image of what the brain intends to encode, but the student keeps "forgetting" how to write specific symbols. Certain letters and numerals are made with backward or upside-down finger motions. Handwriting generally is so awkward and unsatisfactory that dysgraphic writers avoid situations that require them to engage in penmanship. When students with severe dysgraphia are taught to use alternate ways to write, such as keyboard writing at a computer or dictating to a scribe or a tape recorder, handwriting disability can be removed as an educational or workplace problem. If educators and job supervisors insist that all students must have manuscript or cursive penmanship skills, then dysgraphia continues to be a frustrating educational and workplace handicap.

Dysgraphia Syndrome

In classrooms and workplace situations where literacy is judged by the legibility of one's handwriting, individuals with dysgraphia are at a serious disadvantage. Not all persons who write poorly are dysgraphic. There are many reasons why an individual might not develop attractive penmanship skills. A main cause for poor handwriting is lack of structured practice with penmanship skills in elementary school classrooms where other curriculum interests crowd out writing practice. Chapter 1 describes the critical role that structured stimulus plays in "hardwiring" neuron pathways to become competent in such skills as handwriting. Having "sloppy" handwriting does not always mean that a person has dysgraphia. However, among those who are dyslexic are certain individuals whose neural wiring in the primary motor cortex failed to develop fully. These persons face lifelong inability to write legibly by hand.

Checklist Signature of Dysgraphia

Dysgraphic writing includes unique differences that set it apart from lack of training in handwriting skills. The following patterns identify dysgraphia:

_____ Manuscript and cursive styles mixed together.

_____ Capital and lowercase letters mixed together.

_____ Lack of spacing between words and lines of writing.

_____ Words and lines jammed together in meaningless lumps.

_____ Letters or numerals made backwards.

_____ Letters or numerals rolled halfway over (turned sideways).

_____ Letters or numerals made upside down.

_____ Letters or numerals constructed from small fragments of pencil strokes.

(continues)

> _____ Writing floats above the line, then cuts down
> through the line.
> _____ Writing wanders away from the left margin.
> _____ Writing skips lines and fails to follow numbered
> lines.
> _____ Size of writing changes from small to very large
> on the same worksheet.

Difficulty Learning Alphabet Forms

The primary characteristic of dysgraphia is difficulty remembering how to write certain letters and numerals. Instructors might not identify this flaw unless they watch the student write. Both manuscript and cursive writing styles must flow from left to right with each letter or numeral facing the correct direction. Dysgraphia involves the tendency to make backward strokes (right to left). Because letters are not connected in the manuscript writing style, instructors might not see an underlying tendency to make backward finger motions. Dysgraphia is more easily seen when cursive writing contains backward circular strokes or loops facing the opposite way. Chapter 4 explains the perceptual confusion dyslexic learners face when, by age 9, they must become fluent with 104 written alphabet symbols. Shifting from manuscript to cursive writing style is impossible for most students who have dysgraphia.

Figure 6.2 shows the struggle of a bright 10-year-old boy to write the alphabet and days of the week. He began formal handwriting training when he was 6 years old. Figure 6.3 shows the effect of severe dysgraphia in the effort of a 14-year-old boy to write the alphabet in cursive style. Figure 6.4 is the work of a 12-year-old girl who learned how to "draw" cursive-style letters as if each symbol is a separate picture. At first she can control letter size to fit between the lines on her writing paper. Midway through this task she no longer can manage to make small letters. Without warning, her fine motor coordination relaxes to the very large size that is comfortable for her fingers to write.

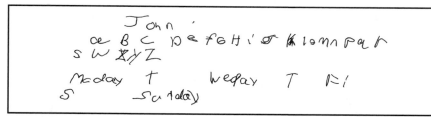

Figure 6.2. This 10-year-old boy struggled for 10 minutes to write the alphabet and days of the week. He has had 4 years of formal handwriting training. Severe dysgraphia makes it impossible for him to develop legible handwriting skills.

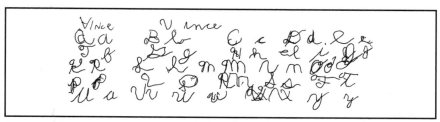

Figure 6.3. Severe dyslexia forces this 14-year-old boy to struggle slowly to write the alphabet. His primary motor cortex cannot develop adequate neural wiring to become skilled with penmanship.

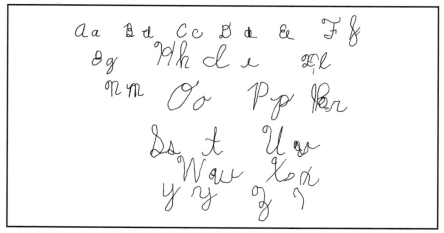

Figure 6.4. A major characteristic of dysgraphia is inability to continue to write small letters. Without warning the motor cortex reaches "burnout" and the student's writing becomes greatly enlarged. As this 12-year-old girl reached her fine motor burnout point, she stopped using small muscles and began to use large writing muscles.

Writing from Dictation

When dysgraphic students write from dictation, they are completely on their own to remember how handwriting should be done. The blank paper on which they write has no print to offer cues about letter forms. A major characteristic of dysgraphia emerges quickly in dictation writing as manuscript style mixes with cursive style. Dysgraphic handwriting does not flow smoothly left to right. Most words are pieced together from unconnected letters. Often individual letters are patched together from short fragments of pencil strokes. Close examination of dysgraphic writing shows the countless times when mental images of words fall apart in the writer's thinking.

Figure 6.5 shows the labored writing of a 12-year-old boy who feels great dread whenever he is required to write. Figure 6.6 illustrates the problem that most dysgraphic writers have in keeping words aligned in columns. This is related to irregular eye tracking and eye teaming, as described in Chapter 3. Figure 6.6 shows the poor eye tracking and eye teaming that frustrates a 9-year-old girl whenever she must write without being reminded to bump the left margin and to follow lines down the writing page.

Writing and Copying Sentences

Students who are dysgraphic have great difficulty writing legibly as they create sentences or copy from textbooks and workbooks. Their difficulty in judging size and space causes writing to wobble up and down, cutting through lines and drifting away from left margins. When several sentences are written in sequence, words become jammed together and space is lost between lines. Soon dysgraphic writing becomes a mass of jumbled shapes that are almost impossible to decipher. Figure 6.7 shows the creative writing of an 11-year-old boy who wrote a holiday note to his teacher. Figure 6.8 is a writing assignment of a 14-year-old boy who cannot maintain adequate spacing as he copies. Figure 6.9 shows the effort of an 8-year-old boy to write an original story. The overlapping layers of severe dysgraphia, auditory dyslexia, and visual dyslexia hide his intelligent thinking. Figure 6.10 is the work of a 17-year-old boy whose English teacher was the first adult to see the depth of talent and language potential this

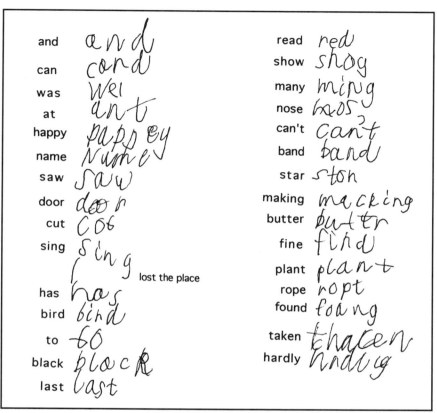

Figure 6.5. This 12-year-old boy struggles hard to write single words during a dictated spelling test. His writing consists of broken, disconnected fragments he cannot always piece together successfully. He constantly mixes manuscript style with cursive style. Each time he forgets what to write next, he is forced to start over. As he begins the next stroke, he inadvertently switches from one writing style to another.

student possessed. Previous teachers had failed to look beneath the surface of tangled penmanship to find the expressive language talent in this bright individual.

Difficulty Copying Simple Shapes

A major characteristic of dysgraphia is inability to copy simple shapes without distortion. Chapter 4 presented the concept of conservation of form (see pages 104–105). To build permanent memory

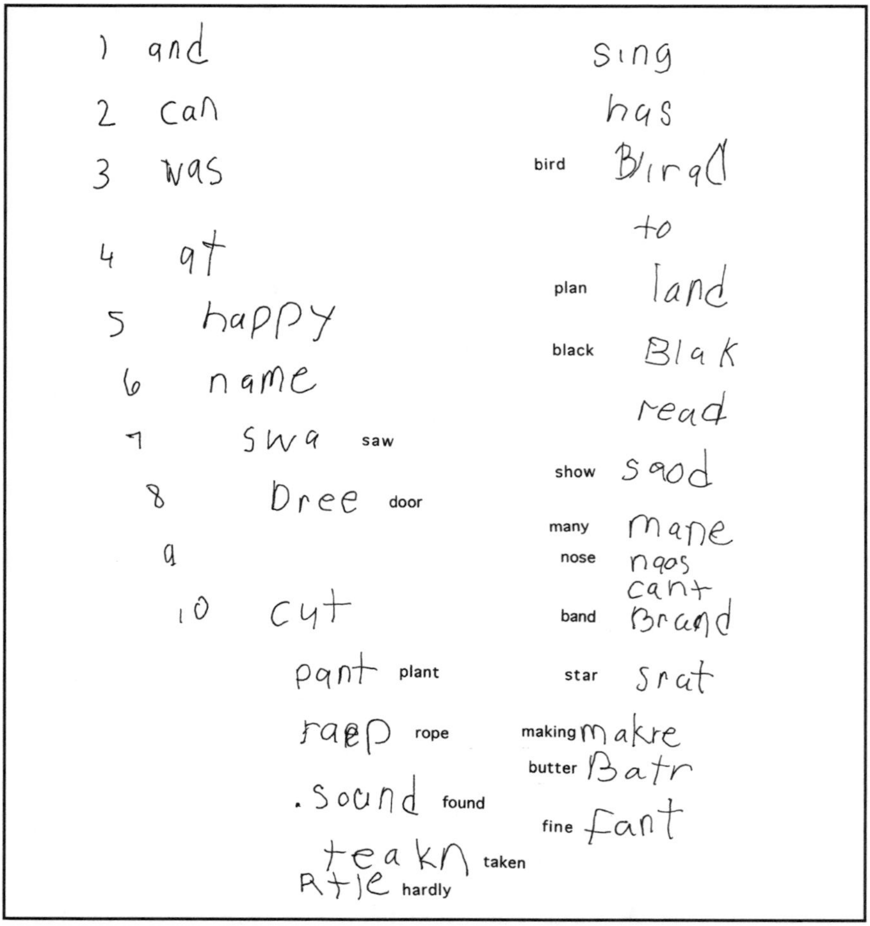

Figure 6.6. This 9-year-old girl cannot keep her writing organized unless someone helps her bump the left margin and stay within lines on her writing paper. Few dysgraphic students can maintain control of pencil placement while writing.

of what one sees, the brain must learn to hold visual mind maps together without scrambling the content or perceiving details out of order. Part of the problem of dysgraphia is having difficulty transferring mind map content onto paper. Individuals who are dysgraphic face major struggles copying shapes, matching shapes, or drawing shapes from memory. Figure 6.11 illustrates dysgraphic trouble copying simple shapes. A major characteristic of dysgraphia is the appearance of "ears" at the corners of diamonds

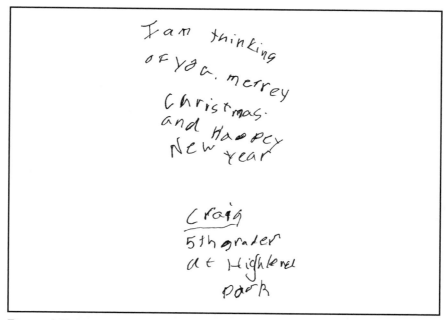

Figure 6.7. This 11-year-old boy wanted to let his teacher know that he appreciated her help and encouragement. This was the first holiday greeting he ever had written.

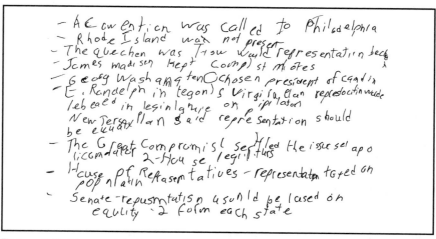

Figure 6.8. Dysgraphia is a handicap for this 14-year-old boy who works hard to do his best. As he copies, it is impossible for him to maintain adequate spacing between words and lines of writing. Countless times his work has been given a failing grade because teachers could not decipher his handwriting. Since first grade he has been accused of not trying hard enough to write neatly.

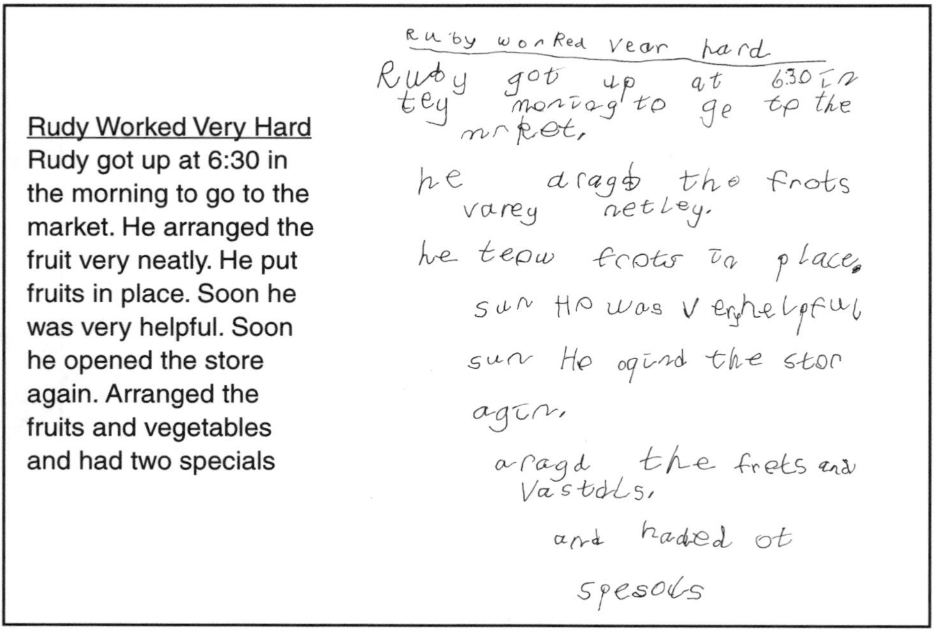

Rudy Worked Very Hard
Rudy got up at 6:30 in
the morning to go to the
market. He arranged the
fruit very neatly. He put
fruits in place. Soon he
was very helpful. Soon
he opened the store
again. Arranged the
fruits and vegetables
and had two specials

> Ruby worked vear hard
> Ruby got up at 6.30 in
> tey moning to ge tp the
> mrket,
>
> he dragb tho frots
> varey netley.
>
> he teow frots in place,
> sun He was verghelpful
> sun He ogind the stor
> agin,
>
> aragd the frets end
> Vastdls,
>
> and haded ot
> spesods

Figure 6.9. This 8-year-old boy learned to talk at an early age. During early childhood his oral vocabulary and language usage were exceptional for his age. Yet when he entered first grade, his handwriting was so poor that no one could decipher what he wrote. Finally his third grade teacher recognized signs of dyslexia and dysgraphia in the child's writing. The boy quickly learned keyboard writing skills and transferred all classroom writing tasks to his laptop computer, which enabled him to compensate for dysgraphia.

and squares. As the pencil reaches the end of a line, the brain reverses direction for the next stroke, causing the fingers to mark a different way. Then the brain corrects by bringing the pencil back in the new direction. As Figure 6.11 shows, it is very difficult for dysgraphic writers to draw or copy circles and curves.

Observation Skills for Teachers

It is not difficult for teachers and parents to develop two skills of observation in order to understand dysgraphia. First, they must watch the struggling writer at work. Individuals with dysgraphia often mask their pencil movement patterns so that the cause for illegible writing may not be apparent when adults scan

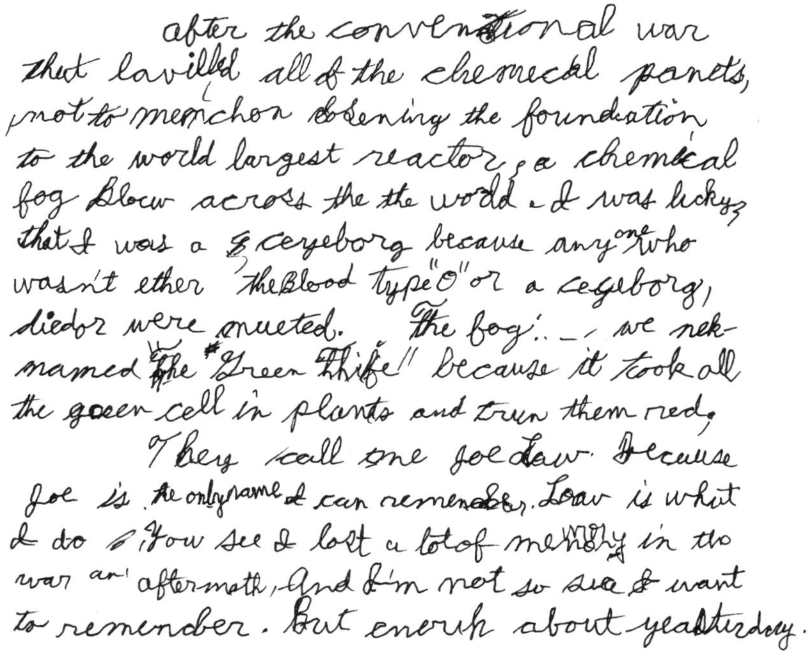

> *[Handwritten text reproduced in print below]*

After the conventional war that leveled all of the chemical plants, not to mention loosening the foundation to the world's largest reactor, a chemical fog blew across the world. I was lucky that I was a cyborg because anyone who wasn't either the blood type O or a cyborg died or was mutated. The fog we nicknamed "the Green Thief" because it took all the green cells in plants and turned them red.

They call me Joe Law because Joe is the only name I can remember. Law is what I do. You see, I lost a lot of memory in the war and aftermath. And I'm not sure I want to remember. But enough about yesterday.

Figure 6.10. This is the introduction to an original story composed by a 17-year-old boy who dreamed of becoming a successful mystery writer. For several years he secretly filled many notebooks with handwritten stories he was too insecure to show to anyone. During his sophomore year in high school, he came to trust a teacher well enough to show him some of the stories. The teacher recognized the student's talent for writing that was hidden beneath the overlay of dysgraphia. The story is translated to reveal the boy's intelligent imagination and mature sentence structure.

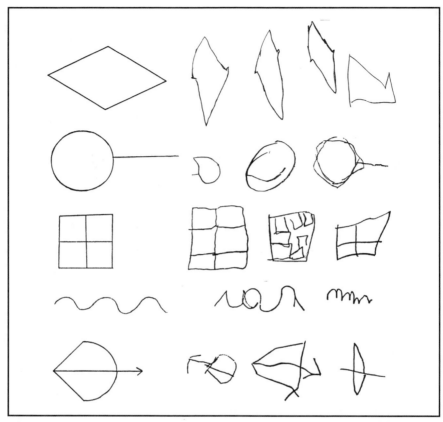

Figure 6.11. This composite shows the kinds of trouble that dysgraphic individuals often have when asked to copy or draw simple shapes. These dysgraphic persons continually erase, change, or write on top of their first pencil strokes. They reverse the direction of pencil strokes, which causes "ears" at the corners of diamonds and squares. These examples are from the Jordan Test for Dysgraphia (Jordan, 2000b). *Note.* From *Jordan Dyslexia Assessment / Reading Program, Second Edition* (pp. 3–4), by D. R. Jordan, 2000, Austin, TX: PRO-ED, Inc. Copyright 2000 by PRO-ED, Inc. Reprinted with permission.

finished assignments. Watching what the writer does with the pencil lets an observer understand why letters, words, and sentences appear as they do. Second, instructors must learn to re-create the student's writing style by slowly tracing over the handwriting. This hands-on experience lets the instructor feel the differences in directionality that guide the dysgraphic person's penmanship.

For example, slowly tracing over Glenda's labored writing in Figure 6.12 re-creates the tactile/kinesthetic feelings of her dysgraphic struggle. Small arrows show the backward strokes that distort left-to-right progression. Small breaks in letters show where her mental image was interrupted. Mixing manuscript and cursive styles reveals how often her mind maps fall apart, forcing her to start again but with a different mental image of what to write next. Tracing Glenda's writing is a quick way to understand why it takes her so long to do assignments and why she shows so much frustration during the school day. Figure 6.13 shows frequent reversed strokes in the writing of a 9-year-old boy who had mastered cursive writing style. His dysgraphic tendencies can be re-created by tracing over his penmanship to feel the places where his mind maps reversed while writing.

Activities for Overcoming Dysgraphia

The first goal for helping dysgraphic writers is to establish a visual framework for all tasks that involve handwriting. Teachers and parents must construct a grid, or template, that shows the

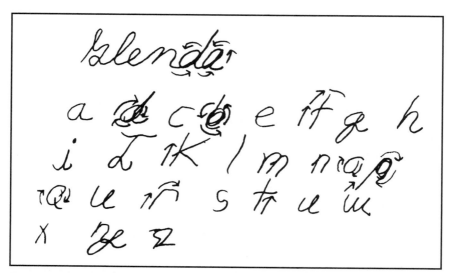

Figure 6.12. Tracing over this 9-year-old girl's handwriting reveals the fluctuations that occur within her brain as she copies or writes. Tracing re-creates the physical stress that triggers frustration and dread in every writing task this child is asked to do.

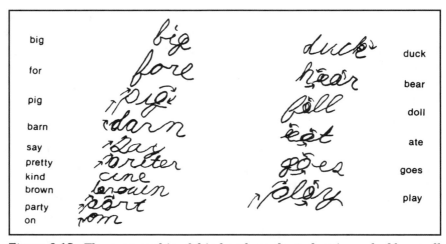

Figure 6.13. The penmanship of this fourth-grade student is marked by small arrows to show backward pencil strokes. Slowly tracing this dysgraphic writing re-creates the physical feeling and emotional frustration this child experiences with every writing task.

student where to write the next word, where to begin the next line, and how to space between words and lines. Whenever handwriting is required, the student must use this grid to increase legibility of what is encoded. Figure 6.14 shows the kind of writing template that will help dysgraphic students produce legible written assignments. Each writing space is clearly defined by dark lines that leave no doubt where next words and lines should go. Persons with dysgraphia need heavy enough boundary markers to trigger visual perception of the work page. Faintly printed lines and borders on writing tablets and notebook paper do not provide enough visual stimulus to show where to write. Sometimes it is possible to find commercially prepared writing paper with heavy enough space-marking lines to guide dysgraphic writers. Usually it is simpler for instructors and parents to provide a supply of writing paper with a grid like that shown in Figure 6.14.

Figures 6.15 and 6.16 show the benefit of teaching students with dysgraphia to use a spacing grid. This 13-year-old boy was asked to write a story about his favorite memory of his grandparents. Proudly he presented his teacher with the dysgraphic "mess" shown in Figure 6.15. As usual, the boy's work was re-

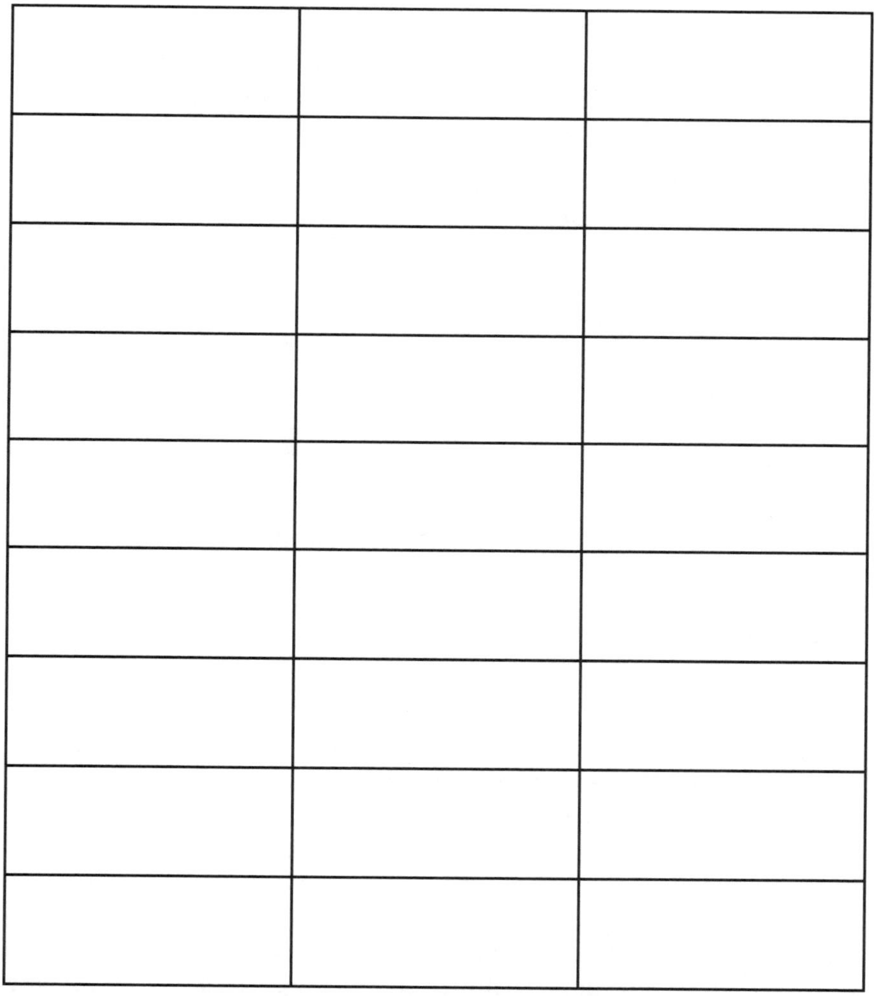

Figure 6.14. This kind of spacing grid is essential for dysgraphic writers who cannot control spacing between words and sentences.

jected with the bright red note: "You did not try hard enough to be neat. I cannot read your writing." An intuitive teacher took time to decode the dysgraphic story by copying each word in its separate place on the spacing grid. She was amazed as an intelligent story emerged from the illegible thicket of dysgraphic pencil strokes.

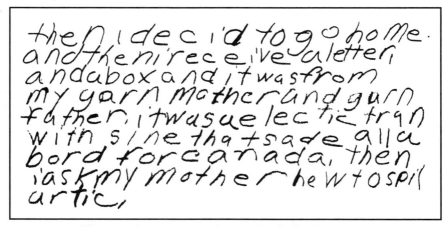

Figure 6.15. A severely dyslexic 13-year-old boy worked hard to write this story, only to have it rejected by adults because it made no sense. An intuitive teacher copied it onto the spacing grid shown in Figure 6.16. She was surprised to see an intelligent story emerge as the words and lines were separated.

Establishing Directionality

The primary writing disability underlying dysgraphia is the brain's inability to deal with directionality. When the dyslexic learner attempts to write symbols on paper, he or she does not have an automatic habit of proceeding left to right or top to bottom. Instead, the writer tends to mark circular strokes clockwise, which is backward from what educators call correct. The writer with dysgraphia also tends to start at the bottom of the letter or numeral and mark upward, which also is backward from the standard orientation. There is nothing wrong with backward orientation as such. If left alone to adapt to reading, writing, spelling, and arithmetic in their own way, most students with dysgraphia would devise ways to cope with literacy requirements. The major obstacles around which they cannot move are stereotyped expectations regarding handwriting. When these unnatural, invented penmanship restrictions are laid aside, these learners are as able as most others to do the work of educated persons.

Instructors who work with dysgraphic learners must follow certain procedures to help them think of directionality:

1. *Avoid soft pencils.* Individuals who are dysgraphic should write with a hard lead pencil that does not become dull

then	i	dec i'd
to	go	home.
and	then	;
receive	a	letter,
and	a	box
and	it	was
from	my	garnmother
and	garnfather.	it
was	a	electic
trqn	with	sine

Figure 6.16. Separating words and sentences reveals the message that the dysgraphic writer of Figure 6.15 wanted to convey. Extra space around each word lets the writer correct errors before writing the story again.

    quickly. Using a 4-F pencil instead of a Number 2 pencil prevents smudged, messy writing.

2. *Double-space all writing.* All handwriting must be double-spaced. It also may be necessary to teach dysgraphic students to lay a finger between words to make sure that the writer does not inadvertently write words too close together.

3. *Mark the starting place.* Learners who are dysgraphic must be reminded where to start on each work page. A starting mark, such as a brightly colored dot or a star, should be placed where writing should begin. Students are taught always to touch the starting place before they begin to write.

4. *Practice directional orientation.* Individuals who are dyslexic must be coached repeatedly in left-to-right, top-to-bottom orientation. As they write, these students must be reminded to move the pencil systematically from left to right. Then they must be reminded to check their work for anything they may have written backwards or upside down.

5. *Mark the margins.* Margins on writing paper must be clearly marked with heavy enough lines to stimulate visual perception of boundaries. The spacing grid shown in Figure 6.14 is marked with heavy enough lines to keep the student's attention at the right place. If other writing paper is used, instructors must use a felt-tip pen to draw margin lines down the left and right sides of the paper. Then dysgraphic learners must be coached in "bumping the margin" as they write.

6. *Assign study buddies.* Each student who is dysgraphic must have a study buddy who patiently coaches the dyslexic writer in reviewing each written activity. Together they find anything that is backward, upside down, or rolled on its side. Quietly they talk about pencil strokes that cut downward through the line or float above the line. As a team they practice bumping the left margin and keeping the pencil inside the correct space. Over time, these coaching strategies teach dysgraphic learners how to monitor their own work and correct most of their directional errors.

Mastering Handwriting Skills

Regardless of the student's age or grade placement, the essential starting place for correcting faulty directional concepts in writing is cursive style. This suggestion may contradict the philosophy of most educators, who, for half a century, have insisted that manuscript printing must come first. The reader should keep in mind that this book concerns expectional learners, not those who have neurological talent for literacy skills. Although most children prosper when they learn manuscript printing first, a different approach must be used in teaching handwriting to those who have dysgraphia.

Many elementary schools in the United States use one of the most effective handwriting methods created during the 20th century. In the 1950s, an intuitive elementary school teacher, Donald Thurber, realized that children with dyslexia/dysgraphia cannot become fluent with the traditional ball-and-stick manuscript writing style, as the figures in this chapter illustrate. Dyslexic individuals who manage to learn legible printing face great difficulty transferring to cursive writing later on. Thurber developed a unique handwriting system based on continuous, single-stroke pencil movements instead of isolated ball-and-stick motions that require several pencil lifts (Thurber, 1993). Thurber named his different approach to handwriting the D'Nealian Writing Program. The acronym D'Nealian was derived from the author's name: Donald Neal Thurber. Many dyslexic children, adolescents, and adults now write legibly with great pride, thanks to Thurber's creative work. The D'Nealian penmanship system gives the student a simple, dependable way to write in cursive style with only a few instances where the pencil must be lifted to make certain letters. Continuous, single-stroke writing solves penmanship problems for students who cannot master handwriting skills in the traditional manner.

Coping with Irregular Eyesight

Chapter 3 described several kinds of irregular eyesight that frustrate most individuals who are dyslexic. Chronic patterns of broken letter formation, irregular spacing, ragged margins, losing the place, and poor placement of writing on the page often signal problems with eye tracking and eye teaming. When irregular vision is corrected, teachers often see dramatic disappearance of dysgraphic symptoms within a short period of time. For example, Figure 6.17 shows the cramped, illegible writing of a deeply frustrated 9-year-old boy. Only he could decipher what he wrote. His teacher kept a diary of the boy's behavior in an effort to understand why he struggled so hard with written

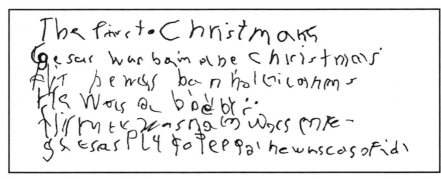

Figure 6.17. This illegible story was written by a shy 9-year-old boy who rarely spoke in the classroom. Alone with his teacher, he talked freely with advanced vocabulary and oral language skills. His written work appeared to be dysgraphic.

language expression. Over time she noted the following signs of vision stress:

_____ Continually squints both eyes hard.

_____ Continually turns away from bright light.

_____ Tries to shade his work from bright light.

_____ Starts to work well, but quickly gives up.

_____ Complains of headache several times each week.

_____ Often lays head down on his arm to shield his face from bright light.

_____ Every day becomes too tired to finish tasks.

_____ Stops paying attention to his work before he finishes.

_____ Continually rubs his eyes.

In a quiet time together, the teacher asked the student to help her copy his story onto the spacing grid she had prepared. Then she asked him to tell the story that the separated words revealed. Figure 6.18 shows the intelligent story that emerged. The teacher suggested that the boy's parents show her checklist to a vision specialist who worked with many dyslexic persons. The vision evaluation diagnosed poor eye tracking, very slow accommodation (delay in changing focus to new distances), extreme sensitivity to bright light, and moderate astigmatism. Within 3 weeks after receiving his new glasses, which were color tinted to reduce stress to bright light, the student's handwriting showed dramatic improvement.

The	first	Christmas
The	*fåret.*	*Christmaks*
Jesus	was	born
Gesus	*nur*	*baind*
on	Christmas	night
ane	*Christmas*	*þÿt.*
He	was	born
be	*nås*	*ban*
in	Bethlehem	He
kn	*olkiLohms*	*Hs*
was	a	baby
Wrois	*a*	*bpëibkr'*
flis His	mother	was
	Hek	*was*
named	was	Mary
nam	*Wpcs*	*(mke-*
Jesus	preached	to
ghcsas	*PLy*	*to*
Pepqal people	He	was
	hew	*whsc*
crucified		
cosofidi		

Figure 6.18. With the student's help, the teacher decoded the dysgraphic writing of Figure 6.17 to reveal sophisticated oral language skills that could not be expressed through his handwriting.

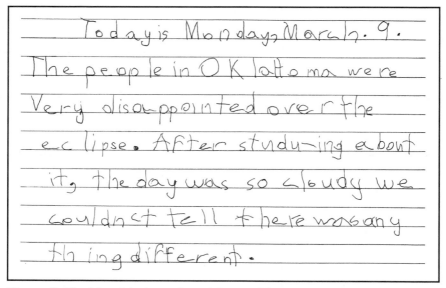

Today is Monday, March 9.
The people in OK lattoma were
Very disappointed over the
eclipse. After studuing about
it, the day was so cloudy we
couldn't tell there was any
thing different.

Figure 6.19. After his irregular vision problems were corrected, the dysgraphic student of Figure 6.17 had daily practice writing on this well-marked paper. Within 3 weeks he produced this moderately dysgraphic work without help. His writing became legible enough to let adults see his advanced language expression talent that had been hidden beneath poor vision and dysgraphia.

Figure 6.19 shows the reduction in dysgraphic symptoms when vision problems were corrected and he had learned how to space his writing.

Dyscalculia Syndrome

Figure 6.20 shows the regions in the left and right brain where skills emerge for arithmetic computation and higher mathematic reasoning. Earlier chapters reviewed two subtypes of dyslexia that often overlap to cause severe learning difficulty. Visual dyslexia prevents fluent processing of printed symbols. Auditory dyslexia makes it impossible for individuals to hear soft/slow speech sounds in the right sequence. This chapter has described a third subtype of dyslexia, dysgraphia, that causes illegible handwriting. The fourth subtype of dyslexia that often exists beneath the layers of poor reading, spelling, and handwrit-

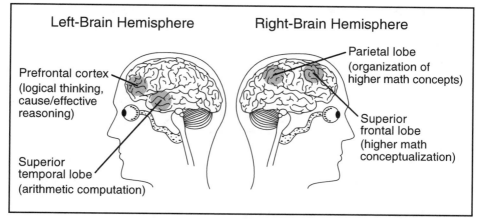

Figure 6.20. Arithmetic computation that requires fluent encoding and decoding ("reading") of printed math symbols occurs mainly in the left brain where the temporal lobe joins the frontal lobe. Higher math reasoning that depends less on reading printed math symbols occurs mostly in the right-brain frontal and parietal lobes. Dyscalculia is caused by incomplete neural wiring in the left temporal lobe. Many dyslexic individuals who cannot learn left-brain concrete arithmetic later become talented with right-brain abstract mathematics.

ing is dyscalculia. This type of dyslexia makes it impossible for many intelligent persons to learn or remember arithmetic information (addition, subtraction, multiplication, division, fractions, decimals). Ironically, some individuals with dyscalculia become talented with higher mathematics that does not require much symbol decoding or encoding.

For example, Chapter 9 presents the biographies of several prominent adults who were or are dyslexic. Among those individuals was Albert Einstein, who did not become a competent student until his early teens. At one point in his childhood, he was dismissed from school with the label "dunce." As he entered adolescence, he experienced the late "hardwiring" of neuron pathways that is described in Chapter 1. Einstein never learned arithmetic computation. In spite of his genius-level intellect, he could not develop the math skills required to do simple problem solving. However, by his early 20s he had extraordinary right-brain higher math talent that conceptualized the formula $E = MC^2$, which opened profoundly important new areas of science and mathematics. Instructors and counselors who work with dyslexic students often wonder how many "Einsteins" our culture has lost through unreasonable assumptions that all students must become proficient in left-brain arithmetic.

Checklist Signature of Dyscalculia

Students who struggle with dyscalculia present unique behaviors as they try to do arithmetic computation. Below is a simple checklist that allows teachers, tutors, and parents to document daily patterns of dysgraphia:

_____ Cannot remember simple facts about addition, subtraction, multiplication, division, fractions, or decimals.

_____ Cannot build long-term memory for arithmetic functions.

_____ Must use a multisensory method to work arithmetic problems. Must see/say/touch at the same time.

_____ Must use scratch paper to practice, rehearse, or doodle in order to figure out number relationships.

_____ Handwriting often is too large to stay within work spaces.

_____ Must count fingers while whispering over and over to recall arithmetic information.

_____ Often writes clusters of marks on scratch paper, then counts them to find sums or totals.

_____ Continually loses the direction of arithmetic functions.

_____ Misreads math signs. Thinks "times" for + or "add" for ×.

_____ Reverses numerals while writing answers.

_____ Continually erases or writes over first answers.

_____ Sometimes can do satisfactory problem solving if given enough time to work at own pace.

_____ Becomes overly frustrated when pressed to work problems in a hurry.

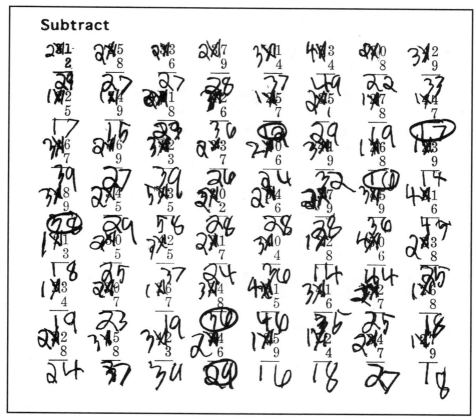

Figure 6.21. The awkward, overly large handwriting of dysgraphia often appears in the work of students with dyscalculia. This 10-year-old student cannot control the size of his writing to fit numerals into the space provided on worksheets.

Dysgraphia Overlaps Dyscalculia

Many students with dysgraphia also have dyscalculia. When this overlap exists, arithmetic worksheets become illegible. Figure 6.21 shows the work of a student with dysgraphia and dyscalculia. It is impossible for him to condense his writing to fit the crowded spaces provided by this worksheet. When the double problems of dysgraphia and dyscalculia exist together, instructors must provide extra space with only a few problems presented on a page. Wide spacing between problems is the only page format with which these struggling learners can succeed.

Dyscalculia Prevents Permanent Memory for Math Facts

Dyscalculia is the least understood form of dyslexia. Many instructors and parents find it hard to believe that intelligent youngsters cannot remember math information. Dyscalculia presents the same problems in decoding and encoding math information that visual dyslexia brings to the act of reading. Different regions of the left brain process reading information and arithmetic computation. It is not unusual for talented readers to have little or no talent for arithmetic or math. Likewise, it is not unusual to find a talented mathematician who is poor at reading or spelling. Dyscalculia creates lifelong "math illiteracy" that is beyond the control of those who struggle over arithmetic information. Figures 6.22 and 6.23 show how dyscalculia appears as those students labor over assignments. Each of these students achieved IQ scores within the superior range of mental ability, yet they cannot build permanent memory for basic arithmetic in-

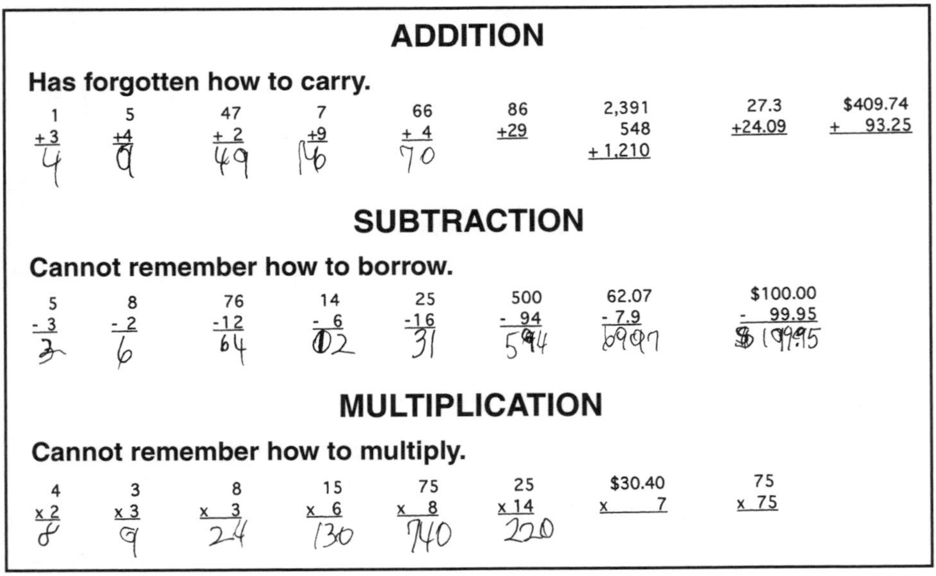

Figure 6.22. This 13-year-old dyslexic boy also has dyscalculia. In spite of a high IQ, he cannot build permanent memory for arithmetic computation. No matter how much he drills on basic arithmetic skills, he continues to struggle to recall how to work simple number problems.

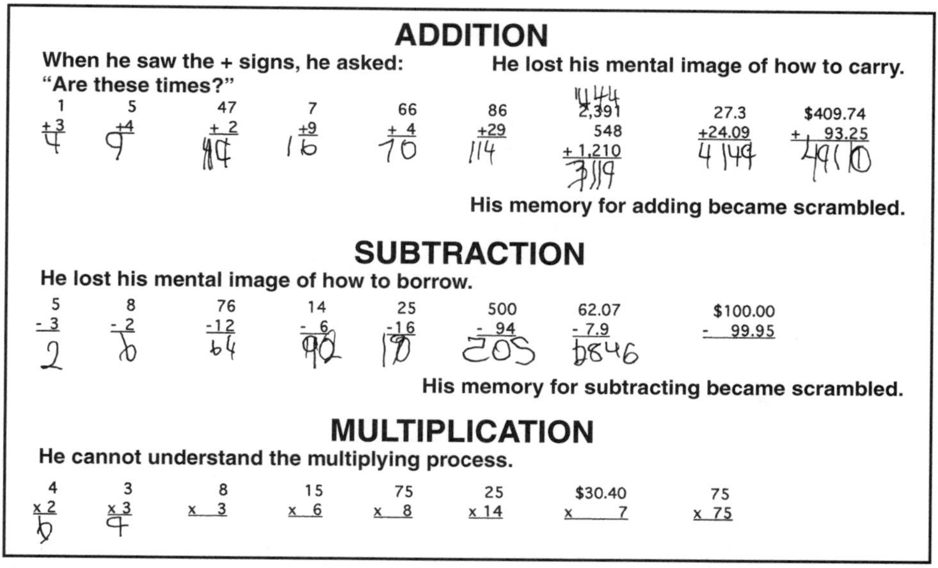
ADDITION
When he saw the + signs, he asked: "Are these times?"
He lost his mental image of how to carry.
1 +3
5 +4
47 + 2
7 +9
66 + 4
86 +29
2,391 548 + 1,210
27.3 +24.09
$409.74 + 93.25
His memory for adding became scrambled.
SUBTRACTION
He lost his mental image of how to borrow.
5 - 3
8 - 2
76 -12
14 - 6
25 -16
500 - 94
62.07 - 7.9
$100.00 - 99.95
His memory for subtracting became scrambled.
MULTIPLICATION
He cannot understand the multiplying process.
4 x 2
3 x 3
8 x 3
15 x 6
75 x 8
25 x 14
$30.40 x 7
75 x 75

Figure 6.23. This 12-year-old boy tries very hard to learn arithmetic skills. His life goal is to become an electrical engineer like his father. Visual dyslexia combines with dyscalculia to frustrate this bright student's effort to do arithmetic problems correctly.

formation. Figure 6.24 shows the kind of scratch paper rehearsal that is essential if students with dyscalculia are going to have any chance to work problems correctly.

Overcoming Dyscalculia

All subtypes of dyslexia are lifelong patterns that tend to diminish in severity as the brain becomes fully mature in early adulthood. However, the dyslexic patterns seen in childhood always will exist to some degree.

Well-Defined Work Spaces

Overcoming dyscalculia requires large enough work space along with scratch paper to let the individual experiment, make changes, practice multisensory techniques, and use a process of elimination until answers appear correct. The greatest need of students with dyscalculia is to have clearly marked boundaries

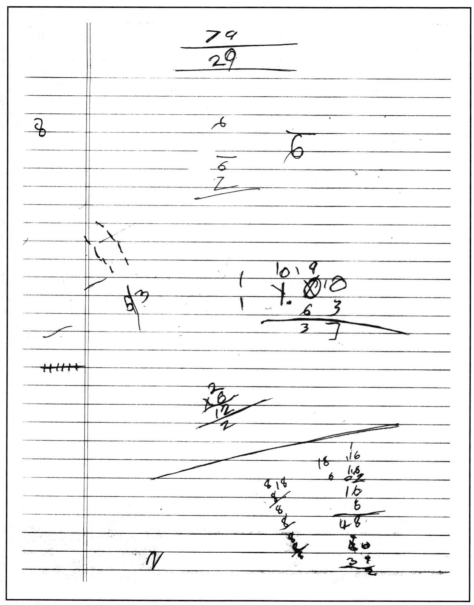

Figure 6.24. Dyscalculia makes it impossible for students to "work problems in their heads." To develop complete mental images of number relationships, they must use a multisensory method in which they see it/say it/write it over and over. These students must have scratch paper on which to practice various possibilities as they do arithmetic assignments. They must have all the time they need without feeling pressure to hurry.

for working problems. Figure 6.25 shows the type of grid that removes overcrowding while providing unmistakable space boundaries. This well-defined structure removes confusion about where to write answers and where number groups begin and end.

2 + 9	17 + 4	14 + 13	76 + 36
12 9 + 14	91 8 + 65	121 10 + 78	56 13 + 109
9 − 7	11 − 4	33 − 27	58 − 49
991 − 66	234 − 29	1177 − 200	333 − 123

Figure 6.25. This work page format is ideal for students with dyscalculia. Each work space is clearly defined. There is ample room for writing inside each grid. This open format removes a major source of frustration that is triggered when the person lacks enough space to work in his or her own best way.

Using a Calculator

Chapter 4 discussed the value of teaching dyslexic individuals to write at a keyboard. Joyce Steeves (1987) demonstrated that teaching dyslexic learners to use whole brain keyboard writing strategies increased their written language skills 15 times above what they could do with a pencil. A similar benefit occurs when students with dyscalculia work math problems on a calculator rather than struggling to do so the paper-and-pencil way. A calculator is a math keyboard. As students with dyscalculia follow multisensory strategies of seeing/saying/hearing/typing numbers with a calculator, many more brain regions become involved than when only a pencil is used. Suggesting that dyslexic learners use a calculator to practice arithmetic always triggers controversy among instructors. Teachers and parents worry that if a child uses a calculator, he or she will not learn math principles. Actually, using a calculator enables those with dyscalculia to learn math principles more successfully than they can the traditional way.

Chapter 7 discusses the critical role that emotions and feelings play in learning new skills. Students with dyslexia, dysgraphia, or dyscalculia bring powerful negative emotions and feelings into all learning experiences. They live under the cloud of the fear of failure. Learners who lack talent for reading, spelling, handwriting, or arithmetic are cut off from normal success and praise. If their best is not good enough, they are helpless to cope with strong negative emotions that trigger the fight-or-flight reflex in threatening situations. Transferring arithmetic practice from pencil writing to a calculator keyboard is a liberating experience for most individuals who struggle with math concepts. A calculator brings the same relief for students who are poor at math that keyboard writing brings to those who are dyslexic. If it is neurologically impossible for certain persons to do well with math principles and functions, it makes no sense to withhold a calculator that fosters more success than failure.

Checking for Dysgraphic/Dyscalculiac Writing Differences

An essential survival skill for individuals with dysgraphia and dyscalculia is knowing how to edit their own writing for dyslexic differences. As Chapter 7 explains, it is important for teachers and parents not to label these differences as "mistakes." The process of "marking mistakes" or "grading your paper" results in extremely sensitive emotional issues for those who have dysgraphia or dyscalculia. It is critical that instructors help students learn to edit their own work first before anyone else scans it for differences. It takes only a few minutes for instructors to prepare models of assignments that contain no writing, spelling, or computation differences. Then dyslexic/dysgraphic students can use those models to check their own spelling tests, arithmetic assignments, social studies exercises, science quizzes, and language activities. If students are taught how to use answer keys and other scoring devices, they can protect personal territory and pride by being the first to see their differences.

Once dyslexic students have checked their work, they do not mind so much when a study buddy or teacher scans it. Chapter 1 described the proto-self that emerges from the midbrain during early childhood (see page 27). From the earliest moments following birth, infants begin to build self-image (proto-self) in response to how adults approach them. If infants and toddlers grow up in a positive environment filled with praise and encouragement, a strong image of self emerges that gives each child courage to face new challenges. If, however, youngsters grow up in negative environments filled with criticism and rejection, they do not develop the courage and self-confidence needed to face new challenges. Most children who are dyslexic enter formal learning dreading criticism they have learned to expect. Instinctively they cringe and pull back when adults mark "mistakes" and send the strong message: "You did it wrong again!" Having dyslexic differences labeled mistakes and errors brings new emotional pain that destroys one's desire to try again. The sight of red ink all over a paper triggers intense negative emotions that interfere with classroom performance and erodes self-esteem.

Many instructors raise the question, "Can I trust students to be honest in grading their own work?" The risk of cheating is no greater among dyslexic learners than among honor students who have no learning difficulty. In fact, cheating is a signal that students feel pressure to be accepted by the system. If instructors discover dishonesty as individuals do self-checking, they should reexamine their educational values regarding the importance of grades. The presence of cheating signals that too much emphasis has been placed on achieving good grades. Insecure students may resort to cheating if that is the only way they can find acceptance within a learning situation. If the pressure to make good grades comes from the student's home, the teacher's options may be limited. If, however, pressure for good grades comes from within the school's curriculum and attitudes, procedures for success must be adjusted for those with learning difficulties so that they have a fair chance at being successful.

Principles for Overcoming Dysgraphia and Dyscalculia

In spite of recent prophecies that new technologies will soon make handwriting and arithmetic computation obsolete, classroom teachers remain very much concerned about each student's ability to communicate through penmanship and to be skilled in basic math. It is essential that all persons develop enough handwriting skills to cope with the workplace. Also, it is essential for everyone in the workplace to have skills in adding, subtracting, multiplying, dividing, using fractions, and using decimals. In spite of personal keyboard writing systems and pocket calculators, literacy for writing and math computation remains a vital issue as the American culture enters a new millennium.

Earlier in this chapter it was mentioned that students with dyslexia usually know what they want to write. However, if there is no model from which to copy, their dilemma is how to transfer those ideas and information into a legible handwritten code. Overcoming dysgraphia in the classroom is possible if certain principles of instruction are observed. Teachers must keep in mind that dysgraphic writers are not just being messy or careless. Unless they become bitter and hostile through repeated failure and blame, individuals with dysgraphia will do their best each time they write an assignment. The teacher's attitude sets the tone for how each student's attitude and self-confidence (proto-self) will grow or decline. If struggling learners do their best, but it never is good enough, serious damage will occur to vulnerable self-esteem and low self-confidence. If, on the other hand, the teacher practices patience and demonstrates long-range optimism, dyslexic learners can learn to enjoy enough success to earn praise for their effort and willingness to try.

Principle 1: The Learner Is Doing His or Her Best

I learned a painful lesson about dyslexia the second year I taught school. I asked my sixth-grade students to write stories built around "trigger words" I wrote on the chalkboard. Wayne seemed especially interested in this project because the trigger words suggested a science fiction theme, his favorite fiction form. As my university preparation had taught me to do, I graded the stories with my usual thoroughness, marking every error in spelling, grammar, punctuation, and penmanship with a blood-red pencil. Wayne's story content was unusually good, but the writing mechanics were awful. At that time, I had no knowledge of dyslexia or dysgraphia. I believed firmly that every child had the ability to learn to read, write, and spell as well as I did. I believed that every student could do good writing if he or she tried hard enough. At the end of school one day I handed back the graded papers, then dismissed the class. As Wayne passed me, I saw tears in his eyes. "Wayne, I liked your story," I said. "Then why did you bleed to death all over it?" he sobbed as he ran from the room.

As a teacher, I had failed to understand a vital fact: *Wayne had done his best*. The messy, smudged paper I had rejected was the best he could do at that time. In "bleeding to death" all over his writing differences, I had failed to perceive that he had done his best for me, and I had rejected him. Most competent grown-ups tend to think of children as miniature adults, which blinds us to many vital elements in educational growth. Because we assume that what we see is what really exists, children are judged by the surface characteristics of neatness, punctuality, quietness, dignity, poise, and how well their work fits the mold. The stereotypes by which we judge student achievement can be cruel, if we mistakenly assume that imperfect papers are evidence that the child has not tried. Such rigid expectations may have some validity for students who are talented for learning literacy skills. However, sensitive children like Wayne are hurt day after day, year after year, because their lack of talent to fit the literacy mold brings false judgment on them. The truth is they usually try harder than their peers who always make good grades.

That afternoon it broke my heart to learn how deeply I had hurt Wayne. He had trusted me with his best. He had taken me at my word when I asked the class to put their imagination on paper. When he turned in his story, he was proud and happy that finally he had a teacher who liked what he could do. My rigid grading system was a dreadful betrayal of Wayne's trust in me. As I left the school that afternoon, tears were in my eyes as I remembered a painful moment of humiliation in my own educational experience. A rigid, unimaginative professor had given my graduate class an assignment to critique the writing of a famous educational philosopher. Instead of writing a traditional term paper, I had created an imaginary dialogue between that writer and me. Through that make-believe discussion I commented on the value of the philosopher's concepts, as my instructor asked me to do. At our next class meeting, I was stunned when the professor held my essay before the class and ridiculed my work. He made scathing remarks about my inability to follow instructions. He stated that he had doubts that I should become a teacher because I failed to do assignments correctly. I recalled the bitter emotions that overwhelmed me. How dare that teacher be so critical of this creative work that made me proud? What right did he have to embarrass me that way in front of the class? I thought he was my friend, but I was so wrong. Suddenly I was inside Wayne's devastated feelings and emotions. Then I knew why he sobbed as he ran away from me that afternoon.

The next day I took Wayne to a private place where we could talk this over. As he turned his back and refused to look at me, I could feel his anger and resentment. I explained to Wayne that I had made a terrible mistake when I bled on his story. I told him about my own humiliation in the university class. I asked him if he could forgive me for being so thoughtless. There was silence as he thought it over. Suddenly he turned and embraced me in a tight hug as he sobbed from relief. Figure 6.26 is a copy of a letter I received from Wayne after helping him develop an award-winning science project. That experience taught me a priceless lesson about the power of emotions and feelings when learning difficulty exists.

How does an instructor or parent determine whether a struggling learner is doing his or her best? The only feasible way to make such a judgment is to note indicators of improvement. For example, if Wayne always has disregarded (failed to perceive) small details in copying from the board or from a book, his work would have poor punctuation, failure to indent for paragraphs, disregard of capital letters, and word chunks left out. The instructor will know that Wayne is doing his best when he begins to perceive minor details that affect the quality of his work. In other

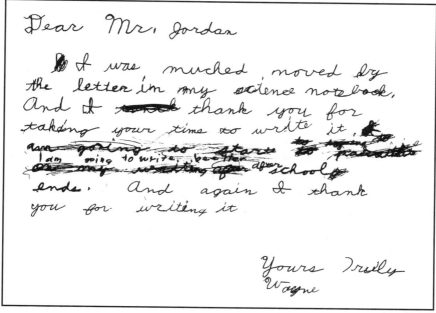

Figure 6.26. This letter from a dyslexic student marked a critical turning point in my attitudes toward teaching. As a student in my sixth-grade classroom, Wayne taught me to respect the emotions and feelings of struggling learners who do their best, but their best seldom is good enough.

words, improvement must be judged by the small self-corrections students begin to make on their own, after these differences have been pointed out by the teacher or study partner. If over a period of time Wayne's finished papers show fewer and fewer dyslexic differences, this is proof that he is doing his best.

Chapter 1 described the critical role played by the emerging brain stem during the first trimester of fetal development. As early as the fifth week of gestation the basal brain begins to ask the vital question: *Is this safe?* At any age, before the higher brain can process new information, the basal brain must determine whether each new experience is safe. If the brain stem and midbrain sense danger, the fight-or-flight reflex triggers a rapid sequence of safety decisions that must come before learning or processing new information is possible. Chapter 7 explains the critical role that emotions and feelings play in learning, or in failure to learn.

The most essential factor in overcoming dysgraphia is emotional safety. That day when I returned Wayne's story on which I had "bled to death" by marking every error, my criticism triggered intense emotions and feelings that caused him to feel unsafe. He ran from my classroom that afternoon because he was overwhelmed by the threat and humiliation of failure. I learned that before I could guide Wayne toward more accurate writing skills, I must help him feel safe in doing so. Although mercy, patience, understanding, and forgiveness are not directly related to spelling or handwriting, these safe attitudes are of critical importance in engaging the trust of students like Wayne. The merciful teacher who is safe to be with begins to look for bits and pieces of improvement, instead of continuing to "bleed to death" over the multitude of writing errors. When learners like Wayne begin to observe capital and lowercase letters, this represents a tremendous stride in achievement for them. What might be 1 inch forward for the teacher may represent 100 feet of progress for students who are dysgraphic. It is cruel and harmful always to judge progress by large increments. If struggling students must leap all the way from C to B to demonstrate that they have done their best, there is no hope for them in the classroom or the workplace. When instructors learn to accept small tokens of progress as being giant steps, then mercy begins to heal bitter attitudes and calm lifelong fear, thus allowing progress to be made.

The first step toward overcoming dysgraphia is not more handwriting practice—it is for the instructor to believe that even the messiest, grubbiest papers may represent the best the student can do under the circumstances. Far too many educators are biased against students with dysgraphia solely because the written work is messy.

The secret is to scan Wayne's written work for molecules of improvement: certain letters no longer reversed, punctuation marks now being used, and/or capital letters where they should be. Many teachers have reversed their marking systems, using the student's favorite color to mark only the points of progress. A paper with no marks would signify no improvement. From this point of view, Wayne cherishes the days when marks cover his work, heralding the fact that his instructor sees improvement.

Principle 2: Handwriting Is Intensely Personal

It would be profitable if every parent and classroom teacher could relive his or her most sensitive experience in which personal writing was criticized. Most adults, especially those enrolled in graduate courses, are extremely sensitive when their written work is judged. Any professor who returns research papers, essay test responses, or written reports can testify to the acute pain experienced by adults who find critical notes on the margins of their work. It is not unusual for grown-ups to burst into tears over criticisms professors have made. None of us is immune to feeling sensitive about what we have written. Editors are especially aware of the problems new authors face in learning how to accept editorial suggestions. Of all the sources of dread that professionals feel, having one's writing criticized, misunderstood, or belittled is among the most acute.

This universal emotional sensitivity toward one's writing is reflected in the way adults carefully guard personal diaries and intimate letters. Although schoolwork by no means is as personal as one's private notes, there is a common feeling of caution when individuals are required to commit themselves to written form. Oral communication is not remembered verbatim. A speaker's clever use of intonation and mannerisms often distract listeners from personal revelations that might be uttered. But thoughts put into writing become permanent. An intimate part of the writer's self becomes vulnerable once it is on the page for all the world to see. Feeling safe is critical for those who express their private thoughts in writing.

Sensitive instructors are aware of how this timidity in writing affects classroom behavior. From the earliest grades through graduate school, insecure students slip up to the instructor to ask, "Do you want to see what I wrote?" Instructors do emotional harm when they impatiently send these students away without glancing over the written material. Professors who do not take time to scan a nervous student's first draft inflict similar pain. When students reach out this way, they actually are pleading, "Please don't be too critical. This is the best I can do. Is it good enough yet?"

As students achieve success, they need less reassurance from instructors and others. Repeated success with writing, especially if one is talented in language usage, brings enormous emotional satisfaction. Teachers always look forward to having students who write well with an interesting style. This kind of success seldom is available to individuals with dysgraphia. By nature, persons like Wayne are overly sensitive and fearful. Those who struggle in the classroom often compensate by appearing indifferent to praise. In reality, they are hungry for the acceptance experienced by more talented individuals. When forced to commit themselves to writing, those with dysgraphia are left in the emotionally dangerous position of being defenseless. For them, writing becomes a threatening experience in which their weaknesses are fully exposed. Their choices are to muddle through or to become defiant and refuse to try. If they hand in messy papers, adults "bleed all over them." If they choose not to write, then they are publicly branded as lazy, careless, uncooperative, or even "dumb." No matter which way they turn, they cannot win, from their point of view.

This book began with a review of the vast knowledge now available about what happens during brain development to cause learning difficulties. It is clear that having a learning difficulty is beyond the choice or control of those who struggle to learn. According to what science has shown us about differences in brain development, no one gets to choose his or her learning style or the degree of talent he or she has for reading, spelling, or writing. From this point of view, learning differences are not a matter of choice. From this perspective, there can be no such thing as the "correct" way to hold one's pencil, slant the paper, or sit in one's chair while writing. Nor can educators logically dictate the angle at which handwritten letters must slant. The penmanship standards imposed by earlier educators were based more on bias than on perceptual reality.

In recent years, handwriting has come to be recognized as a unique signature of the writer's personality. Wayne slants his letters toward the left, not because he is "incorrect," but because of unique ways in which his brain pathways were formed. The size of a writer's script can have a definite correlation with his or her intelligence, just as the way Julia dots the letter *i* or crosses a *t* indicates specific character traits or dispositions of mood. It is terribly presumptuous for a teacher to declare that a student is wrong just because the person's script does not flow like the instructor's. A great deal of ignorance has been involved in handwriting methodology, especially where children with dysgraphia have been concerned. Fortunately, the term *correct* is being replaced by the more realistic term *acceptable*. Having one's best efforts accepted does not imply that further progress is not necessary. Being labeled acceptable allows room for growth, a step at a time.

If writing indeed is a sensitive, personal affair, then parents and teachers should handle the subject accordingly. The rule of thumb should be a practical one: *So long as the student's writing is legible, and so long as it is the best he or she can do, I will accept it without making the writer feel threatened or inferior.* As Wayne demonstrated for me, dysgraphic students who feel safe will learn to write more maturely.

Principle 3: Respect the Learner's Territory

During my final year as a classroom teacher, I learned a lesson that has shaped my professional life for the the past 35 years. A dramatist turned popular science writer, Robert Ardrey, wrote two books that fascinated me: *African Genesis* (1961) and *The Territorial Imperative* (1972). Ardrey drew hundreds of examples from the animal world to support his thesis that human beings, like lower animals, possess a strong territorial imperative that we will defend at all costs. Ardrey contended that this instinct to stake out one's territory, then defend it against threatening intruders, explains human behavior. According to his idea, every aspect of human civilization—religion, education, politics, family life, recreation, technology, war—is governed by the driving need for territory. From his observations, Ardrey inferred that, to be a wholesome individual, every person must have a certain degree of privacy (territory) in which he or she feels safe from intrustion by outsiders. The theory holds that, when human beings are deprived of private territory, they become neurotic and cease to be emotionally well balanced.

Ardrey's concepts have suggested some useful applications in education. Numerous studies have documented excellent learning results when territorial needs have been provided for in the classroom. There are critically important lessons for educators, parents, and workplace supervisors within the concept of territoriality.

If we are to help students who are struggling to overcome learning problems, close attention must be given to the interactions between these frightened, insecure individuals and confident, sometimes overbearing instructors and supervisors. Few educators realize that one talented, self-confident instructor alone with one apprehensive, low-talented learner is not a one-to-one relationship. If the instructor is overbearing and the student is insecure, the relationship often is overwhelming for that student. This explains why some struggling learners often do not respond when tutored by well-educated instructors. When viewed through the perspective of territorial imperative, dyslexic behavior does indeed appear defensive because the person feels that his or her territory (inner privacy) is threatened. This accounts for much of the disruptive behavior encountered by teachers of students who have learning difficulties. Most adults do not hesitate to defend their rights (territories) against outside threats. Walkouts, strikes, professional holidays, and other forms of protest have become common among educators. If professional adults react this way when their workplace territories are violated, then certainly one would expect overly sensitive students with dyslexia to do the same.

My experience with Wayne illustrates this principle. As his teacher, I had carefully "motivated" him to respond to the creative story assignment. I wish I could say that I coaxed him out of his shell. What actually happened was that he let me enter his private world of make-believe. I was proud of the expertise with which I manipulated the class into writing stories from my trigger words. After all, did they not decide to use my words instead of theirs? Until I saw Wayne's angry tears, it did not occur to me that I had made an unspoken contract with my students:

> If you will write a story as I have suggested, I will read it carefully. I know that it's hard for you to spell and punctuate accurately. But don't worry about that. The main thing is for you to express yourself. Be creative! You can trust me to appreciate the part of yourself you put on paper. I won't betray your trust!

Then I "bled to death all over it," as Wayne so accurately stated.

The fact that I was a young teacher was no excuse for my violation of that boy's trust. As a sensitive adult, I certainly knew the pain and embarrassment of having my own writing (territory) violated by stern graduate professors. Not 6 months prior to that day with Wayne, I had driven home in tears of rage when a professor had belittled a paper I had written for his graduate course. The mistake I made with Wayne was not to respect his territory. I betrayed his trust by "bleeding" on his dyslexic differences. Then I compounded the injury by saying, "I liked your story." He reacted as any healthy person should react—by thrusting me out of his inner territory. It was several weeks before he let me back in. There are times when teachers never regain a comfortable relationship with students whose territories they have failed to respect.

Develop a Contract

If educators are to gain entry into the inner space of students with dysgraphia, they must establish ground rules that will govern the behavior of both parties. Often this is called a contract. The teacher has a frank, private conversation with the student, explaining the skills that must be developed. The teacher presents a checklist of the trouble spots in the student's work, along with samples of work that illustrate these differences. Then the teacher proposes alternatives, naming the kinds of activities available for correcting the problem. This contract specifies the amount of individual attention the teacher can give and who study partners or tutors will be. Also, the contract explains the grading system and spells out how much homework practice will be expected. The student is encouraged to suggest changes that would make the contract more comfortable or less threatening. Finally, both teacher and student sign the agreement that will guide each of them in this skill development project.

Approach with Patience

At first, not all struggling learners are mature enough or interested enough to receive this much information. The instructor must use good judgment to determine when enough has been discussed at one conference. The point is to present a simple outline of the student's needs, explain what can be done about it, and specify his or her responsibilities in overcoming the skill challenges.

There are many reasons why a student like Wayne might be reluctant to admit a teacher into his confidence (territory). In the first place, Wayne probably will not trust the outsider to keep this new bargain. A wise teacher does not push to get inside Wayne's territory. There is nothing more devastating to students who have difficulty expressing ideas than for an articulate, outgoing educator to bombard them with personal questions. The teacher must not try to pry answers from the student. If no interaction is forthcoming, the instructor takes the initiative by making direct statements about how, when, and where the corrective work will begin. As Wayne digests this offer of help, he will realize that the instructor is genuinely ready to accept his efforts, dyslexic differences and all. At this point, Wayne and his teacher begin to have a more open dialogue. In fact, one of the dilemmas of tutoring students with dyslexia is how to persuade them to stop talking in order to accomplish drill work.

The gist of this principle is simple and direct. The teacher does not overwhelm the apprehensive learner by entering private, personal territory before the student is ready to allow the outsider in. Until Wayne offers cues that he is ready for a more personal relationship, the teacher should confine the relationship to simple drill routines, explaining whatever Wayne seems interested in knowing. Above all, written work must not be condemned, even when it is illegible. Tactful ways to require the unacceptable work to be done again must be devised. One of the best methods is to let Wayne evaluate his own work against a model. Most of all, the teacher must not write all over Wayne's paper to the point where he becomes hurt, overly discouraged, or too afraid to try again.

When the instructor genuinely respects Wayne's territorial boundaries and is careful not to betray the subtle trust he begins to show, great strides toward improvement will be seen. Abrupt, impatient, or domineering educators see virtually no growth among the dyslexic students in their charge. Persons with strong, forceful personalities seldom realize the effect they have on sensitive individuals. Most domineering teachers perceive themselves as excellent instructors because their rooms are quiet and their students are busy. Rarely should such teachers be in charge of individuals with dyslexia. Territorial boundaries are so fragile in these fearful students that a heavy-footed instructor tramples down the fences many times each day without realizing the emotional devastation this aggressive behavior is causing. Teachers should be chosen for corrective work because they are skilled in sensing territorial boundaries. Strong-willed adults work best with outgoing, self-confident individuals who thrive on competition for territorial dominance in the classroom.

The Emotions and Feelings of Being Dyslexic

7

Dyslexia is black and a rainbow.
It tastes like fear.
It sounds like a growl.
And smells like a problem.
It makes me feel weird but hopeful.
> —Chris, age 10, after he received helpful counseling and tutor-
> ing for dyslexia following an episode of deep depression

Success is red, bright red.
It sounds like everything and nothing,
but it sounds good to me.
It tastes like sweet triumph, sweeter than cherries.
It looks like a flower
Because everything is coming up roses for me.
> —Cindy, age 36, following her success at passing the GED
> exam that was preceded by an attempt at suicide

The Brain's Design To Regulate Emotions and Feelings

Chapter 1 summarized the natural role that emotions and feelings play in every person's life, beginning during the first
trimester of fetal development (see pages 10–11). Figure 7.1 shows
the brain regions that work together throughout an individual's
life to regulate emotions and feelings. As neural pathways emerge

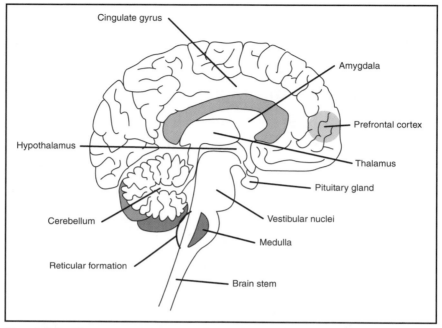

Figure 7.1. These regions of the brain stem, midbrain, and higher brain begin to regulate feelings and emotions as early as the 10th week of fetal development. As neurons mature, these brain regions form a lifelong network that balances emotions, feelings, and moods.

in the brain stem, two specialized neuron clusters begin to ask the question, Is this new event safe? By the 10th week of fetal development, the medulla and reticular formation are starting to filter new experiences for emotional safety. During the second trimester of fetal development, at the top of the brain stem the vestibular nuclei begin to check the safety of all new sounds and noise. During the third trimester of gestation, the limbic system (midbrain) becomes the final control region for strong emotions and feelings. At this early stage of life, the hypothalamus and pituitary gland begin to safeguard the emerging brain from too much stress. The cingulate gyrus, hypothalamus, and thalamus link together to filter sensations and emotions associated with pain and pleasure. At the same time, the amygdala begins its lifelong work of controlling socially destructive emotions such as fear, anxiety, rage, terror, hatred, urge to kill, lust, desire for revenge, depression, and impulse for self-destruction. For the rest of each person's life, these brain structures stand guard over emotional issues, ready to trigger the fight-or-flight reflex that protects individuals from harm while keeping destructive emotions and feelings under control.

During the first 2 years of early childhood, the prefrontal cortex begins to generate higher emotions and feelings, often called socially constructive emotions. Figure 7.2 shows the emotional balance that normally emerges when brain development follows normal growth patterns. By age 6 in most children, the prefrontal cortex becomes the executive function center that maintains a stable balance between basal and higher emotions and feelings.

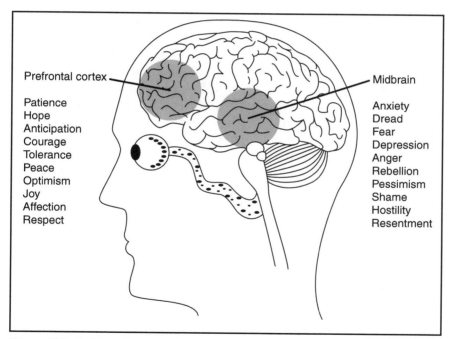

Figure 7.2. Individuals who do not have dyslexia or other types of LD usually maintain a balance between the higher emotions and feelings that originate within the prefrontal cortex and the basal emotions and feelings that arise from the midbrain. When dyslexia exists, negative basal emotions and feelings, such as dread, fear, and anxiety, often overwhelm the person to make successful classroom performance impossible.

The Lifelong Power of Emotions and Feelings

A surprising result of recent brain research has been the discovery of the vital role that emotions and feelings play in shaping every person's life. In his book *The Feeling of What Happens: Body and Emotion in the Making of Consciousness* (1999), Antonio Damasio describes the types of emotions and feelings that govern every aspect of human behavior. According to Damasio, feelings are the private inner thoughts and reactions that individuals conceal from the world. Emotions are the manifestations of inner feelings as seen by others. Emotions and feelings occur in various patterns. At times, emotions and feelings occur in "burst" patterns that begin suddenly, escalate quickly to a peak of intensity, then fade rapidly away. Intense feelings such as rage, jealousy, surprise, disgust, or sudden joy burst into emotional action, then quickly fade away. Other types of emotions and feelings emerge gradually, finally reach peak levels, then persist over long periods of time. These long-range emotions and feelings include worry, anxiety, shame, contentment in relationships, and satisfaction with one's life. Sometimes long-range emotions and feelings become moods that take control of one's attitudes and reactions. A growing body of brain research supports Damasio's assertion that emotions and feelings are the most powerful forces that influence each person's life (Adolphs & Damasio, 1998; Damasio, 1994, 1999; Ekman, 1992; Jordan, 1998, 2000a, 2000b; Sutherland, 1992; Tranel & Damasio, 1993).

The Emotions and Feelings of Dyslexia

As previous chapters have explained, it is impossible to understand dyslexia without also understanding the lifelong emotions, feelings, and moods of those who are dyslexic. Chapter 3 described the multiple layers of learning difficulty that often accompany dyslexia. To understand dyslexia in the classroom, it is critical that each layer of LD be identified so that dyslexic patterns are seen accurately. To understand dyslexia fully, it is critical that the person's feelings, moods, and emotions also be recognized and modified enough to permit the struggling learner to feel safe. A person cannot learn if he or she does not feel emotionally safe.

The Devastation of Shame

Of all the emotions and feelings linked to dyslexia, the most devastating is shame. The destructive role of shame has been summarized as follows:

> At least 20 percent of all children have difficulty due to learning disabilities. The first casualty is self-esteem. They soon grow ashamed as they struggle with a skill their classmates master easily. (National Institute of Child Health and Human Development, 1998)

> Being illiterate in our culture is a devastating condition. Enormous emotional problems develop early in nonreaders who suffer from low self-esteem and anger over being isolated from the rest of society. Being illiterate spawns disruptive behavior that often leads desperate individuals into addictions, emotional imbalance, or even mental illness. Being illiterate is degrading and a constant source of shame. (Jordan, 2000a, p. 1)

Loss of Emotional Balance

In describing how regions of the brain work together to establish functions that are well balanced, Chapter 1 presents the concept of *homeostasis*. Figure 7.2 shows the brain regions where emotions and feelings originate. For the brain to work effectively, the higher emotions from the prefrontal cortex must be well balanced with the basal emotions from the midbrain. If neurotransmitters that regulate one's sense of well-being are out of balance, it is impossible for the higher brain to learn new facts and skills. The brain depends on a balance (homeostasis) of emotions and feelings so that mood swings do not disrupt normal brain processes. The many faces of dyslexia, including poor vision for reading, inability to learn phonics, poor spelling, illegible writing, and low reading comprehension, threaten the balance of emotions and feelings in persons who are dyslexic. Lack of emotional homeostasis keeps dyslexic individuals feeling upset, anxious, resentful, fretful, and ashamed. Only occasionally do dyslexic persons feel happy, satisfied, or proud of themselves. Over time, lack of emotional balance implants strongly negative moods and feelings that do not go away. It is rare for individuals who are dyslexic to feel joy in the classroom.

Shame Is the Absence of Self-Love

James Gilligan, a psychiatrist who specializes in treating inmates serving life sentences for violent crime, has proposed a model that demonstrates the devastation of shame and how shame can be eliminated from one's moods and feelings. Gilligan (1996) states,

> I believe that violence—whatever else it may mean—is the ultimate means of communicating the absence of love by the person inflicting the violence. . . . The word I use to refer to the absence or deficiency of self-love is shame. Its opposite is pride, by which I mean a healthy sense of self-esteem, self-respect, and self-love. When self-love is sufficiently diminished, one feels shame. (p. 47)

In presenting his model of rehabilitation for those who are overwhelmed by shame, Gilligan uses the rather unusual terms "love," "death of self-esteem," and "resurrection of self-esteem." Figure 7.3 shows the first step of Gilligan's concept of homeostasis that fosters healthy self-esteem, which leads to a productive, satisfying life. Figure 7.3 illustrates the wholesome balance between success and failure that children achieve when they are reared in a positive culture that nurtures their growth through respect, support, and praise. Figure 7.4 shows Gilligan's model of what causes the death of self-esteem. When a child grows up in an unsafe culture that overwhelms his or her emotions with too much failure, self-esteem dies from the toxic emotional stress of shame. Figure 7.5 illustrates Gilligan's model of how it is possible to resurrect self-esteem that has been crushed by shame. As the shame-filled person experiences success, along with affection, love, and support, positive self-esteem comes to life again as emotional homeostasis is restored.

Gilligan's model for resurrecting crushed self-esteem has been criticized because of its "soft" attitude toward adults serv-

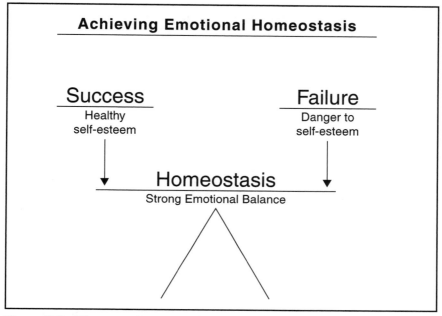

Figure 7.3. When a child's culture provides positive nurture, praise, love, and language stimulation, constructive social emotions begin to emerge in the pre-frontal cortex region of the left brain. Children within this positive culture learn to share, wait their turn, notice the needs of others, and extend kindness. By elementary school years, self-esteem is strong enough to let the child cope with occasional failure without permanent harm to self-image or self-confidence (also called proto-self). The child's personality is well balanced between healthy self-esteem and handling occasional failure or embarrassment. This balance is called *homeostasis.*

ing life sentences for violent crimes. However, the long-range success of his approach that replaces shame with success is beyond question, as Gilligan (1996) has summarized below:

> When one of the Harvard teaching hospitals was awarded a contract . . . to provide psychiatric services at a newly opened prison mental hospital in the late 1970s, I became its medical director. . . . Four years later, I became the clinical director . . . of psychiatric services throughout the (Massachusetts) state prison system . . . from 1981 to 1991. Perhaps the most encouraging thing I learned from that experience is that it is indeed possible to prevent violence. In the Massachusetts state prison

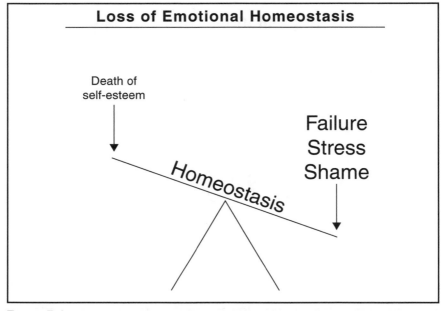

Figure 7.4. If a child's culture is overloaded by the negative emotions and feelings of stress, shame, failure, anger, and lack of love, self-esteem becomes stunted, causing loss of emotional homeostasis. Death of self-esteem occurs when children experience more shame than success during developmental years. These youngsters do not learn to share. They act out in socially disruptive ways through anger, revenge, impatience, impulsivity, self-centeredness, anxiety, fear, intolerance, and explosive tantrums.

> system, the level of lethal violence, both homicidal and suicidal, was reduced to nearly zero, while some other types of violence. . . such as riots and hostage taking . . . simply became nonexistent. (p. 47)

Dyslexia in Prison

As Gilligan and others work with prison populations, they encounter dyslexia among most of the incarcerated juveniles and adults. Since the early 1970s, numerous studies have been done of learning patterns and levels of literacy among prison inmates (Brier, 1989; Jordan, 1974, 1989a, 1996a, 1996b; Payne, 1994; Pollan & Williams, 1992). On average, three out of four males serving prison sentences show significant signs of dyslexia. The

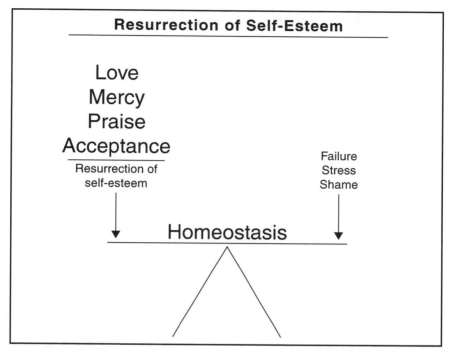

Figure 7.5. When children grow up without praise, love, affection, and positive support, they live in a world of blame, criticism, humiliation, and failure. These negative emotions and feelings "hardwire" the brain to view one's self as shameful. It is possible for "dead self-esteem" to become "resurrected." This new life attitude begins when affection and love begin to generate new hope. As the defeated person experiences the safety of being loved, accepted, and praised, hope begins to replace shame. Step by step, individuals with crushed self-esteem learn to succeed. Each step of success is surrounded by praise and affection from a special person who knows how to replace shame with love. The higher brain begins to absorb facts and new information, which brings a new level of success. Emotional homeostasis comes back into balance. Formerly defeated individuals learn to believe in themselves as "dead self-esteem" becomes "resurrected."

average level of literacy skills within the prison population is below fourth grade. Few of these individuals were identified during their school years as being LD or dyslexic. The issue of shame and crushed self-esteem is a critical factor in understanding why poor readers might become involved in adolescent or adult crime. As Gilligan has demonstrated, violence of any sort usually arises from shame that fosters disruptive or dangerous lifestyles.

The Shame of Being Dyslexic

During the 43 years I have worked one to one with dyslexic individuals, I have learned that the most prevalent emotional state within this population is a lifelong sense of shame. From early childhood, those who are dyslexic live with an inner feeling of shame that threatens to extinguish self-esteem, erode self-confidence, and distort self-image through chronic emotional pain. Before literacy skills can be achieved, shame must be replaced by steps of success that transform the sorrow of failure into the joy of achievement. When instructors press struggling learners with facts about phonics and reading techniques without heeding their hidden feelings of shame, great damage is done to already injured self-esteem. Far too often, well-meaning instructors contribute to the death of self-esteem by imposing threatening or impossible expectations on those who are dyslexic.

Causes of Shame in Individuals Who Are Dyslexic

There are myriad causes for shame in individuals who are dyslexic. Many of those who lack neurological talent for literacy harbor unresolved guilt that often is based on a misunderstanding of what is right or wrong behavior. Others are shamed by physical differences that make them the object of teasing or ridicule. Still others are victims of abuse that convinces them they are "no good" and unworthy of praise or affection. Virtually every person who is dyslexic harbors the feeling that he or she is "dumb" or "stupid," which fosters deep shame as classmates quickly learn new skills while dyslexic individuals lag behind. As Chapter 3 describes, more than half of those who are dyslexic also struggle with poor vision for reading along with difficulty maintaining full attention. Undiagnosed "tagalong" learning problems add to the sense of shame when struggling learners do their best, but their best never is good enough to satisfy parents or instructors.

Shame from Guilt

I met Julian when he was 21 years old. At his mother's insistence, he came to me to find out why he always had struggled with classroom learning. On the surface, Julian appeared self-assured and confident. He was tall, muscular, and well groomed. As we worked through a series of diagnostic activities, I became aware of his barely concealed anxiety toward reading and spelling. After a few minutes of decoding and encoding activities, Julian broke into heavy perspiration from emotional stress. While we took a break, I turned off the overhead lights, leaving my office in an indirect glow from a lamp. Julian visibly relaxed and became calm. Later we discovered that he had moderately severe scotopic sensitivity syndrome. In telling me about himself, he described his father's death when Julian was 2 years old. His parents were in their late teens and did not have a formal wedding. There were no wedding or graduation pictures for the son to cherish. The only picture Julian had of his dad was a faded snapshot showing a young man who closely resembled Julian. "I tried to go to college," he said quietly. "But my high school grades were too low for me to get a scholarship." Without warning, his eyes filled with tears. He clenched his teeth to keep from sobbing as he gripped his chair. Julian bowed his head to cut off eye contact. On a hunch, I asked, "Julian, is it possible that you are having some feelings of shame?"

Suddenly this intense young man exploded into deep sobs. It was obvious that he was in severe emotional pain. Through his tears he gasped, "I'm no good. I can't do anything right. I'm nothing but a cheat. My daddy would be so ashamed of me!" Then his sobs became too intense for him to talk. Finally he said, "I miss my daddy so much! But I know he would be ashamed of me if he were still alive."

In my work with struggling adolescents and adults, often I add touching or holding to exploratory talking that triggers such deep emotions. I knelt beside Julian's chair and put my arms around his shoulders. Suddenly he turned and grasped me in a crushing embrace. He buried his face on my shoulder and continued to sob for several minutes. "I miss my daddy so much!" he repeated. "I've dreamed so many times about him holding me like this. I've dreamed about what it would be like to hug my daddy and have him hug me." Then Julian straightened and turned me loose. "But he would be too ashamed of me. I can't read. I can't spell or write. I've cheated to get through school. I'm nothing but a fake and a cheat. My daddy would be so ashamed of me!" He sat quietly for a few minutes to recover his emotional control.

As we finished the evaluation, I showed Julian his test results and explained what I had discovered in his learning patterns. He was fascinated to know that he was dyslexic, which I explained by showing dyslexic patterns from other adults like those presented in Chapters 4, 5, and 6. For the first time, he understood why he could not learn to spell, sound out words, or write correctly. He could not believe the dramatic way in which two layers of purple overlay stopped print distortions on book pages. With the print stabilized and clear, and with the room in soft, indirect light, Julian began to read, and read, and read. He started to cry again, but this time he shed tears of joy. As we finished our work, his sense of shame was replaced by joy. "I can't believe what you've done for me," he said several times as he embraced me in giant hugs of affection. "I'm not dumb! I'm dyslexic, and I'm scotopic. But I'm not dumb!" he marveled. Then he asked, "Is it possible my daddy was dyslexic? Do you think that's why he dropped out of school?" We discussed the likelihood that his father might have been dyslexic. For the first time, Julian had a positive link with the dad he loved so deeply.

Not all struggling learners achieve this kind of emotional homeostasis so quickly. However, it is not unusual for new self-knowledge within the context of safe affection to bring rapid emotional freedom from shame. As Gilligan (1996) has shown, strongly antisocial behavior often turns around quickly when talking therapy is frank, honest, safe, and straightforward. When shame is replaced by information that explains one's life-long learning difficulty, individuals like Julian seldom need pro-longed psychotherapy to develop new self-esteem that is based on hope and success.

Shame from Guilt About Personal Behavior

A majority of the dyslexic children, adolescents, and adults I have known have suffered from unresolved guilt. Occasionally, I have met individuals so intensely guilt-ridden they have become neu-rotic. Usually the level of guilt is more a nuisance, like a low-level toothache that never quite goes away. This pervasive guilt comes from several sources, all of which stem from the person's failure to live up to moral codes presented by family or society. The family of a child with dyslexia need not be religious to instill feelings of guilt and sin. Most parents and members of the extended family hold certain strong beliefs of what is right or wrong. Sometimes these values are expressed through racial bias that teaches a young child not to associate with certain groups. Religious values often are implanted within the context that a child should not associate with others who believe or practice different faiths. Many children who are dyslexic grow up hearing moral teachings that implant vivid mental images of God's wrath or punishment for certain activities. Most children gradually work out their own interpretations of moral teaching as they begin to read for themselves and develop broader understanding of truth and doctrine. Those who are dyslexic cannot do so for themselves. Few readers who are dyslexic can study scriptural sources for themselves to find out what sacred writings actually say about specific issues. The tone-deaf barrier of auditory dyslexia creates continual misperception that makes it difficult for poor listeners to remember what they hear in sermons, lessons in religion, and family discussions of moral issues. I seldom have met a dyslexic person who had accurate or fluent knowledge of what his or her religion teaches. This special population often lives at the level of superstition, growing up with incomplete understanding of religious doctrine or scriptural truth. It does not matter in what religion the child receives instruction. Individuals who are dyslexic cannot go to printed source materials to find out for themselves what sacred literature says. They must rely on others to interpret moral and spiritual values for them.

Daniel is typical of many dyslexic men I have known. We first met when he was a child. At age 10, he had deep dyslexia at level 8 in severity (see page 38). It was impossible for him to read, spell, do arithmetic computation, or maintain clear central vision without constant help and supervision. He grew up in a devoutly religious home where spiritual values were interpreted in a strict fundamental way. When Daniel's learning problems were identified, he was enrolled in a church-sponsored school where issues of right and wrong were spelled out in a rule book. He could not read the rule book, nor could he read the Bible from which his family and school took their articles of faith.

I saw Daniel frequently through his years in middle school and high school. Then he disappeared. One day he reappeared as one of the most troubled young adults I have seen. His face was contorted by grief, and his body was slouched and disheveled. This young man in his early 20s fell into a chair in my office and began to sob his heart out. After several minutes of weeping, he looked around my office where he had been many times. Finally he said, "It's always so peaceful here. I always feel so safe." Like many others through the years, Daniel had "come home" to a sanctuary where he knew that he would not be judged or criticized.

As Daniel poured out his feelings, I learned that he had attempted suicide a few days before his return to my office. It was his third suicide attempt since his 16th birthday. He hid his face in shame as he whispered his story. He could not look me in the eye. He tried to tell me what was causing such deep grief, but he could not choke out the words. Finally I embraced him and said, "Daniel, you're about to die from guilt, aren't you?" He clung to me and sobbed, "How did you know?" I replied, "Are you feeling this terrible guilt because you believe you've sinned?" As he bowed his head and wept, he nodded yes. Finally I asked, "Is this about sex? Are you feeling guilty from something sexual you've done?"

Suddenly it all came gushing out. For the next hour I listened to Daniel's confession of secret guilt. What a miserable sinner he always had been! What a dirty hypocrite he had turned out to be! Now there was no hope of salvation because God could not love anyone as dirty as he. This litany of guilt went on and on until Daniel was exhausted. Finally I asked what his awful secret sin had been all those years. "I want to have sex with girls," he blurted out. "But that's a sin. The Bible says a man will go to Hell if he thinks about having sex with girls. But I can't help it. It gets so strong sometimes I jerk myself off. Then I want to die because that's a sin and God hates any man who does that to himself. I can't go on living like this. I'm so dirty and filthy. I can't do anything right. I've disappointed you, and if my mom had any idea, she would throw me out of her house."

When Daniel's emotional storm was over, we carefully reviewed his concepts of sin and evil, right and wrong. Like so many other dyslexic persons I have known, he had locked onto several misunderstandings of what his religion taught regarding sexuality. Those misperceptions had colored his entire life. As he entered puberty, his strong sexual drive had overshadowed everything else, creating a neurotic condition that made it impossible for him to function successfully in school or on a job. He could not bring himself to date girls because of his "terrible secret." He isolated himself from normal society because of his belief that spiritually he was filthy for thinking certain things about girls. During his late teens, Daniel began to drink heavily and take drugs to escape his haunting guilt. He began staying up all night because he was afraid to go to sleep. While asleep, he frequently had erotic dreams he thought would doom him to Hell. Many times he tried to read the Bible, but he could not find scriptural passages that dealt with morality and sexuality. He had driven himself into the emotional corner of believing himself to be a vile man, filthy in his Creator's eyes, and unfit as a member of society. This extreme level of guilty suffering had gone on for several years.

Eventually I asked Daniel, "When you look at yourself in the mirror, what do you see?" His reaction was astonishing. "I never look at myself in a mirror!" he exclaimed. "How do you shave?" I asked. "I hold a towel over my face," Daniel said. "I use an electric razor and I feel where it is on my face. If I have to see part of my face, I move the towel just a little. I have no idea what my face looks like. But I know I'm very ugly." In astonishment, I gazed at this handsome young man who easily could have become a fashion model. "What does your body look like?" I asked, referring to his athletic build and good muscle tone. "I have no idea," Daniel replied. "I work out to stay in shape, but I don't know what my body looks like. I can't look at myself. I'm too filthy and ugly."

This story is, of course, an extreme illustration of guilt. Yet most individuals with severe dyslexia harbor some level of unresolved guilt that partly disables their ability to function in society. Few dyslexic adolescents or adults I have known could describe themselves realistically or accurately. Virtually all of these individuals put themselves down when they talk about their physical appearance, attractiveness, appeal to others, or how righteous they might be.

Those who listen to secret stories from dyslexic individuals hear litanies of guilt from sin, inadequacy, failure, and unworthiness. This underlying sense of guilt is like smog over the landscape of a beautiful city. The natural beauty of the person is partially masked by a dark cloud that blots out his or her sense of personal worth. After ancient Israel's King David broke his religious laws with Uriah and Bathsheba, he wrote these poignant words in Psalm 51: "My sin is ever before me." Often this is true with those who are dyslexic. Their perceptions of right and wrong, adequacy and inadequacy, holiness and unholiness, or being worthy and unworthy often are skewed and incomplete. They enter adulthood carrying unresolved burdens of guilt that never have been discussed or analyzed with someone whom they can trust.

It is critically important that supervisors of dyslexic children take care to make issues of morality, sin, and righteousness fully clear. It requires much patient teaching and reteaching to help them comprehend the full meaning of a balanced sense of morality. Whatever the child comprehends about right and wrong, that is what he or she believes to be the truth. When overly sensitive youngsters like Daniel misperceive such vital issues as normal sexuality, that misunderstanding sets into motion lifelong consequences that can disable the person emotionally and spiritually. This adds enormous stress to the already stressful life of growing up with dyslexia.

Shame from Being Different

Few people would win a prize at a beauty contest. Most of us, of whatever age, must make the best of the physical endowments we inherit. How one's body is shaped, the characteristics of one's eyes and ears, the structure of one's face, the quality of one's teeth—all of these factors are part of one's self-image (proto-self). The level of a person's self-esteem is closely tied to personal appearance. This is especially critical for individuals with dyslexia. These sensitive individuals must deal continually with the risk of failure and the stress of probably making a mistake within the next few minutes. If the body is not attractive, it becomes all too easy to slip into the pit of low self-esteem that is so difficult to escape. Young people who do not have dyslexia also have trouble with poorly aligned teeth, slightly crossed eyes, severe acne, large ears, obesity, and so forth. Thoughtful parents do what they can to overcome these physical differences as children mature. If a dyslexic child also has physical differences that diminish appearance, shame causes the self-image to suffer heavily in a culture that emphasizes good looks.

I remember many intelligent, overly sensitive dyslexic youngsters whose parents did not have the wisdom to recognize the importance of their child's physical appearance. For example, countless times during his teen years, I had to calm Mark when he became enraged over his "crooked teeth." This physically attractive boy did have poorly aligned teeth that could have been corrected easily through orthodontal care. But his father saw no need to spend money for that kind of thing. Mark grew up watching his dad drive expensive luxury vehicles and park expensive boat-and-trailer rigs in the driveway. Yet there never was any money for Mark's dental care. At age 36, he still is angry over his "ugliness" that he blames on his dad's ignorance and stubbornness. It has colored all of Mark's self-image and self-esteem. His proto-self is that his mouth is "ugly" and that his smile is offensive to others. In reality, he is a good-looking man, but his inner view of himself is the opposite. Mark lives under a cloud of shame caused by his perceived personal appearance. The lack of parental concern for this boy's sensitivity about his physical appearance instilled a lifelong attitude of being shamefully "ugly" and unattractive. During his school years, this wall of shame made it difficult for teachers to reach Mark on an academic level. The anger embedded within this shameful proto-self has made it impossible for him to succeed in marriage or in lasting personal relationships.

I met Jill when she was 15 years old. She had spent several miserable years in school before her dyslexia was identified and explained to her parents. All her life she had been chubby or obese. By the time she entered high school, her parents concluded that their daughter was "just fat and lazy." Discovering that Jill had a brain-based learning dysfunction did not change their attitude. During her critical teen years, lifelong shame drove her into gorging on foods until she was more than 100 pounds overweight. In addition to being dyslexic, Jill was shy. In the 20 years I have known her, I have never seen her look anyone in the eye. When she talks with me or others whom she trusts, her eyes look elsewhere. As we talk, she looks at me frequently with rapid, darting glances to make sure that I am listening. Whenever her eyes contact mine, she blushes deeply and turns away. As Jill entered adulthood, her self-confidence and self-esteem remained so low that she could not tolerate the normal interaction that comes through eye contact between friends. She made a meager living working in low-paying childcare jobs that reinforced her self-image of "being too dumb" to earn a higher income.

Shortly after her 25th birthday, Jill met a man who liked her and wanted to know her better. She was astonished that any man could be interested in her, given her obesity and the fact that she was so "dumb." As that friendship progressed, Jill joined a weight reduction club and lost 100 pounds. She began to use makeup attractively and dress in better fashion. Yet her self-image remained very low. No matter how good she looked, she could not make eye contact while talking with friends. Finally her special friend gave up trying to build a relationship. There were too many ghosts from Jill's past, too much shame, and too many "old voices" still criticizing her appearance and intelligence to let her believe that anyone could find her attractive or interesting.

Looking One's Best

It is of critical, lifelong importance that children with dyslexia be encouraged to look their best and make the most of their attributes. The brain-based differences that complicate life through learning difficulty need the best possible packaging to allow these individuals to overcome their limitations and enter society successfully. It is false economy for families to save a few dollars during childhood years by not providing orthodontal care, acne treatment, diet or body chemistry control, or good-grooming instruction. From early childhood, self-esteem is too easily fractured in these sensitive, insecure young persons. To face life with deficits in physical appearance in addition to coping with cognitive differences is too much for many fragile ego structures. Of all our children, those who are dyslexic are the most urgently in need of support in developing strong self-image and positive self-esteem that is free from shame.

Shame from Chronic Failure

In societies that stress literacy skills, the most destructive factor for the self-esteem of dyslexic individuals is chronic failure. To have dyslexia in a reading-based society is to risk failure at every turn. From their earliest childhood experiences with language, dyslexic individuals live with invisible moments when their memory "shorts out," causing them to stumble over speech, lose their words, or misunderstand what they hear. Outwardly, persons with dyslexia mask much of their language failure through strategies that divert attention away from their expressive or receptive language problems. By making jokes, clowning for a moment, or changing the subject, they often succeed in hiding dyslexic "blips" that trip up their mental activity. However, these insecure individuals constantly feel the discordant emotional "twang" of another experience of failure or near failure. These lifelong invisible dyslexic failures occur without warning, keeping the individual on edge and feeling uncertain. As early childhood language failure progresses, dyslexic youngsters grow up with low self-confidence in communication skills. By the time they enter school, they have begun to feel "dumb" as they watch their peers become fluent in language activities. As handwriting is introduced, dyslexia no longer is invisible. There on daily papers for all to see is the "proof" that these youngsters must be "dumb" or "stupid," as they have suspected. Failure occurs without warning as individuals who are dyslexic become confused while turning corners or suddenly losing their sense of body-in-space orientation. Mind maps of north, south, east, and west vanish, leaving them lost in familiar places. Awareness of left or right disappears, causing dyslexic individuals not to know which way to turn. These invisible stumbling points may not be observed by others, but inwardly, persons who are dyslexic once again have failed to carry out a normal procedure.

Speaking to others is hazardous for individuals who are dyslexic. The tongue may catch on certain words or strings of syllables, causing another "tongue twist" moment when the flow of articulation gets stuck. The needed word may be lost altogether, creating another awkward moment when the dyslexic speaker cannot continue his or her flow of speech. When dyslexia is below level 5 in severity (see page 38), these chronic oral language "blips" usually are managed well enough so that no one else pays attention. But when these dyslexic patterns are at or above level 6 in severity, the moments of stumbling over words, reversing details, or losing one's body in space become obvious and embarrassing. Early in the dyslexic child's life, he or she begins to feel shame from chronic failure. When dyslexia is at or above level 7, the person continually is being corrected or scolded impatiently by a tone of voice that implies, if it does not say, "Why can't you ever get it right? How many times have you been told how to do it right?" As time goes by, the smog of chronic failure engulfs the person's developing ego structure, blocking out the warmth of praise, affection, and admiration required for the growth of healthy self-esteem.

No Good Stories To Tell

I became acutely aware of lifelong shame from chronic failure during a counseling session with Eric, who was 19 years old. He never had been able to attend a full year of school because of severe fear of failure, called school phobia. Chronic dyslexic failure during his childhood always triggered harsh scoldings and punishment from his father. This punitive family pattern implanted an acutely neurotic personality structure too fragile to cope with group participation. Three times during elementary school years, Eric erupted into violent frenzies at school while trying to defend himself. Three times he was committed to mental health facilities for treatment of pervasive personality disorder. None of those teachers or mental health professionals recognized Eric's severe dyslexia or the depth of shame that permeated every feeling and emotion.

I first met Eric when he was 17. For the first time in his life, he felt safe enough to open himself to someone like me. He trusted me to be gentle with his disabilities and not to criticize his weaknesses. Over time, he cautiously shared extraordinary poetry and song lyrics he had composed during his years of social isolation. We began to talk about his secret thoughts regarding himself and his failure to relate to the outside world. By age 19, Eric was living alone in an apartment that was funded through a program for adults with disabilities. I asked him if he ever visited places where he could meet young adults his age. He said that he had gone to a few singles bars, and occasionally he had gone to church. When he failed to impress others in those social occasions, he decided never to try socializing again. "Why not?" I asked. Without hesitation, he responded with one of the most profound statements I have heard a dyslexic person make: "Because I don't have any good stories to tell."

Those nine simple words gave me a tremendously important piece to the puzzle of dyslexia. After working for 20 years with this special population, finally I understood a major reason why self-esteem is so difficult for individuals who grow up with dyslexia. Chronic failure makes it difficult, often impossible, for them to develop good stories to tell. I had not thought about that before. What do all of us do when we get together? What happens when adults meet at church or synagogue or mosque? What do we do while we visit the barber shop or hair salon? What do friends and neighbors do when they meet in the supermarket? What goes on continually as we work and when we travel? We tell stories. All kinds of stories. Most of our stories are good as we chat about nice things that happen. We tell good stories about the weather, our children, and problems we have solved. Sometimes we tell difficult stories about sorrow or misfortune. We spend a great deal of our social time telling stories.

Individuals with dyslexia often do not have good stories to tell. As Eric explained so clearly, "Sure I have stories to tell. But who wants to hear my stories about getting kicked out of school, or being committed to a mental hospital three times, or being put on drugs to make me calm, or how my dad yelled and cussed me out? What kind of girl wants to go out with a guy who tells stories like that? And you know the weird sex fantasies I have a lot. I sure can't tell those stories to decent people. Nobody wants to hear my stories about being afraid all the time and being paranoid about strangers. I sure don't have any good stories to tell about school. Who wants to spend an evening listening to my stories about flunking third grade and being kicked out of elementary school? You're the only person I ever met who will even listen to my stories and not think I'm crazy."

Developing Good Stories To Tell

Earlier this chapter described Gilligan's success at teaching violent criminals how to develop good stories to tell. By replacing shame with success along with praise and safe affection, violent habits are transformed into productive behavior that quickly generates a repertoire of good stories to tell. Although Eric's unfortunate life is a rare result of being dyslexic, his chronic failures at school, at home, and in society are a mirror of what most dyslexic individuals experience to some degree. It need not be this way. Children with dyslexia who are blessed with patient, observant relatives develop good stories to tell. Students who are fortunate enough to spend several years with intuitive, flexible teachers develop anthologies of good tales about ways in which they succeeded within the school environment. They did not make top grades, but they were given opportunities to earn praise, which is what good storytelling is all about. When athletes who are dyslexic have thoughtful, caring coaches, they develop many good stories about athletic success and achievement. Dyslexic individuals with strong right-brain talents for drawing, painting, tool handling, and computer skills emerge into adulthood with many good stories to tell and show. When young adults with dyslexia meet caring romance partners who accept left-brain limitations without rejection, they learn good stories about love, affection, and the fun of a good relationship. The key to replacing shame with good stories to tell is patient, affectionate relationships that instill trust surrounded by success. When leaders are thoughtful, patient, and careful to make things clear, bright dyslexic youngsters like Eric develop a repertoire of good stories to tell.

Coping with the Lifelong Stress of Being Dyslexic

The most critical challenge a person with dyslexia faces is coping with stress. From their first language experiences until the end of their lives, dyslexic individuals wrestle with the ever-present factor of stress. Youngsters who will become dyslexic students begin life failing to comprehend the flow of oral language that surrounds them. They fail to remember details accurately. They misinterpret countless social signals that must be understood correctly if one is to be a functional member of society. Children who are dyslexic continually mishear words, misperceive instructions, misinterpret jokes and conversations, and misunderstand the complex world in which they live. Having dyslexia means experiencing the never-ending stress of trying to do one's best but continually disappointing key people in one's life.

The chronic social and academic stress experienced by dyslexic individuals is similar to living with chronic pain. On better days the pain can be ignored, but it still is there whenever the body makes certain movements. In a similar way, on better days those who are dyslexic almost forget their language-processing awkwardness, but always it is there, ready to trip them up without warning. This haunting insecurity in language processing colors all relationships with a depressing shade of gray. As dyslexic children mature into adolescence, and as adolescence becomes adulthood, this invisible pressure from stress takes its toll. Self-image, self-esteem, and self-confidence must grow in a rocky soil that never is free from the arid influence of stress.

Levels of Stress

Earlier chapters have shown that dyslexic patterns range widely from mild (an occasional nuisance) to severe (a serious disability). To understand how lifelong stress influences individuals with dyslexia, it is necessary to review the severity scale. Stress follows this continuum closely.

1	2	3		4	5	6	7		8	9	10
	mild				moderate					severe	

Mild Dyslexia

When dyslexic symptoms are mild, a person occasionally reverses certain symbols and sometimes tangles the tongue saying longer words. Mild dyslexia forces individuals to consult a dictionary for accurate spelling. This level of dyslexic stumbling creates mild stress that comes and goes with circumstances. Mild dyslexic episodes trigger momentary frustration that is stressful. However, these moments of feeling the stress of mild dyslexia rarely handicap a person's emotions or trigger moodiness. Occasionally, mild dyslexic "blips" bring criticism from a teacher, parent, or job supervisor who wishes the person would be more careful. Momentary stress occurs as feelings of embarrassment and frustration surge, but this level of stress is neither chronic nor harmful to one's sense of well-being. Most individuals who have mild or occasional dyslexic patterns handle this degree of stress with no damage done to self-confidence or self-esteem.

Moderate Dyslexia

Stress becomes a lifelong challenge when dyslexic symptoms are within the moderate range of severity. Individuals whose dyslexic patterns are at levels 5, 6, or 7 make continual mistakes. Spelling never is fully accurate, and details continually scramble out of sequence. Listening comprehension is faulty and unpredictable, causing continual misunderstanding, and reading is slow and labored. Persons with moderate dyslexia have difficulty taking accurate notes rapidly enough to keep up with the flow of new information. They confuse or reverse body-in-space directions (east/west, north/south, up/down, top/bottom, left/right). They continually forget important things unless they keep written lists and daily schedules, and they habitually are late for meetings and appointments. These individuals usually are slow doing certain kinds of activities that require recall of specific information. As they speak, they lose their words and cannot always remember what to call familiar objects. They are socially awkward, hesitant, slow, and prone to make many more "care-less" mistakes than others their age. Moderately dyslexic individuals live under a constant weight of stress because they cannot meet society's expectations without continual pangs of shame when they fail. These persons rarely find safe places or circumstances where they are accepted without some kind of judgment or criticism coloring the relationship.

Severe Dyslexia

When dyslexic symptoms are at the severe range, individuals live in a constant state of heavy stress. Few persons at levels 8 and 9 know what it is to be free from social, educational, economic, or family stress. Those who are at level 10 often do not survive without serious mental health problems because their developmental years are so heavily saturated by stress that crushes self-esteem through shame. Individuals with severe dyslexia grow up under a dark cloud of constant criticism. Throughout childhood and adolescence they hear, "You messed up again!" or "Why don't you ever do it right?" or "Don't you ever listen to what I tell you?" If these strugglers are fortunate enough to have parents who are compassionate and supportive, reduction of stress at home often is offset by teachers who do not provide compassionate support. If a brother or sister seems to understand, grandparents or other relatives may not. If a boss is tolerant and forgiving, other job supervisors are critical and demanding. If adolescents or adults with severe dyslexia allow themselves to seek romance through dating, they run the risk of being rejected once that special friend finds out about dyslexia.

Individuals with severe dyslexia also face overwhelming emotional trauma trying to find work. If they reveal their condition, few employers will hire them, and they are denied admission into military service. If they say much about having dyslexia, they are told, "Well, we all have our problems," or "You just use your dyslexia as an excuse." These insecure individuals continually meet adults who believe that dyslexia is linked to mental retardation, or that there is no such thing as dyslexia. Everywhere these persons turn, they face the stress either of dealing with the problem alone or of being rejected and criticized because of it. From the earliest childhood years when toddlers begin to interact with their larger world, youngsters who struggle with language development feel the stress of being different and not being correctly understood.

No one can develop normally and wholesomely if he or she cannot find respite from stress. Even in persons who are not dyslexic, stress takes a heavy toll in heart disease, digestive problems, anxiety, mental health, ruptured personal relationships, and so forth. It is impossible for anyone to be a whole person if stress exists day after day, year after year. The irony of dyslexia is that the language-processing deficits that trigger stress cannot be removed through counseling or psychotherapy. This genetic life pattern is built in from the moment of conception, as Chapter 1 describes. Severe dyslexia is a lifelong factor that cannot be removed. Dyslexic individuals must develop ways to cope so that stress can be reduced as much as possible, as Chapter 8 suggests.

Multiple Brain Differences and Dyslexia

A major outcome of recent brain research is the concept of dual diagnosis when two or more differences come together. This is called *comorbity*. For example, Russell Barkley's (1990, 1995) research with attention deficit disorder discovered that 65% of those with attention deficit with hyperactivity (ADHD) also have a personality dysfunction called oppositional defiant disorder (ODD). Thirty percent of those with ADHD also have conduct disorder (CD). Barkley determined that 20% to 30% of ADHD individuals also have some type of specific learning disability. Barkley's research demonstrated why making dual diagnosis is critical in treating ADHD. If ADHD is treated alone with cortical stimulant (Ritalin, Cylert, or Adderall), 30% of those individuals show improvement in paying attention, listening effectively, finishing tasks without supervision, and practicing positive social skills. However, if a second type of medication also is prescribed to treat comorbid mood or conduct disorders, 55% of ADHD patients treated for dual disorders show improvement.

Research by Helen Irlen (1991), Dale Jordan (1996a, 1996b, 1998, 2000a, 2000b), and Laura Weisel (1992, 2001) has revealed that more than half of those with dyslexia also have central vision disorders, such as scotopic sensitivity syndrome or Aubert–Foerster syndrome. My clinical experience with struggling learners indicates that as many as 65% of those with dyslexia also have some degree of attention deficit disorder (ADHD or ADD) (Jordan, 1989b, 1996a, 1998, 2000a, 2000b). Research by Nancie Payne (1994), Laura Weisel (1992, 2001), and Carolyn Pollan and Dorothy Williams (1992) found 45% overlap of dyslexia/ADHD or ADD/behavior disorders among adolescents and young adults who read poorly and have difficulty with classroom performance.

Mood Disorders and Dyslexia

Less well documented is the frequent coexistence of mood disorders and dyslexia. The process for diagnosing dyslexia has been explained in Chapter 4. However, if only these assessment strategies are considered, it is easy to overlook comorbid problems with chronic moods that afflict many who are dyslexic. The growing trend for dual diagnosis focuses on looking beneath the surface of whatever problem brings an individual to be diagnosed for learning difficulties (Damasio, 1994, 1999; Jordan, 1998, 2000b; Ratey & Johnson, 1997; Schacter, 1996). Figure 7.6 presents the Jordan Social–Emotional LD Mood Index, which summarizes the range of mood disorders often seen in individuals who are dyslexic. If these underlying emotional factors are ignored or are not diagnosed, then treatment for dyslexia is mostly ineffective.

Depression and Dyslexia

The mood disorder that most frequently accompanies dyslexia is chronic depression that often has existed for several years. Most individuals experience brief bouts of depression that are triggered by ill health, job loss, financial difficulty, breakdown in important personal relationships, death of a friend or relative, or academic failure. This type of mood dysfunction is called *situational depression* because it comes and goes in reaction to changes in one's life. Chronic depression that lingers for long periods of time is caused by imbalance in the brain's neurotransmitters dopamine, serotonin, and acetylcholine. These brain chemicals regulate emotions and feelings that originate in the higher brain and midbrain (see Figures 7.1 and 7.2). The tendency for chronic depression often is inherited along with dyslexia. If underlying depression is not recognized, it is impos-

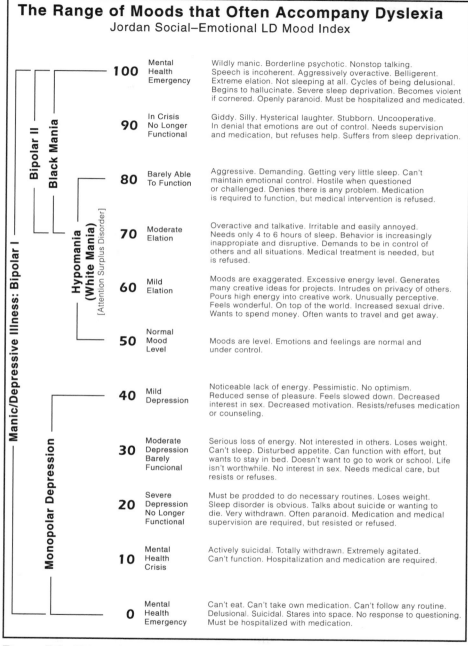

The Range of Moods that Often Accompany Dyslexia
Jordan Social–Emotional LD Mood Index

100 — Mental Health Emergency — Wildly manic. Borderline psychotic. Nonstop talking. Speech is incoherent. Aggressively overactive. Belligerent. Extreme elation. Not sleeping at all. Cycles of being delusional. Begins to hallucinate. Severe sleep deprivation. Becomes violent if cornered. Openly paranoid. Must be hospitalized and medicated.

90 — In Crisis No Longer Functional — Giddy. Silly. Hysterical laughter. Stubborn. Uncooperative. In denial that emotions are out of control. Needs supervision and medication, but refuses help. Suffers from sleep deprivation.

80 — Barely Able To Function — Aggressive. Demanding. Getting very little sleep. Can't maintain emotional control. Hostile when questioned or challenged. Denies there is any problem. Medication is required to function, but medical intervention is refused.

70 — Moderate Elation — Overactive and talkative. Irritable and easily annoyed. Needs only 4 to 6 hours of sleep. Behavior is increasingly inappropiate and disruptive. Demands to be in control of others and all situations. Medical treatment is needed, but is refused.

60 — Mild Elation — Moods are exaggerated. Excessive energy level. Generates many creative ideas for projects. Intrudes on privacy of others. Pours high energy into creative work. Unusually perceptive. Feels wonderful. On top of the world. Increased sexual drive. Wants to spend money. Often wants to travel and get away.

50 — Normal Mood Level — Moods are level. Emotions and feelings are normal and under control.

40 — Mild Depression — Noticeable lack of energy. Pessimistic. No optimism. Reduced sense of pleasure. Feels slowed down. Decreased interest in sex. Decreased motivation. Resists/refuses medication or counseling.

30 — Moderate Depression Barely Funcional — Serious loss of energy. Not interested in others. Loses weight. Can't sleep. Disturbed appetite. Can function with effort, but wants to stay in bed. Doesn't want to go to work or school. Life isn't worthwhile. No interest in sex. Needs medical care, but resists or refuses.

20 — Severe Depression No Longer Functional — Must be prodded to do necessary routines. Loses weight. Sleep disorder is obvious. Talks about suicide or wanting to die. Very withdrawn. Often paranoid. Medication and medical supervision are required, but resisted or refused.

10 — Mental Health Crisis — Actively suicidal. Totally withdrawn. Extremely agitated. Can't function. Hospitalization and medication are required.

0 — Mental Health Emergency — Can't eat. Can't take own medication. Can't follow any routine. Delusional. Suicidal. Stares into space. No response to questioning. Must be hospitalized with medication.

Left-side bracketing labels: Manic/Depressive Illness: Bipolar I; Bipolar II; Black Mania; Hypomania (White Mania) [Attention Surplus Disorder]; Monopolar Depression

Figure 7.6. This wide range of mood disorders often coexists with dyslexia. The diagnostic tests used most often to identify dyslexia are not designed to reveal underlying moods that interfere with learning and group participation. *Note.* From *Understanding and Managing Learning Disabilities in Adults,* by D. R. Jordan, 2000, Malabar, FL: Krieger. Copyright 2000 by Krieger. Reprinted with permission.

sible for the person to benefit from tutoring or classroom instruction. Depression keeps the brain in a state of elevated emotional stress that robs the higher brain of its ability to translate new data into permanent memory.

The Effect of Chronic Depression with Dyslexia

The most important effect of long-term depression is the way that very low moods rob individuals of positive self-esteem and self-knowledge. Persistent depression distorts emotional reality so that it becomes impossible for the person to be realistic about his or her self-worth. Like a constant voice in the background, depression whispers, "You're dumb. You're ugly. No one thinks highly of you. There's no use trying because you will fail anyway. You're nothing but a failure. No one loves you because you're so unlovely and undesirable." This destructive emotional litany never ends when depression is in control. The victim of depression hears only negative brain language with no hope that life ever will improve.

Deeply depressed individuals are immersed in worry and grief that remain out of proportion to reality. If money is a little short, the individual in depression believes that financial ruin has occurred. If a friend or loved one offers a compliment, the person in depression is offended, believing that others are lying. An active ingredient of depression is paranoia that is suspicious of others, distrustful of all situations, and unable to cope with any stress that emerges within relationships. Without hope, the depressed person sees only gloom, sorrow, and futility. The brain's inner voice mutters sadly over and over: "Why try? It won't make any difference. Why bother? I'll only fail again. Why be polite? They don't really like me anyway. Why take a shower and do my hair? I'm too ugly to be attractive, no matter what I do. Why go to work? I'm going to be fired anyway. Why go to class? I'm too dumb to learn. . . ." This negative self-perception of depression is dangerous because it coaxes the person into thinking about death. Suicide becomes more attractive than continuing to live like this. When dyslexia also exists, depressed individuals often make the attempt to destroy themselves.

Paul was one of the most depressed young men I have ever met. He never had done well in school, in spite of continual encouragement and support from his parents. His years in school were so miserable that he grew up thinking about how to kill himself. Only his intense fear of going to Hell kept him from making a suicide attempt. During primary grades he became withdrawn, sullen, and angry. No matter how hard his parents and teachers tried to cheer him up and encourage him, Paul's attitude snarled back, "Leave me alone!" He entered high school with few academic skills, no close friends, no hope, and a constant wish to die. A few weeks after he entered 10th grade, one of Paul's teachers took special interest in this lonely, withdrawn student. With exceptional intuition, she looked beneath Paul's sullen surface and saw signs of language disability and deep sadness. She convinced his parents to have their son evaluated for possible learning disability and emotional problems.

I first met Paul when he was 16 years old. He entered my office sandwiched between his mother and father who always walked beside him as human shields, protecting him from the world that he perceived to be threatening and unfriendly. Paul sat between them around my circular conference table. Never before had I seen such a grief-stricken adolescent. At age 16 he was 6 feet, 5 inches tall with an athletic build and such a handsome face he reminded me of several movie stars. His immaculate grooming surprised me as I saw the depth of his depression. In that first meeting, he scarcely spoke, and he avoided eye contact with me. His mother did most of the talking on his behalf. I learned that as he reached age 15, Paul had begun to talk openly about wanting to die. He had stopped trying to do school assignments without his mother's help. He no longer attended religious services with his family. When visitors came, he shut himself in his room. He had no friends, he avoided all social events, and he refused to read. He spent many hours sitting before his television with the sound turned off. His parents could not tell if he watched the shows on his screen.

As his parents and I talked quietly, Paul began to glance at me, then quickly look away. Whenever I spoke his name, he looked my way but refused to make eye contact. He sat with head bowed, hands folded tightly in his lap, and body stiff in a rigid posture. As our conference continued, I saw Paul's body begin to relax. Finally his posture was normal, and he separated his hands in a comfortable way. He listened intently to what his parents and I discussed, but he did not take part in our conversation except to nod "yes" or shake his head "no."

I was surprised when Paul agreed to come again so that he and I could work alone. During our first private visit, he chose to sit beside me close enough to let our arms touch now and then. I placed a tablet and pencil on the table and asked him to write the alphabet, days of the week, and months of the year. Figure 7.7 shows his work. As he wrote, I noticed that his face became flushed and he was breathing harder. I asked if he would mind writing some words I would dictate. He said it would be OK. Figure 7.8 shows the dyslexic patterns that emerged on that dictated spelling activity.

As Paul finished writing the last word, he was trembling. His eyes were filled with tears, and he was breathing rapidly with shallow gulps of air. Suddenly he cried out and clutched at his chest. To my surprise, he fell to his knees and bowed his head low. I knelt beside him and encircled his shoulders with my arms. "I'm having a heart attack," Paul choked. "No, Paul," I said. "You aren't having a heart attack. You're having a panic attack that makes your chest feel tight." Slowly he relaxed in my embrace, then he began to cry. I held him for several minutes while his sobs released the tension that had triggered those physical signals of too much emotional stress.

When Paul was relaxed again, we talked about times when such panic attacks occurred. "They started when I was in third grade," he remembered. "I didn't tell anyone because I was afraid they would make me go to a doctor. But all my life, sometimes it drops me to my knees and makes me feel like I'm about to die. It hurts so much. And I'm all alone and nobody knows what's happening to me."

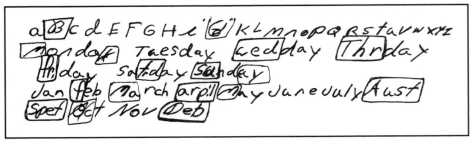

Figure 7.7. This 16-year-old boy reached 10th grade before a teacher recognized signs of dyslexia in his writing. From primary grades he had lived in a state of deep depression that was not recognized by his pediatrician, teachers, or parents.

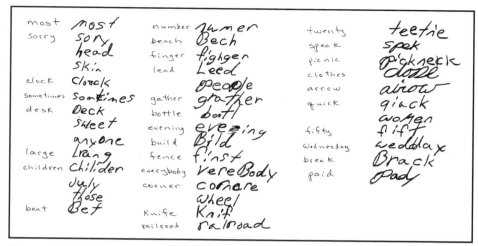

Figure 7.8. Writing these dictated spelling words triggered frightening physical sensations for this 16-year-old student who had severe chronic depression. His face flushed, his eyes filled with tears, his heart beat faster, and his rate of breathing increased. He was engulfed by pains in his chest that caused him to fear he was having a heart attack.

I showed Paul a map of the brain to let him see where emotions come from. He was fascinated with the information shown in Figures 7.1 and 7.2. Then we talked about dyslexia and how it had made reading, spelling, and writing so hard and fearful for him. "Will I ever get over all this?" he asked. I explained that a certain kind of medication called an antidepressant might help his brain chemistry become normal. He agreed to see a psychiatrist who specialized in treating mood disorders in children and adolescents. That doctor was himself moderately dyslexic. Paul was amazed that a doctor could be so understanding. After taking antidepressant medication for 2 weeks, Paul came to see me again. He entered my office with a broad smile. Then he laughed. He lifted me off the floor in a huge embrace while he laughed and chuckled. Finally he put me down so we could talk. "I'm like a new guy," he said with a twinkle of joy in his eyes. "My brain works better than it ever has before. I've decided that life isn't so bad, after all. I had no idea that this is the way most people feel all the time."

With his feelings of depression replaced by new self-confidence, Paul was eager to find out how intelligent he was. He was fascinated as we worked through the *Wechsler Adult Intelligence Scale–Third edition* (WAIS–III; Wechsler, 1994a). Figure 7.9 shows the very wide subscore scatter that usually signals dyslexia. Paul was intrigued as I explained the concept of different neurological talents. He touched his IQ profile, feeling the high IQ areas as well as the lower IQ subtests. "So this is why I've never felt good at school," he said quietly. "I just thought I was too dumb to learn. I've always been so ashamed of being dumb. Now I guess I'll have to change my mind about myself." For the first time in his life, through correct medication, Paul experienced the joy of emotional peace as dopamine and serotonin became balanced throughout his brain. He rapidly caught up in academic learning and later earned a university degree in computer science.

Bipolar Disorder (Manic/Depressive Illness) with Dyslexia

The first time I saw 13-year-old Phil was like standing outdoors in a hailstorm. Half an hour before he was scheduled to meet me, his father shoved the screaming boy into the reception area of my office, then fled down the elevator. When I came out of my office to investigate the commotion, I was confronted by a violently angry boy who had no intention of cooperating with this forced situation. I stopped just out of arm's reach and looked at Phil. Like a trapped wild animal, he snarled at me, "I hate being here. You can't make me do anything." His arms were crossed over his chest in a classical stance of defiance. I absorbed his violent feelings without comment. "I mean it!" he screamed. "You can't make me do anything!" I said nothing, which surprised him. Like most overly angry youngsters, Phil's strategy was to start a fight in order to keep adults off balance and out of control. When I refused to fight, he had no alternative course of action. For several minutes we stared at each other. Then I smiled. "You can't make me!" he declared again, but he unlocked his arms and shoved his hands into his pockets. I smiled again. Phil was too bewildered to keep on being angry. "Let's find someplace to sit down," I said as I turned away. To let me know that he would not be conquered, he stomped his feet as he followed me into my office. Phil was surprised with what he saw. Nothing looked like school or like a doctor's office. Everywhere he looked he saw a comfortable, quiet

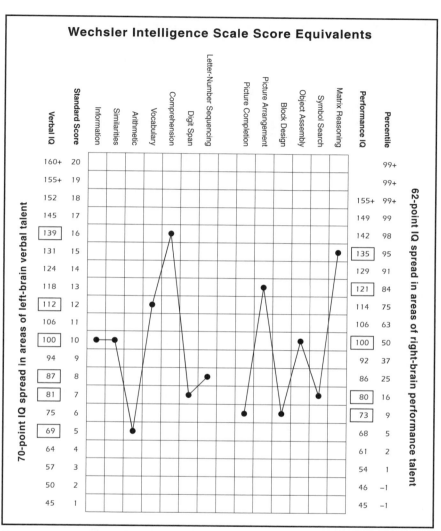

Figure 7.9. This kind of very wide subscore pattern usually signals the presence of dyslexia. This imbalance among an individual's neurological talents triggers constant stress in academic activities and often induces long-term depression.

place that was safe. I sat at my large round table and smiled again. In the middle of the table was a large dish of hard candy and chewing gum. He watched as I unwrapped a piece of candy. Without a word, he grabbed a piece of candy, than flopped down on a giant bean bag across the room. "I don't want to be here," he said quietly. His anger was gone. "I know you don't want to be here," I said, as I sat on the floor near the bean bag. "But I also know you don't want to be at school. Why not?"

For the next half hour I listened to a torrent of pain as Phil lashed out at school, teachers, his parents, and all the "weird kids" who hated him. It was the first time an adult had listened to his feelings without interrupting or criticizing him. Finally Phil trusted me enough to let me in. When I asked him to tell me why he felt such negative things, he burst into tears and spent the next several minutes sobbing with his head behind his arms. Through his sobs he choked out enough words to let me understand: "I can't read. . . . Can't spell. . . . I'm stupid. . . . Hate school. . . . Makes me feel so dumb. . . . Kids are mean to me. . . . Everyone hates me. . . . Life sucks!" It was midmorning before Phil's emotions and feelings were calm. With his anger gone, he began to talk about himself. He told me that sometimes he went crazy and climbed onto the roof and tried to fly to the moon. Several times he had climbed more than 100 feet to the top of the city water tower and wondered what it would be like to jump off. Then he described times when he felt so sad he crawled to the back of his clothes closet and hid beneath a pile of blankets. Sometimes he ran away from home just to make his parents angry. Other times he would not get out of bed for 2 or 3 days on end. "I'm crazy," he confided to me. "I've never said this before to anyone, but I'm crazy. I'm no good, and I'm crazy."

That extended talking released Phil's anger and caused him to relax. Finally he was ready to do some work with me after I promised not to make fun of his writing. "I'm a lousy writer," he said. "It drives my parents nuts when I make an F on spelling tests." I let Phil sit on the bean bag to write the alphabet, days of the week, and months of the year. "This is a dumb thing to do," he said. I explained that it would help me answer some important questions about why schoolwork was hard for him. With a very skeptical expression, he wrote what is shown in Figure 7.10. "You promised me you won't laugh," he said. "I hated doing that."

By then Phil and I had been together for 2 hours. He paced my office, examining everything in the room. My office was filled with pictures, sculptures, and other handmade art objects. He wanted to know where I had gotten all of those things. I explained that each art object was a gift from someone who had spent time with me finding out how school could become better. I commented that all of this art was done by intelligent individ-

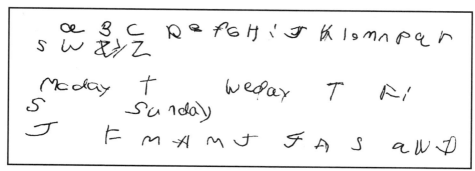

Figure 7.10. This was the best an intelligent 13-year-old boy could do writing the alphabet, days, and months. Later dual diagnosis revealed that he was severely dyslexic along with suffering from bipolar disorder (manic/depressive illness, bipolar I).

uals who had found out about themselves by working with me. Finally I asked Phil if he would let me find out how intelligent he was. "I'm stupid," he snapped. "I told you I'm dumb." "What if I find out you're actually very bright?" "You can't do that," he said defiantly. "Yes, I think I can," I said. "Will you give me the chance to find out?" Phil decided it would be OK. We spent another hour working through the *Wechsler Intelligence Scale for Children–Revised* (WISC–R; Wechsler, 1974). He was stunned when I showed him the results: verbal IQ, 124; performance IQ, 132; full-scale IQ, 130. Phil sat down on the bean bag and stared at me. Then his eyes filled with tears. "You're not joking me, are you?" he asked. Suddenly he was sobbing as he beat the floor with his fist. "I've spent my life feeling so dumb. You don't know how much I've hurt over being stupid. Now you tell me I'm very intelligent. This makes me so mad! Why didn't anyone ever tell me this before?"

At that moment my receptionist rang to tell me that Phil's father was there to take him home. "I don't want to leave," Phil said. "I want to stay here. Can't you tell my dad that you need me to stay this afternoon? I'll do a lot more work. Just tell him I need to stay." As I had seen so often, unexpected hope had begun to replace deep shame in a bright person who is dyslexic. That morning was the first experience of joy that Phil could remember. At last he had tasted success, and he craved much, much more. Later an intuitive psychiatrist diagnosed a serious mood disorder called *manic/depressive illness: bipolar I* (see Figure 7.6). The dual diagnosis of dyslexia and bipolar disorder is not unusual in low-performing students whose moods swing from manic high to depressive low. Eventually Phil and the psychiatrist discovered the right medication called SSRI (selective serotonin reuptake inhibitor) that stabilized the neurotransmitters throughout his brain. The wide mood swings disappeared, allowing Phil to have access to his high intelligence to learn how to overcome dyslexia.

Building a Positive Self-Image

For persons who are dyslexic, positive self-image develops through "baby steps" over a period of time. Those who are not troubled by left-brain language limitations judge success by long strides forward, but individuals with learning differences gain success a little at a time. Dyslexic youngsters who are fortunate enough to live within compassionate, observant families make small steps of progress all of their lives because self-esteem continually is supported and nurtured. Language gaps are gently supplemented, not criticized. Directional confusion becomes part of a funny family game as everyone thinks of ways to help the dyslexic individual master left and right, north and south, east and west. All kinds of memory tricks are developed through rhymes and simple ways to keep things straight. Dyslexia is managed through good humor, not by scoldings and punishment when awkwardness or forgetfulness occurs.

Every "baby step" of progress is praised, the way star pupils are praised for outstanding achievement. Moments of fear that cause the child to freeze are treated thoughtfully, not with criticism. Impulsiveness or lapses of good judgment are absorbed by the family as the dyslexic child is guided through the family standards of right and wrong. Tongue twisters that all dyslexic individuals create are treated with delight, as the child makes a contribution to the family's fun and joy. John runs into the house to show his mom the "sliver dime" he found in change from the store. From that moment everyone looks for "sliver dimes." One day Jerri told her dad, "I'm too trier to play any more Uno," and ever after her family had a wonderful way of saying "I'm tired." Through this kind of gentle, humorous praise, a dyslexic person's contribution is honored, not criticized.

Parents and other relatives actively look beneath surface dyslexic patterns to find the child's natural bent and talents. During childhood and adolescence, adults look for special skills or talents that set the child apart in spite of chronic trouble with reading and spelling. Then the family helps this child to grow in his or her unique ways. Over a period of years, all of these "baby steps" carry the child through adolescence and into adulthood with a healthy ego structure, strong self-image, and positive self-esteem. Such a fortunate person enjoys looking into the mirror because the image looking back is good and worthy of being praised. This individual with good stories to tell is strong, intelligent, interesting, and alive with hope. Always it must be remembered that good stories come gradually over time. Unless at least one parent figure honors the child's differences as being strengths, it is very difficult for a dyslexic youngster to become a confident adult with good stories to tell. By the time I met Eric, it was too late. For the rest of my life, I shall wonder what difference it could have made had I met him and his parents when he was a child. Perhaps his overly angry father could have learned to deal with his son's differences more positively. If that highly sensitive boy had learned a few good stories to tell along the way, perhaps his adult self-esteem could have been salvaged and restored.

Developing Social Skills and Independence

8

This book began with a review of current knowledge of how the brain learns and remembers. Chapters 1 and 2 summarize the milestone neurological discoveries since 1869 that support the concept that dyslexia and other types of LD originate within specific regions of the brain when neurons, dendrites, and axons fail to mature on schedule. Chapters 3 through 6 describe the often devastating consequences of visual dyslexia, auditory dyslexia, dysgraphia, and dyscalculia. These forms of learning difference (LD) arise from anatomical differences in left-brain structure. For more than 100 years, attention has been focused mainly on left-brain learning difficulties related to language processing.

Professionals of my generation, who began working with struggling learners in the 1950s and 1960s, were aware that many persons with dyslexia display irregular, often disruptive patterns of immature emotions, exaggerated feelings, mood swings, and a lack of commonsense reasoning. In my first classroom teaching experiences with adolescents who were illiterate, I had to cope with a continual overlay of emotionality that kept many of them in conflict with peers, parents, and leaders. I have met children, then grandchildren, of the first dyslexic individuals I encountered in 1957. This three-generational involvement has let me observe the impact of combined immaturity and negative feelings and emotions on the lives of those who have dyslexia. In the early years of my professional experience, a well-defined model of the emotional side of learning disabilities did not exist.

Nonverbal Learning Disabilities

In 1971, Doris Johnson and Helmut Myklebust published their landmark analysis of what they called *nonverbal learning disabilities* (NVLD). They defined this dysfunction as the inability to comprehend the significance of what occurs in the social world surrounding the person. Johnson and Myklebust pinpointed three primary characteristics of NVLD. First, they noted a major social deficit: *NVLD individuals are very poor at pretending.* For example, suppose that several friends are having fun with a make-believe situation. Spontaneous jokes are flying, everyone is laughing or giggling at silly words and outrageous ideas, and the group is having a wonderful time teasing each other. Individuals with NVLD do not get the point. They are puzzled and out of the loop in this kind of pretend socialization. Second, *persons with NVLD cannot anticipate.* A major part of socialization involves guessing ahead, predicting what probably will happen next, speculating about what maybe lies ahead, and making small talk about what might be. NVLD individuals do not have this quick ability to look ahead or anticipate what might come next. Third, *NVLD individuals cannot read nonverbal social signals.* They are "socially blind" to facial expressions, hand gestures, body language, friendly touching, and tone of voice. Persons with NVLD do not comprehend these paralanguage components of successful socialization. Johnson and Myklebust concluded that such individuals fail to read nonverbal social signals the way that dyslexic persons fail to interpret printed symbols. In the 1970s, NVLD often was called "social dyslexia."

Right-Brain Influence

In 1978, Martha Denckla, pediatric neurologist at Johns Hopkins University School of Medicine, expanded the concept of NVLD to include visual perceptual deficits as part of the social–emotional difficulties generated by NVLD. During the 1980s, new brain imaging technologies made it possible to explore deeper and more complex regions of the brain. New knowledge of right-brain functions led Drake Duane (1985), a neuroscientist at the Mayo Clinic, to develop the concept he called *right-hemi syndrome.* Right-hemi syndrome described individuals whose lifestyles manifested the following irregular behaviors:

_____ Often is well educated.

_____ Cannot maintain eye contact while conversing.

_____ Speaks in an irritating sing-song way (prosody).

_____ Smothers friends and relatives with inappropriate displays of possessive affection.

_____ Triggers such intense dread in others that friends, peers, and relatives find excuses to avoid the individual.

_____ Is blind to social signals.

_____ Cannot comprehend the issues of personal privacy and personal space.

In 1986, Kytia Voeller, psychiatric specialist in childhood disorders, described the *right-hemisphere deficit syndrome.* This concept linked two pervasive childhood patterns to right-brain damage or dysfunction: *stubborn / resistive behavior* (now called oppositional defiant disorder) and *failure to interpret social cues.* The youngsters Voeller studied could not express their feelings in typical ways, yet they seemed aware of emotions in others. Voeller concluded that right-brain differences relate directly to the ability to enter into appropriate social relationships. In 1987, a team of neurologists led by Daniel Tranel studied maladaptive social behavior and erratic school performance in patients who had sustained injuries to the right brain (Tranel, Hall, Olson, & Tranel, 1987). Tranel and his colleagues adopted the term *right-hemisphere learning disability* to describe poor socialization patterns of NVLD individuals. Tranel's team concluded that lesions along neural pathways throughout the right brain contribute to chronic disturbances in social skills and emotional balance. In 1988, Robert Joseph at the Neurobehavioral Center in San Jose, California, published a comprehensive review of what had been learned about right-brain influence on emotion, visual/spatial skills, body image awareness, dreams, and awareness of social processes. His research pulled together a large body of knowledge of how neural development within the right cerebral cortex determines how well individuals interpret and interact with the social world around them.

In 1990 Margaret Semrud-Clikeman and George Hynd reviewed the latest evidence that right-hemispheric dysfunction is directly related to behaviors called NVLD. That study covered a broad range of behavioral, emotional, and perceptual dysfunctions that are linked to differences in right-brain structure and development. Denckla (1991a, 1991b) estimated that 10% of all persons with left-brain LD (dyslexia, attention deficits, aphasia) also manifest right-brain NVLD characteristics.

In 1993 a further piece was added to the puzzle of right-brain involvement with poor socialization skills and inadequate commonsense reasoning. Vilayanur Ramachandrian (1993) at the University of California in San Diego discovered what he called *unidentified bright objects* (UBOs) along axon pathways within right-brain regions involved with mood control. New brain imaging techniques allowed him to see extremely small breaks in the myelin sheath surrounding axon segments (see Figure 1.1). These "cracks" allow brain fluids to seep into the axon pathway, the way moisture enters electrical lines through broken insulation. This creates tiny "blisters" that trigger "short circuits" within neurons. UBOs cause incomplete processing of information and thought patterns throughout the right brain. These right-brain lesions are commonly seen in individuals with NVLD.

Range of Severity of NVLD

To understand nonverbal LD (NVLD), it is important to consider how severe each person's symptoms appear to be.

1	2	3		4	5	6	7		8	9	10
	mild					moderate				severe	

Mild NVLD

Individuals with mild NVLD often are successful students who become specialists in one or two skill areas. They seldom achieve the social skills of attractive grooming, pleasant small talk, or working cooperatively within groups. Their sense of humor is different enough to be called "weird," and their idea of fun often is considered strange. They are self-focused in that they do not pay attention to the needs or wishes of others. Their own desires come first. These individuals never quite fit into the mainstream of their peers. They "march to a different drum beat" in how they dress, how they play, and how they learn and work. Within a classroom or workplace, mildly NVLD persons trigger complaints about being untidy, making too much noise, creating too much clutter, and failing to follow schedules or meet goals set by the group.

Moderate NVLD

Individuals who fit Duane's right-hemi syndrome profile are within the moderate range in severity of NVLD symptoms. Moderate NVLD causes an individual to be eccentric or "weird," too overbearing in relationships, ritualistic by repeating the same behaviors over and over, and jealous when others receive more attention. Moderately NVLD individuals do not make good work partners or committee members. They spend too much time splitting hairs and arguing instead of getting on with tasks. They enjoy baiting others into arguments just for the entertainment of creating conflict. These individuals rarely pay attention to personal hygiene and grooming. Often they offend others through body odor or unwashed clothing. However, these persons often are well educated with graduate degrees and may have established a reputation as being a specialist in some area of expertise. Moderately NVLD individuals often are dyslexic, which compounds their difficulties in achieving success.

Severe NVLD

During the 1970s and 1980s, Denckla researched the brain structures of NVLD individuals whose symptoms were within the severe range on the 1–10 scale. Their social behavior was so odd, eccentric, and irregular it was impossible for them to fit into groups or succeed on most jobs. In 1991, Denckla reported her conclusion that severe NVLD actually is a form of very high-functioning autism called *Asperger's syndrome* (Denckla, 1991b). In 1994, the fourth edition of the *Diagnostic and Statistical Manual of Mental Disorders* (DSM–IV) included Asperger's syndrome as a type of psychological disability called *pervasive personality disorder* (American Psychiatric Association, 1994).

During the four decades I have followed the lives of several thousand struggling individuals, I have observed lifelong symptoms of Asperger's syndrome that make it very difficult for these persons to function within school groups, in the workplace, or within personal relationships. Appendix E presents the Jordan Asperger's Syndrome Scale, which provides a comprehensive index for evaluating this behavior. The following checklist presents the NVLD behaviors usually seen when symptoms are severe:

Checklist Signature of Asperger's Syndrome

_____ Awkwardness in gross motor development.

_____ Pedantic (lecture-like) speech.

_____ Flat, monotone voice.

_____ Awkwardness at making small talk.

_____ Too slow at thinking of something to say during conversation.

_____ Restricted, strange sense of humor.

_____ Stiff, awkward body posture.

_____ Excellent recall of trivial details within a narrow range of interest.

_____ Narrow, inflexible range of interests.

_____ Obsessive habit of splitting hairs, arguing, and correcting others.

_____ Boring personality.

_____ Inappropriate, obnoxious social habits.

_____ Obsessive ritualized behavior.

_____ Blindness to social signals.

_____ Obsessive about controlling others.

_____ Stubborn and resistive toward change.

_____ Automatic rationalizing of own mistakes.

_____ Works best when alone.

_____ Is creative within a narrow range of interest.

_____ Is obsessively self-focused.

Social–Emotional Learning Disability (SELD)

In 1975, John Wacker, a founding member of the Association of Children and Adults with Learning Disabilities (ACLD, now called LDA, Learning Disabilities Association), wrote an intriguing account of his daughter's struggle with socialization skills and learning disability. In his monograph *The Dyslogic Syndrome,* Wacker presented the first detailed description of the disruptive lifestyle that came to be called *social–emotional LD.* During the 1980s, the term *social–emotional LD* (SELD) was adopted by most specialists (Denckla, 1985; Duane, 1987; Osman & Blinder, 1982; Silver, 1985). In 1993 Keith Stanovich proposed the term *dysrationalia* to describe this lifestyle that is devoid of logic and commonsense reasoning. In 2000, Jordan listed the following characteristics of this disruptive, often destructive lifestyle (Jordan, 2000a).

Checklist Signature of SELD (Dyslogic Syndrome or Dysrationalia)

Appendix F presents the Jordan Scale for Social–Emotional LD (SELD). This assessment tool provides a comprehensive profile of the characteristics of SELD, along with guidelines for managing this disruptive lifestyle.

_____ Pays no attention to consequences of one's behavior.

_____ Displays no commonsense reasoning in making decisions.

_____ Lives by impulse.

_____ Is mostly self-focused.

_____ Makes aggressive, insatiable demands for instant wish fulfillment.

_____ Is insensitive to needs and interests of others.

(continues)

_____ Explodes in tantrums when challenged or denied.

_____ Makes irrational spur-of-the-moment decisions without regard to costly consequences.

_____ Is prone to panic attacks that trigger violent behavior.

_____ Cannot be relied on.

_____ Views the world through personal biases and prejudices.

_____ Does not learn from mistakes.

_____ Does not change habits because of moral or spiritual teaching.

_____ Is overly generous to members of peer group.

_____ Lives recklessly.

_____ Engages in high-risk behavior.

_____ Refuses to be responsible in a traditional cultural sense.

_____ Lives an unconventional, nonconformist lifestyle.

_____ Is an irregular person in social behavior and lifestyle.

_____ Is loyal only to the peer group of the moment.

_____ Is ritualistic/obsessive in following current social fads.

_____ Is superstitious.

_____ Lives by gossip rather than fact.

_____ Thrives on rumor.

_____ Is a shallow, superficial person.

_____ Has volatile feelings, emotions, and moods.

_____ Is too sensitive to accept criticism.

_____ Usually is diagnosed ADHD, ODD, bipolar I, character disordered, or borderline personality disorder type.

Failure of Executive Function in SELD

Chapters 1 and 3 present the concept of executive function. The left-brain prefrontal cortex is designed to stay in charge of higher level thinking while keeping strong basal emotions under control, the way an executive stays in charge of a successful organization. When the prefrontal cortex is functioning well, individual lives are governed by logic and commonsense reasoning that are balanced by constructive feelings and emotions. When neurotransmitters throughout the brain are well balanced, the prefrontal cortex and limbic system cooperate as a well-coordinated executive team. Too little or too much dopamine and serotonin tips the balance (homeostasis) to cause the prefrontal cortex to lose executive function.

The brain is designed to function as a highly organized community. As Chapter 1 describes, the brain stem stands guard against threats to the community's safety (see Figure 1.6). The midbrain and parietal lobes are receiving/distribution centers where incoming data are sorted, classified, and sent on to specialized destinations throughout the brain. The occipital lobes handle vision tasks, and the temporal lobes do the listening, language processing, and time keeping. Left and right sensory cortexes monitor taste, odor, and body sensations to make sure that the brain is not overloaded by too much stimulus. The cerebellum and motor cortexes make sure that muscle movement is balanced. Both frontal lobes oversee thinking, problem solving, and creativity. The executive in charge of all this community activity is the prefrontal cortex located "upstairs" in the higher brain. The power station that regulates energy flow, emotional surges, and the community alarm system is housed "downstairs" in the limbic system. Like all successful communities, brain activity must stay organized, correctly synchronized, well maintained through good health, and protected from threatening events. All of this is accomplished through collaboration between the executive function of the prefrontal cortex and the limbic system.

The brain's executive function involves three major processes that, in most individuals, work in harmony: *organization, inhibition* (self-control), and *attention*. It is impossible to evaluate intelligence, quality of education, or a person's neurological talents if these three executive functions are out of balance. When the higher brain fails to do its work properly, socially disruptive feelings, emotions, and moods are out of control. Such an individual has a very poor sense of organization along with little self-control over impulses and sudden urges. The person's lifestyle shows too little logic and commonsense reasoning that keeps the individual in continual conflict with others. When executive function fails, disruptive behavior takes charge of the person's lifestyle.

Chronic Irritability of Moderate SELD

Listing the characteristics of SELD only hints at the disruptive impact this socialization disorder can impose on a community. Many SELD individuals are within the moderate range of the 1–10 severity scale. Their daily behavior creates continual conflict with relatives, colleagues at work, instructors, job supervisors, sales representatives, and everyone else whom they encounter. By nature, moderately SELD persons are irritable, overly sensitive, prone to "jump the gun" without pausing to think things through, and prone to have tantrums when they do not get their own way. They are too quick to feel insulted over differences of opinion. They have no patience to wait or take their turn. Their first thought is of themselves and how each situation will benefit them. They are impulsive, rude, aggressive, and always on the defensive. Moderate SELD behavior is a social nuisance that brings stress into all relationships, but it can be managed well enough to allow these individuals to earn a living and have partly successful social and workplace experiences.

Outrageous Behavior of Severe SELD

Those whose impulsive/compulsive SELD behavior is at the severe level often place others in grave danger. For example, in March 2000 my community was assaulted by a very disruptive episode of SELD behavior. A 30-year-old man whom friends called the "outlaw superstar" was stopped in a line of traffic where police officers were conducting a vehicle safety check. As an officer approached the man's car, he suddenly wheeled around and sped away at 80 miles per hour with a police car in pursuit. As other officers raced to block the road ahead of the speeding driver, a motorist was injured when his van was struck by a pursuing squad car. During this high-speed chase, several other vehicles were damaged and pedestrians injured as people scrambled out of the way. This wild chase accelerated to 110 miles per hour up and down city streets. Inside the fleeing car were the driver's fiancée, her teenaged daughter, the daughter's boyfriend, and a pet dog, all screaming from fear of dying. Finally the fugitive vehicle was stopped and the driver arrested. The man's fiancée told the police, "We asked him to stop, but he wasn't saying anything but 'Oh God, Oh God!' He looked wild. He looked so scared. You don't want to distract somebody like that." Later a reporter interviewed the driver about running from the police. "I was real concerned about people getting in my way," he said. "I had just met the lady I'm in love with. I'm going to get married, and it's a lot harder to run from the cops with someone you love. But I'm so used to running from them it's become a habit" (Branstetter, 2000).

As this story unfolded, it was learned that the driver had a long history of high-speed traffic violations. During an interview he said, "I've been driving fast all my life. I've gone as fast as 160 miles an hour running from the police." His driving record revealed that he had outrun police vehicles five times during the first 3 months of 2000. His record showed a string of arrests for eluding police officers, resisting arrest, driving without a license, and driving with a suspended license. This driver stated that he flees from police because they have beaten him several times following his arrest. Witnesses have testified that when he is apprehended, the man becomes so violent that several officers must wrestle him to the ground to subdue him. Police files also showed an arrest for attempted burglary and driving a stolen vehicle. An investigative reporter asked the man about that charge. "I wasn't trying to burglarize," he said. "I lived there. I lost my keys and was climbing in through the window when the cops came. They had their guns drawn on me so I jumped in my neighbor's truck and I ran." The reporter stated that this man seemed almost proud of his driving record. "I ain't never hit nothing," he told the reporter. "I ain't never wrecked a vehicle I've been in." When the reporter reminded him that he had crashed a truck a few years earlier, the man replied, "The motor locked up in that truck. It was not my fault."

The Impact of Social Disability

In viewing the life of someone with dyslexia, probably we would conclude that if a person had to choose between success in school or success in life, it would be more important for one to be socially successful. It is possible for someone with limited literacy skills to earn a living and be a contributing member to family and society. However, it is virtually impossible for a person who is socially disabled to establish and maintain a successful life beyond the sheltered years of school attendance.

Social disability is a heartbreaking pattern for those who must live with such a person. The individual who is socially disabled is oblivious to the protocols that must be followed if one is to love and be loved. Those with the dual challenge of dyslexia and socialization disorders cannot read the subtle signals that tell most people how to respond to others. Persons who are NVLD or SELD do not see boundary markers that say, "Not just now. Give me some space." These individuals are self-centered in that their major concern is for themselves. They do not have the sensitivity to realize when they are being overbearing, too shrill, or unreasonably demanding. They are too unaware socially to recognize when their behavior has offended someone or when their habits are embarrassing and inappropriate. These irregular individuals do not blend into the normal give-and-take that must occur in any successful relationship. Often they display deep stubbornness that makes them impossible to influence, even when they are wrong and must change their ways. These socially different individuals tend to have poor manners that grate on the nerves of those who must share their space. They do not perceive how their decisions create problems for others, even when they spend money impulsively or waste precious resources on trivial or immature things.

Persons with NVLD or SELD cannot accept or comprehend constructive criticism because they tend to be overly sensitive and too easily offended. They do not follow through on plans, do not see how poor punctuality affects coworkers, and cannot understand why they are unpopular on the job. Usually, they keep moving from job to job, unable to learn from their mistakes. Individuals who are socially disabled and also have dyslexia seldom are sensitive to the needs of a spouse or children. Even though these adults with NVLD or SELD show affection during moments of shared love, the long-range business of building a marriage and rearing children is beyond their understanding. Most have "tunnel vision," seeing only a few issues clearly while failing to comprehend social issues that also must be considered. As spouses they are self-centered and blind to the needs of loved ones. As parents they are overly demanding and narrow in how they discipline. As workers on the job, they tend to be stubborn and inflexible when it comes to following instructions. As citizens they generally are uninformed on issues that affect society. Teenagers with these disabilities tend to become strongly opinionated adults who harp on the same few issues over and over. As they leave their 20s and move on toward middle age, they settle into narrow, shallow lifestyles that become rigid and inflexible. As time goes by, any spouse or companion must do most of the adapting and changing to keep the relationship going. Persons who are dyslexic along with having NVLD or SELD are somewhat paranoid, never fully trusting anyone but themselves. Habitually they flare into angry confrontations when their points of view are challenged or criticized. To emerge into one's adult years as a person who is socially disordered is costly to everyone involved in that person's life.

Changing SELD

When young children show early signs of SELD, is it possible to guide them in such a way that they will not become socially disabled teenagers or adults? Earlier chapters explain the plasticity of the brain that permits "rewiring" of certain neural pathways through the right kinds of stimulus. If academic and social intervention through creative stimulus occurs early enough, many LD symptoms can be diminished. For example, Russell Barkley's research (1990, 1995) with early intervention of ADHD has shown that when medication and counseling therapy are provided before adolescence begins, 8 out of 10 youngsters diagnosed as ADHD "outgrow" enough attention deficit and behavior disorder patterns to become nearly normal young adults. Apparently early intervention can stimulate changes in the brain's neural wiring so that more mature, less disruptive lifestyle habits can be acquired. Research reported by reading specialists who use the intensely multisensory Lindamood–Bell ADD reading method (see pages 134–135) report lasting improvement in how dyslexic learners process written and oral language. Apparently intensive stimulus of left-brain neural wiring alters dyslexic pathways enough to permit permanent growth in talent for reading, spelling, and writing. During my 40 years of diagnosing and treating dyslexia, I have seen lifelong changes occur when one-on-one tutoring and nurturing are provided for young struggling learners. My experience has shown that if dyslexic patterns are identified by age 7, and if good remedial teaching and home guidance begin at that point, 85% of younger children who are diagnosed as dyslexic can be taught how to achieve "normal" academic success. If dyslexic patterns are not identified until age 9, with remedial teaching and guidance not begun until that age, 70% of those youngsters can overcome enough dyslexic tendencies to become normally successful in the classroom. If dyslexia is not identified and treated until age 13, only 5% of those struggling learners can achieve normal academic success (Jordan, 1989a, 1989b, 1996a, 1996b).

Early identification and treatment of left-brain, right-brain, and midbrain LD *can* change the academic and social patterns that characterize dyslexia, attention deficit disorder, and the socially disabling behavior of NVLD and SELD. However, as time goes by, this becomes increasingly difficult to do. Each passing year of academic failure and social struggle "hardwires" the brain, making it less possible for deeply embedded patterns to be modified. Those who struggle with the dual differences of dyslexia and NVLD or SELD often reach a point of no return.

Social Disability Profile for Individuals with Dyslexia and SELD

The syndrome called socialization disorder is composed of several overlapping factors, all of which interact like the roots of a tree to support the complex structure of SELD, or social dyslexia. By looking at each factor separately, we can see how NVLD and SELD lifestyles develop. This also provides clues about how to remediate dyslexia at the same time the lifestyles of NVLD and SELD are modified.

Self-Centeredness

The taproot of social disability, whether NVLD or SELD, is self-centeredness. This basic orientation of self-focus supports the rest of the SELD syndrome. In psychiatric terms, extreme self-centeredness is called *narcissism*. In ancient mythology,

Narcissus was a handsome young man who could not take his eyes or thoughts off himself. He spent long hours gazing at his reflection in pools and mirrors, losing all contact with the outside world as he gazed at himself, loved himself, groomed himself, and thought only of himself. As the ancient myth tells, eventually Narcissus disappeared inside himself and was transformed into a lovely flower that looked at itself all day by the side of a pool. In modern terms, a truly narcissistic person would be mentally ill, incapable of normal emotional interaction with others. Persons with dyslexia and SELD or NVLD are not mentally ill, except in isolated cases when true mental illness emerges. However, they are self-centered. Their primary concerns are "What do I get out of this situation? What's in this for me? What can my friends and family do for me? What does my roommate owe me for all I've done?"

This type of thinking dominates the waking hours of individuals with SELD and NVLD. They simply do not see the needs of others. When occasionally they do recognize that someone else has a need, the tendency is to do something impulsive for that person at the moment, then get back to the business of satisfying self. It is impossible for such a person to keep his or her attention focused very long on others.

Joseph is a striking example of this socially disabled, dyslexic self-centeredness. I met him when he was 10 years old. He was so frustrated in an elementary school classroom that he was having tantrums that disrupted everything the teacher tried to do. He and I formed an immediate bond because I was the first adult ever to give him the quality of attention he was hungry to find. Joseph loved me intensely in his self-centered way. As his advocate and counselor, I was able to absorb his self-centeredness so that he felt great joy when we were together. His family could not help me with Joseph's dyslexic tendencies because their deeply embedded family style was one of confrontation. The relationship between mother and father was based on competition to see which adult could outsmart the other. This often-fierce rivalry was absorbed by the children, who carried this competitive spirit into their sibling relationships. This toxic family environment included finding fault with each other, seeking ways to dominate and control each other, and reminding others of past mistakes that never were forgiven or forgotten. Joseph entered this socially combative arena unable to cope. To survive, he had to become a little gladiator, slashing his opponents before they slashed him. This intelligent but aggressive lifestyle was an emotionally abusive, poisonous environment for a sensitive child who had dyslexia.

Professionals who work with dyslexic students see a critically important survival paradigm: If individuals like Joseph can find two sources of positive support, they can change enough from being socially disabled toward becoming at least moderately successful academically and emotionally. If the home cannot give such support, but the child receives affirmation and help at school and from another important source, the negative influence of the home can be largely overcome. If the school cannot provide positive support, but the child finds it both at home and from another important source, then the youngster can overcome enough of the negative classroom influences to become successful. Unfortunately for Joseph, he was isolated from positive change both at home and at school. The stubbornness and self-centeredness of his parents kept them from agreeing on the best school placement where their son's academic and emotional needs could be met. If one parent suggested one place, the other disagreed.

Joseph went through school in a learning environment that matched his home life in terms of competition, criticism of failure, and lack of support for positive self-esteem. By the time I met him, Joseph was filled with shame. At home he was regarded by parents and siblings as a problem child. At school he was regarded as a "lazy, disruptive boy" who would not try. His relationship with me was the only safely positive oasis in his emotionally arid life. That one source of approval and affection was not enough to prevent him from becoming socially disabled. To survive, this bright child with LD had to become self-centered. To be thoughtful of others at home or school was to expose himself to criticism and ridicule that overwhelmed him with shame.

During his teen years, Joseph discovered a talent for writing poetry. He filled many notebooks with poems that expressed his complex feelings, emotions, and moods. His dyslexic spelling patterns and incomplete language skills produced rather primitive writing, but the poetry was warm and beautiful. However, it was self-centered material. Joseph was madly in love with many girls in a self-centered way. It was impossible for him to understand when I explained the give-and-take required in love. He developed the habit of buying each new girlfriend a single rose, which he presented over a candlelight dinner at a luxurious restaurant. At first, each girl was overwhelmed and delighted. However, within a few days or weeks, Joseph would tell me about how still another girl had rejected him for "some jerk not nearly as smart as I am." I read the poems he had composed for each new girl, reminding her of what she had forfeited by refusing his love. It was impossible to make a dent in Joseph's narcissistic patterns. He could not comprehend what I said about turning his attention from himself to others. "But I'm one of the most thoughtful guys in town!" he would shout at me. "What do you mean, I'm self-centered? I buy them roses. I take them to the nicest places to eat. I treat them like royalty!" "Yes, you do," I replied. "But why do you do all these things?" "So they will like me!" Joseph always exclaimed. He could not recognize his self-centeredness in all those brief relationships.

Joseph's social disabilities reached a peak in something he did one day. He brought me a set of photographs he had taken with an automatic camera. As he proudly watched me look through the stack of pictures, he kept asking, "How do you like my photography? Don't you think I'm good with a camera?" I was astonished as I kept turning to the next picture. Every shot was of Joseph. He had used three rolls of film to photograph himself. By setting the timer, he could settle into a new pose before the camera snapped yet another picture of himself. Joseph had brought me 108 snapshots he had taken of himself, and he could not comprehend why I was not delighted. He was baffled by my questions: "Why did you take pictures of yourself? Why not take pictures of others?" He slammed out of my office in a rage. "There you go, criticizing me! You're just like my parents!" After his first year of college, Joseph took a vacation trip with a friend. When he returned, he showed me a lot of snapshots of their trip. I soon realized that every picture was of Joseph. "Where is your friend?" I asked. "Oh, I threw away all the pictures he was in," Joseph said with a shrug.

Individuals who are socially disabled and also have dyslexia do not always take pictures of themselves, but their lives are centered on themselves. Rarely are they aware that this is so. In fact, most of the persons with social disabilities whom I have known think of themselves as being thoughtful, considerate, and generous. Their blind spot is that they cannot see why they give gifts, do courteous things, or remember birthdays. Everything they do is designed to get something back in return. Their generosity is a means of receiving praise and satisfaction for themselves. If they do see a real need in others, they immediately turn that need back toward themselves. For example, if Joseph saw a friend crying, he would take the friend into a warm embrace. However, instead of listening to the friend's need, Joseph would say, "I know how you feel. I've cried a lot myself. Why, last week I cried when a girl broke up with me. You know, there sure are a lot of immature girls in this town. They just aren't mature enough to appreciate a guy like me. Yeah, I've cried a lot myself. My mom and dad make me cry a lot, the way they criticize me all the time. You ought to be at my house and hear them yell at me all the time." By this time, the friend with the problem has pulled away from Joseph's self-centered embrace. The reality soon becomes clear that he is not really interested in the friend's problem. All Joseph can think about is himself. Thus, he faces another situation in which he is pushed away by someone who needed more than he could give.

Self-Centeredness Is Based on Brain Structure

Self-centeredness is common in children. In fact, one of the earliest social milestones that children must achieve is learning how to share playthings within a group. Teachers and parents are delighted when youngsters learn this important social lesson of looking beyond themselves with playmates. Chapter 1 described how, during fetal development, the cingulate gyrus within the midbrain prepares for the time when the proto-self will emerge (see page 21). As this vital neurological milestone is reached during early childhood, the developing brain begins to pay attention to others. Children who are behind schedule in learning this important social skill remain self-focused, disruptive, and too irritable to fit into a group. The child with emerging SELD is behind schedule in neurological development.

If the negative characteristics of NVLD or SELD are treated early enough, it is possible to modify self-centeredness at the same time the child learns how to modify dyslexia. To stimulate the brain to make these changes in neural wiring, children like Joseph must have models at home and at school that demonstrate thoughtfulness and consideration of others. Adults cannot model concern for others if they themselves are self-centered.

Youngsters with emerging SELD habits must have at least two sources of instruction if these deep-seated tendencies are to be modified, and they must see these models day after day over a period of years. Training the brain to respond differently to others must begin before "hardwiring" of neural pathways occurs before age 10.

Learning not to be self-centered involves certain basic concepts, including how to read body language and emotional signs. This requires the same kind of careful coaching that goes into teaching phonics and reading when a child cannot "hear" the sounds in words. As children with dyslexia comprehend literacy skills, they also can master social awareness skills, if the instruction begins soon enough and continues long enough.

Noticing Others

Self-centeredness is constantly looking at self and paying attention to self. Social awareness is looking at and paying attention to others. The first step is to change the point of focus from the self to someone else. Over a period of time, children like Joseph are taught what to do when they enter a room. Adult supervisors explain, "Joseph, don't wonder what everyone will think about you. That's a self-centered thought. Instead, look at other people and speak to them. Look for signs that tell you how they are. Is Mary happy this morning? How can you tell? Does her face show it? Do her clothes show it? Is Robert unhappy this morning? How can you tell? How does his face show it? How might his clothes show it? Is Mrs. Jordan happy today? Does she feel well this morning after her cold last week? How can you tell? Why don't you ask her if she feels better today? Did Jason have fun over the weekend with his dad? How can you tell? Listen to what Jason is saying. Is he telling happy stories about what he did with his dad? Or is he not talking about it at all? Look at Janice, the new girl in the class. Has she been crying this morning? How can you tell? Do her eyes look sad? Is there something nice you can say to let her know you're glad she's in your class? Remember how Robert always loses his things? How can you tell if he has his pencil ready for class? Can you help him look for his pencil before the teacher asks him about it?"

These are the kinds of "baby steps" parents and teachers must take to help children with dyslexia and NVLD or SELD learn how to turn their attention away from themselves. Some homes and classrooms have a natural climate of thoughtfulness where children are immersed in caring, thoughtful attention to others. Some children are sensitive enough to follow models and learn to behave that way. Others must be guided step by step, the way they must learn the multiplication tables. Dyslexic children who also have SELD or NVLD often come from homes and class-rooms where such a model of specific, consistent thoughtfulness is not demonstrated or taught. It takes years of careful nurtur-ing with daily practice before the natural bent toward self-centeredness is changed to noticing the needs of others.

Reaching Out to Others

One of the most difficult skills for dyslexic youngsters who also have SELD or NVLD to learn is how to reach out to others. Most children with dual LD patterns are forced to exert a great deal of conscious effort just to get through each day successfully. During academic years, their energies go into doing their best in difficult studies, keeping up with volumes of homework, dealing with the emotional trauma of flunking tests and making low grades, ab-sorbing criticism without being too badly hurt, and so forth. Al-though they seldom have much emotional energy left over for others, they must learn to become socially thoughtful individu-als, at least to some degree. Children like Joseph must see the model of reaching out before they can claim it for themselves. From their early years, these children must see generous social attitudes demonstrated. If the family has a negative attitude to-ward helping others, this lack of generosity is quickly absorbed by youngsters. If parents complain about having to be generous, their children will have trouble sharing.

The lesson of reaching out to others was vividly implanted in my mind at age 7 by a single action by my father. I have only a few clear memories of him. He was stricken with cancer before I started school, which was toward the end of the Great Depres-sion. Like so many parents of the late 1930s, mine were out of work, and our family faced the terror of no income with three children to feed. My father's medical needs were supplied by the Veterans Administration, but he had to live at a VA hospital to receive treatment for the malignancy. My mother moved my sis-ters and me into a very humble apartment in an impoverished neighborhood while she tried to make ends meet on an income of $24 per month. I recall vividly one day when my father came home for a brief visit from the hospital. We were in the tiny backyard near the alley that the apartment faced, enjoying this rare family time together. A shabbily dressed, very dirty man came along and asked for something to eat. As a 7-year-old, I had only a primitive notion of how scarce food was for our family, but I knew that we had to be very careful and that there were no extra helpings or treats. I knew that things were bad and that my mother cried a lot. As the shabby man stood there asking for food, I saw my mother shake her head. Later I would realize how little she had for her own family, let alone anything to share.

Suddenly my attention was drawn to my father's face. My dad smiled at the stranger and asked him to sit down and rest. Then he turned to my mother and said, "Could you fix one of your egg sandwiches for this good man?" My mother's egg sandwiches were among the wonders of the world when I was a child. It was an exceptional treat when we got to have one of her creations with a fried egg, a slice of cheese, and toasted bread. I remember that scene as my dad rubbed the pain in his amputated leg, chatted with the stranger who had no place to go and nothing to eat, and showed me what it meant to reach out to someone beyond ourselves. I have never forgotten the gratitude as that stranger thanked my mother for her gift. An egg sandwich never brought more joy than hers did that day. As I have reflected on that scene many times, I am so grateful for the gift my father gave me that day. He demonstrated what it means to reach out to others instead of feeling sorry for ourselves. That experience set into motion a lifelong pattern of paying attention to others I have followed to this day.

Youngsters with LD often find it hard to reach out to others. Yet they can learn to do so if they see the model and are taught the skill. The crippling limitation of being socially disabled is not having the ability to reach beyond oneself, except for selfish purposes. This essential social skill can be taught if supervisors in the child's life do not wait too long. Reaching out to others can be demonstrated along with practice in reading, spelling, phonics, and math as the child is taught what it means to attend to the world beyond self. For example, as they master encoding and decoding techniques, youngsters also can practice noticing what others need: "Look at Mark. Why is he frustrated? Look at Sue.

She can't get her pencil to draw that circle. Can you help her to do it so she can finish her picture? Look at Joe. He can't see the math book under his jacket. Can you help him find it? Look at Mrs. Jordan. She dropped part of the spelling papers by her desk. Can you help her pick them up? Look at Mr. Jones, the custodian. He can't get all his stuff through the door. Can you help him by holding the door open?"

These small steps in reaching out to others soon turn the self-centered bent another way. The child learns that helping some-one in need brings its own miniburst of joy and its own rewards without needing something in return. The act of being generous is a social skill, part of the "tribal dance" one must learn. If mod-eling is begun early enough, children with LD and social differ-ences can learn this skill, even when their own feelings and emo-tions are exhausted.

Self-Pity

One of the most unattractive faces of SELD is self-pity. The "poor little me" syndrome is a major reason why persons who lack so-cial skills are unattractive. Of course, many who do not have dyslexia, SELD, or NVLD also bog down in the swamp of self-pity. At times it feels good for anyone to "have a pity party," but the person with good self-image and active social skills soon laughs and gets back to the business of being mature. It is espe-cially easy for dyslexic youngsters to develop self-pity. The re-frain often sounds like this: "Nobody else has to do this much work. Why do I have to work so hard all the time? Jason makes good grades and he doesn't have to work all the time! How come my brother gets to ride his bike and I have to finish this home-work? How come I never get to play? I have to work all the time! It's not fair! How come I have dyslexia? I didn't ask to be born this way!"

All of this is true, of course. It is not fair to be born with dyslexia. It definitely is not fair for your siblings to get to play when you have to keep on with unfinished work. It is not fair to have to go to tutors or special classes or summer school. It is un-fair never to have your papers on the bulletin board with gold stars, or never to make top grades when you know that you stud-ied harder than the star of the class. It is not fair when adults say, "If you just tried harder! I know you can do it. You just don't try!" It is not fair to be smarter than a friend, yet he or she can read better and make better grades. It is not fair to lose your words and get tangled up trying to tell stories and look dumb every time you answer in class. It is not fair never to finish a test first, never to get all your work done so that it won't have to be taken home. It's just not fair!

The antidote for self-pity is a good sense of humor, which is not easy for a child with dyslexia to learn. How do you laugh about making poor grades? Where is the funny part of feeling "dumb" all the time? What is there to laugh about when you get lost turning corners and can't remember where you leave things? What is funny about forgetting how to spell your own name, or getting things backwards and read "Altus" when the sign said "Tulsa"?

Wise parents and teachers help these youngsters learn to smile instead of lapsing into self-pity. "OK, so it's not very funny when all these dyslexic things happen, but let's see how we can make the best of it." It helps to start with the really funny things that come along. For example, most dyslexic individuals create marvelous tongue twisters that can be a lot of fun for the family. Relatives of those who have dyslexia actually can be proud of verbal slips that turn into famous family sayings. One day Keith was explaining why he wanted to be alone for a while. "I just need to be synonymous," he said, and his family had a wonderful new way of talking about privacy. There was no criticism or embarrassment, just praise and good humor over this rich contribution to the family vocabulary. One day Judy said that she had three "sliver dimes" in her coin collection, and suddenly her family had a new Judyism. After that, they all looked for "slivers" when they counted their change. Moesha became her "daddy's little gril" when she got her letters backwards, and that grew into her father's tenderest term of endearment for his precious daughter. Erin always said, "Mom, where's my tallow?" when it was time for her shower. Her family adopted the wonderful new Erinism as they used tallows after their showers. I knew that Stan had outgrown his self-pity when he brought me a wooden statue he had carved and painted so carefully. "This is my dyslexic sheriff," he explained with a smile. He showed me the word that he had carved below the sheriff's left foot: WARD. "That's dyslexia for DRAW," he laughed. One day Chris left his mom a note: "My book is no my bed." From then on, the family had a richly funny phrase. When anything was lost, they always said, "Look no the bed."

These are the kinds of "baby steps" adults can take in disarming the trigger of self-pity and turning it another way. But this journey away from self-pity must begin early before the concrete of emotions and feelings hardens into inflexibility. I have seen many children with dyslexia, SELD, or NVLD reach adulthood without a sense of humor. They grew up too overly sensitive, which placed them beyond the reach of others who would have liked to help them loosen up. A lifelong pity party is the reflexive habit of blaming others instead of taking responsibility for oneself by saying, "It's not my fault!" This point of view makes excuses for self and places the blame on others: "I inherited this problem from my dad, so it's his fault I'm dyslexic." "I had lousy teachers who didn't like me, so I never learned to read." "My math teacher was too lazy to do her job, so I never learned my times facts." "They didn't like me in middle school, so I dropped out when I got old enough." "My boss worked me too hard, so I just quit. I won't work anyplace I'm not treated with respect." This litany of self-pity goes on and on until the person finds himself or herself in the position of being a loser. If children with LD are not taught how to take responsibility and laugh at their mistakes, they gradually settle into the self-pity swamp where they become encased in an attitude that is offensive to others and degrading to themselves.

Stubbornness

Individuals who have social disabilities usually are stubborn. Their interpretation of events has a bullheaded quality, and their approach to life is single-minded. They view life through the lens of self, conclude that whatever they think is correct, then cling to that opinion, no matter what.

For most persons with dyslexia and SELD or NVLD, being safe is guaranteed by always being in control. For many individuals, being safe is accomplished by being stubborn, which is a fiercely loyal protection of self. New suggestions are met with disbelief: "If I didn't think of it, it isn't important to me!" New ideas are dismissed with scoffing: "That's the dumbest thing I ever heard!" Skepticism is displayed through the automatic judgment: "That won't work." End of discussion.

These individuals dig in their heels and refuse to budge, which generates all kinds of friction and conflict. A parent who has social disabilities sees no value in the opinions of children or spouse. Any effort to bring up new ideas within the family is met with sarcasm and hostility. The stubborn person with SELD maintains control through verbal browbeating, nagging, threatening, and refusing to listen to anything new or different. If a new idea is brought into the relationship, it is pounded into the ground by verbal attacks and belittling comments until the other person backs off.

This stubborn characteristic is especially detrimental in a culture where change is prevalent and frequent. In the workplace of the 21st century, most workers will change jobs or occupations several times before retirement. During the 1990s, more than half of all families in the United States moved their place of residence more than once. In most occupations, new technology makes old job knowledge obsolete within 5 years unless the worker continually learns and grows. It is not easy for individuals with dyslexia and SELD or NVLD to adapt to change. They tend to cling stubbornly to whatever point of view they brought into adult life, and they fight to keep it that way. They tend to move from job to job, never understanding why boss after boss fires them or lays them off. Yet they believe that they are being strong by defending a principle that gets them in trouble in the workplace. They cannot see the role they play in making it impossible for them to get along with others. Stubbornness locks the door against letting anything new come inside. Being stubborn freezes marriage into a one-sided relationship that gradually squeezes the life out of the spouse while building walls between parent and children so that no communication can occur. Stubbornness drives wedges between coworkers and colleagues, creating division that eventually causes a work group to fall apart. The stubborn person who does not see the situation realistically soon is left behind as society moves forward and new technology makes old ways obsolete.

Chapter 1 explains that stubbornness begins as a defense strategy based on fear. Youngsters freeze when they are too afraid or too unsure to step ahead. When a fearful child is pushed by adults, he or she feels the strong emotions of the fight-or-flight reflex that places the brain on full alert for danger. Under this stress, the child balks or lashes out. This is automatically defensive behavior that wise adults try to understand. Why is this bright child refusing to cooperate? Is he or she afraid? If so, what is causing the fear? Thoughtful parents and teachers find ways to help stubborn youngsters release their fear so that progress can occur.

Children with LD are afraid of many things. Virtually everything they attempt poses a risk of failure. Adults who work with these youngsters recognize how often they freeze and feel immobilized. This defensive behavior protects the child from too much failure, because it is better to be scolded for not trying than to face the scolding that comes from failure. Thus, stubborn habits are established early.

Unfortunately, not all parents and teachers know how to deal successfully with childhood stubbornness. Adults with the mindset that "No child is going to get the best of me!" continue to push too hard. The contest of wills is on. To explain chronic stubbornness in many children, Hugh Missildine and Larry Galton (1972) developed the concept of the "over-coerced syndrome." They described this deeply entrenched behavior as the ultimately stubborn child who digs in the heels and refuses to budge when adults press for obedience. The more adults press, the more stubbornly the child refuses. These extremely stubborn children are believed to have been pushed too hard too many times while they were overly afraid. As a result, they develop the automatic habit of digging in their heels through stubborn resistance whenever adult pressure is felt or anticipated.

Dyslexic individuals with SELD or NVLD tend to fit this pattern of extreme stubbornness even when there is no reason to display such an attitude. For these individuals, being stubborn is an effective form of control. Others must either give in and submit to the will of the person being stubborn, or they pay an emotional price. Stubbornness is one of the most difficult forms of rebellion to manage.

Because this kind of stubbornness originates in childhood fear, it is possible to avoid the problem by guiding children to learn better ways to deal with their fear. The process must begin early. Adults must recognize the signs of fear and quietly, thoughtfully discuss it with the child. "What exactly is causing you to be afraid, John?" "I don't know." "Are you afraid because it's dark?" "No." "Are you afraid because Daddy isn't home yet?" "Yes," John blurts out. Or he may only nod his head. "OK. I'm glad to know how you feel. Come sit on my lap. Let's talk about it. Did you know that Daddy called while you were playing outside? Did you know that he asked how John is this afternoon? Did you know that when the big hand gets to six and the little hand says nine, Daddy will be home?" As John quietly hears all of these facts, he relaxes and no longer is afraid. Now he is ready to eat supper and be ready to give his father a big hug at 9:30. This is the way that thoughtful parents walk children through the moments when fear springs up.

Teachers work in similar ways to disarm fearful students at school. Because handwriting is so difficult for him, John freezes when the class is asked to write the alphabet. He stares out the window and refuses to lift his pencil. The teacher bends down. "You know, John," she says quietly. "I wonder something. Has your pencil forgotten how to write A?" John nods. "Well, that's no problem. Here, let me help you teach your pencil how to write A. Pick up your pencil. That's right. Now I'm going to hold your hand around your pencil. Let's teach your pencil to write A. Oh, yes, that's very good. Now see if your pencil remembers how to write B." And John is at work without being afraid of failing.

It takes great courage for a fearful person to move ahead. "What if I fail? What if I don't know how? What if I look dumb? What if someone laughs at me or criticizes me?" All of these questions must be put to rest before fear can relax and progress can occur. The stubborn portion of SELD is born from this kind of self-questioning. Children can learn how to turn such questions into forward steps if they begin early and are taught how over a period of time. Stubbornness must be faced in so many areas: how one dresses for school, doing chores instead of playing, tasting new food, meeting new people, giving up worn-out clothes and toys, letting Mom rearrange the furniture, sharing things with others, letting brother or sister use your stuff, and so forth. Wise parents and teachers guide youngsters through these developmental steps, one at a time. Over a period of years, stubbornness is replaced by courage and willingness to try because fear has been removed through understanding, not by nagging, yelling, or criticizing.

Arrogance

Perhaps the most offensive SELD characteristic is arrogance. This often is the last straw in causing relationships to break apart. Self-centered persons frequently can be charming, and self-pitying individuals often attract sympathy by appearing cuddly and needing lots of hugs. The arrogant person is abrasive and cold in his or her display of superiority. "I am the best. I am the smartest. If you want to know, just ask me. Anyone who disagrees with me is dumb and stupid." An arrogant attitude places others in the embarrassing position of not being bright or competent. The arrogant person with SELD brags and struts with no regard for the feelings of others. These insensitive individuals control and dominate conversations through a nonstop monologue about self: "I did this. I saw that. I said such and such." The opinions of others are dismissed with a condescending tone because they do not matter. This social bully intimidates others to get his or her own way.

Social Misfit

Individuals who have an arrogant attitude quickly become labeled as a "know-it-all" and are mocked behind their backs. Yet, they are blind to this social reaction. These individuals are social misfits, unable to fit successfully into groups. Because they cannot find acceptance in the usual social ways, these arrogant ones often try to develop their own group whom they control. It is interesting to watch such an individual work out strategies for gaining a network of followers. Relationships are based on the pretense that this person is special or that he or she has something unique that others do not have. Highly charismatic individuals successfully manage for years in such an arrogant role. Within the group, there may be intense loyalty that defends the arrogant leader and explains away all of his or her rudeness.

Using Others

Arrogant leaders view others with contempt, yet they stroke their followers in ways that make them feel important. The person with SELD seeks others who are vulnerable while needing to be associated with someone who represents power. These power groups are seen at every level: the school playground, large-city street corners, corporate boardrooms, religious organizations, the world of politics, and within colleges and universities. Arrogance uses others, devalues their worth, degrades their dignity, and stifles their growth. Such persons are among the least loved of all members of society, but they never understand why. They are blind to the offensive impact of their behavior on others. Worst of all, they do not care what others think of them.

Attitude of Superiority

Of all the elements of social disability, arrogance is one of the most difficult to change. The example of Joseph's behavior discussed earlier in this chapter demonstrated much arrogance. He truly thought that he deserved special treatment because he was bright. He used our friendship to brag to friends that he was "Dr. Jordan's special friend." Joseph could not keep from making cutting remarks whenever he observed a mistake or weakness in others. He could not keep his tongue from blurting "I told you so!" in a manner that angered others. His car was better. His all-weather coat cost more. His gold chain was more valuable. His dad made more money. Girls liked him better than they did other guys. Someday he was going to be a doctor and make a lot of money. Joseph could not comprehend how this arrogant litany provoked others and made him the target of ridicule. He had no friends, and he never knew why. It was impossible for him to accept any level of constructive criticism. His automatic reaction was, "There you go, criticizing me like my folks always do!" When the root of arrogance is not changed during early formative years, it becomes an obnoxious weed that makes the person offensive and unable to fit into normal society. The depth of loneliness is incredible when the arrogant person stops pretending and actually looks for companionship. Individuals like Joseph cannot understand why no one cares to be close to them.

Reducing the Level of Arrogance

How does an arrogant person learn to be humble? In most instances it seems impossible, once that characteristic of SELD becomes deeply embedded. To be arrogant is to be blind to others, seeing only self. How does one see others when one has no social vision? As with all other SELD characteristics, the key to change is beginning the process of teaching good social skills early in a child's life. This transformation from being egocentric to recognizing the worth of others starts with "baby steps" that show the child how to look at others realistically. For example, whenever Joseph blurts out a judgment, "Juan is dumb! He's really stupid!" he is guided through a discussion. "No, Joseph. Juan is not dumb.

He's just as intelligent as you are. Have you ever noticed that certain things are hard for Juan to do? Have you ever noticed how hard he struggles to write well? Watch how hard he must work to write as well as you do." "OK, but I'm better than he is at writing." "That's right, Joseph, you are. But Juan is better than you at math. Have you ever noticed that every person is best at something, but nobody is best at everything?" "Well, OK, but it's still dumb the way Juan writes." "No, Joseph, we aren't going to call anyone dumb. Do you want people to say you're dumb because you can't remember your multiplication facts?" "No, but that's different!" "No, Joseph, it's not different. Writing is easier for you than it is for Juan, but math is easier for him than it is for you. We aren't going to call each other dumb, Joseph. That is not acceptable."

This kind of patient yet firm teaching bears good results over time if the arrogant child receives this model from at least two sources. If Joseph sees this thoughtful model in one person while he continually sees an arrogant, sarcastic, overly critical attitude in others, he will not change his antisocial habits. If two important people in his life demonstrate patience and kindness, this provides enough outside strength to help Joseph understand the social–emotional need to treat others as he would have them deal with him.

Unfortunately, the Joseph I have described did not have this kind of patient guidance at home or at school during his formative childhood years. He followed the stringent, overly critical models of his home and the school he attended. His close, supportive relationship with me was not enough to change his bent toward being arrogant. Had either his home or school presented him with a nurturing, caring model and example, together we could have replaced his arrogance with a much better attitude of tolerance and compassion.

Immaturity

Most individuals with dyslexia and SELD or NVLD are immature. Although they may reach physical maturity ahead of schedule, they remain behind schedule emotionally. They are impatient, flashing into anger at the least irritation. They are impulsive, making decisions and taking actions without thinking of consequences. They rarely fear physical danger, which deprives them of the internal warning signals most of us hear. Because they behave much less maturely than their peers, they are seen as misfits. They have short attention spans, becoming bored too soon to enjoy social activities. They are shallow spiritually because they have no patience for developing a deeper understanding of faith or religious teaching. They are materialistic, wanting all kinds of nice things without having the income to afford them. They are jealous, which makes them impossible partners in romantic relationships or friendships. They are insatiable, never achieving full satisfaction, no matter how much attention or affection they receive. Thus, they burn out personal relationships by being overly demanding and possessive. They are insecure, always fretting over little issues that most people shrug off or ignore. These immature individuals clamor, fret, fuss, beg, demand, accuse, have tantrums, waste what they have, and live dangerously.

Intelligence Ahead of Emotional Maturity

In evaluating the learning patterns of individuals who are dyslexic, professionals usually find wide differences between their highest areas of ability and their lowest areas of performance. For example, most dyslexic individuals are quite intelligent. Mental age usually is higher than chronological age, but reading is well below mental age, and work stamina age is far below mental age. When individuals have dyslexia and SELD or NVLD, emotional maturity age also lags far behind the level of intelligence. The following profile provides a good example:

Mental age	16
Chronological age	12
Reading age	8
Work stamina age	7
Emotional maturity age	6

In a quiet, one-to-one situation, this student who is LD displays the mental ability expected of most 16-year-olds, although his age is only 12. However, in his seventh-grade classroom, his reading skills are stuck at third-grade level. As the teacher works with his group, this youngster, who also has SELD, begins to fidget, squirm, and interrupt as a 7-year-old child would do. Compared with his classmates, this boy is immature and disruptive, never keeping his attention focused on the task. He reacts to stress as if he were 6. He flares too easily, whines too much, complains too often, argues too frequently, and wheedles to get out of work. He bursts into tears at a certain point of frustration. He is like an overwhelmed 6-year-old child trying to cope with middle school expectations.

Immaturity in Adults

Older persons who have SELD have the same kind of wide disparity between their highest abilities and their level of emotional control. Being immature means that they cannot cope with life at their age. Young adults with SELD do not carry out responsibility. They cannot be depended on to keep promises, show up for work on time, help out when they agreed to do so, pay their share of expenses, pay bills on time, save money instead of spending, or deny themselves immediate pleasure so that something can be enjoyed later. They give in to whatever whim or impulse bubbles up at the moment. If they have $50 to pay on the rent, they may spend it all for a good time on Saturday, then be in trouble for not having rent money on Monday. If they promise to meet someone at a certain time, they may not show up or bother to call. Something else more immediate came up and they forgot their appointment. If they have a job interview at 9:00 a.m., they may oversleep and not wake up until noon. They never understand when someone else always gets the job. In the workplace they look for the easy way out and try to avoid doing whatever the boss assigns.

If these loose, immature individuals marry, they are like disorganized children playing house. If a child is born into the marriage, the parent is no more able to cope than a 12-year-old would be. Many cases of child abuse occur when such adults try to rear children. The crying of the child, the mess of changing diapers, and the need to earn a steady income to provide food and medical care for the baby are too much for the adult with SELD. Without warning, he or she bursts into tantrums and tries to make the baby stop crying. A great deal of physical abuse toward the spouse or mate also occurs. All their lives, these SELD individuals have thrown tantrums, slammed doors, squealed tires, and gunned their vehicles at 100 miles an hour when they are angry. They carry these habits into marriage, onto the job, or into any relationship.

Replacing Immaturity with Maturity

How do parents and teachers tame this kind of explosive emotional immaturity? Is it possible to turn this pattern of volatile response a different way? If the process begins early in the child's life, immaturity can be modified enough to the give the SELD child the basic social skill of self-control. When a child has a tantrum, adults face certain choices. One reaction would be to fly at the child and spank, slap, or otherwise punish physically. This often stops the tantrum, but the adult has stooped to the child's emotional level. In effect, the adult's tantrum has won over that of the child. Peace may have been restored, but the child now has experienced the model of hitting when one is angry. Occasionally it will be appropriate for a supervisor to shock an angry child into breaking the tantrum. Sometimes one firm swat on the bottom is appropriate at the moment. However, the habit of hitting the child who is having a tantrum is not the way to teach mature behavior to youngsters who are SELD.

For children to behave maturely, they must see it demonstrated every day. They must see what it means to have patience, to forgive, to maintain self-control, and not to hit back. Adults must demonstrate persistent patience over a long period of time. This does not mean that they should not be firm or decisive. The adult stays in charge in a firm way that guides the child through moments of immaturity, followed by a discussion. "John, why were you so angry?" "He got my toy." "But you have lots of toys. Just look at all of the toys you have to play with." "I want that toy. He can't have it!" "No, John, that is not how we deal with our toys. We have to share. Did Jim jerk your toy away from you?" "No, but I wanted it next." "You mean you weren't playing with it when Jim took it? "No, but it's mine! I want it. He can't have it!" "No, John. It's Jim's turn to play with the toy. You have another toy to play with. Later Jim will let you play with his toy." If this kind of patient rehearsal does not work, then John is taken firmly away from the situation. He may be taken to his room if he is at home or to a different part of the classroom if he is at school. The supervisor does not let him have his own way. Over and over during his developmental years, John receives this kind of firm, reasonable guidance. Whenever possible, the adult gives him something else to do, but the child's temper does not prevail. His tantrum does not make Jim give up the toy because John demands it.

As these children grow up, thoughtful parents and teachers require certain amounts of responsibility from them. Parents make written lists of chores, then guide the child in doing everything on the lists. Teachers write lists of assignments, then show the child how to do every task on the lists. As parents and teachers work together, the child begins to understand that a certain amount of structure must be followed. He or she may not like structure but will learn to accept it. Sometimes a reward is the right way to motivate a child to finish responsibilities. At other times, taking away a privilege is the only discipline he or she will understand. Supervisors may have to ground the immature child if certain rules are ignored or disobeyed. Over a period of time, this type of structure instills a sense of responsibility within the child's emerging set of values.

Dyslogic Behavior

When SELD symptoms are severe, a lifestyle emerges that does not follow logic or commonsense reasoning. Earlier this chapter reviewed the destructive behaviors called dyslogic syndrome, or dysrationalia. When neural pathways within the midbrain (limbic system), the brain stem, and the left-brain hemisphere fail to develop fully, the higher brain loses control of logical function, allowing strong basal emotions to take control. The usual result is a lifestyle that is mostly compulsive and impulsive with little evidence of logical thinking. Many individuals with this SELD lifestyle also are dyslexic.

Irrational Decisions

Dyslogical behavior is very upsetting to anyone involved in the life of the person who displays it. As the label implies, individuals with dyslogical behavior do not do things in a normal, commonsense way. Decisions are unpredictable and irrational. For example, a young adult suddenly might sell his vehicle for $300 in cash after making $1,500 in payments. One Saturday night he decided that he wanted his buddy's flashy vehicle even though it was about to fall apart, so he sold his vehicle to make that purchase. Or a girl with dyslogical behavior might drop out of high school within a semester of graduation to work part-time for minimum wage. She got bored with school and wanted to start her career. It makes no sense that now she is earning $65 a week at a fast-food restaurant. A boy with severe SELD might suddenly quit his job 2 days after being promoted to assistant manager. "I just got tired of it," he explains. "How are you going to keep up your car payments and insurance?" his father asks. "Oh, it will work out," the boy says as he dashes off to party with his buddies.

Unfortunately, these dyslogical young people often marry others with the same social disability, which creates a marriage not based on any structure or logical foundation. They run up debts on charge accounts, buy expensive items on impulse, party all night and sleep all day, and do not clean the apartment or do dishes. They fight all the time, yet they are extremely jealous if one spouse is friendly to another person. It is impossible for parents to reason with young people whose lives are controlled by this syndrome. They do not think in a logical way. They have no regard for tradition that expects everyone in society to be responsible. They have no intention of "dancing the tribal dance," yet they demand to have all the comforts modern society offers. They want their parents to give them money, pay their bills, and bail them out of trouble, yet they refuse to work things out through counseling. These SELD young people are too loose to establish productive lives. They do not follow guidance and cannot live by schedules. They get themselves into astonishing, difficult situations with no plans for resolving problems because they live by the impulse of the moment.

Reducing Impulsivity

Is it possible to turn such oppositional, impulsive behavior another way? Dyslexia is caused by incomplete neural wiring within the left brain. Most of those who are dyslexic gradually outgrow enough of their childhood learning difficulties to become educated. To some degree, for the rest of their lives they will continue to stumble over reading, spelling, and writing. Some individuals are too severely dyslexic ever to attain functional literacy skills, yet they can become successful adults in occupations that do not require them to read or write. Youngsters who display the dyslogic syndrome (severe SELD) face enormous challenges in reducing impulsivity, immaturity, and lack of commonsense reasoning. Because SELD is caused largely by lesions within the right-brain hemisphere, traditional talking therapy cannot change the social disability behaviors of NVLD and SELD.

Firm Guidance with Structure

If dyslogical behavior is recognized early enough, it can be modified somewhat, although the individual always will be prone to impulsive decisions and irregular social behavior. If firm behavior modification is begun in childhood while the youngster is teachable, it is possible to implant enough awareness of cause and effect to enable him or her to succeed by early adulthood. However, it is impossible to erase dyslogical thinking patterns altogether. The key is to maintain very tight structure over a period of years so that the oppositional youngster is kept within certain boundaries. Every restriction and boundary limitation must be clearly labeled as the reasons why are made clear. "No, Jason. You may not ride your bike over to Allen's house." "Why not? Jim gets to ride his bike everywhere he wants!" "No, Jason. Your brother does not ride his bike anywhere he wants, and you know that. The reason you may not ride your bike to Allen's house is that you don't pay attention to traffic. Until you learn to stop and look carefully, you may not ride your bike that far. And that is how it's going to be."

No amount of complaining, threatening, or fussing changes the rule. So long as Jason's behavior is illogical or exposes him to danger, then his behavior will be supervised and controlled. As he matures, he is held responsible for paying for things he breaks. He must apologize whenever he is rude. He must face up to the part he plays when things get out of hand or he creates difficulty. He is not allowed to get away with blaming others, demanding his own way, saying hateful things out of spite, acting out jealous feelings, having money to splurge on whims, and so forth.

Step by small step, Jason learns certain lessons as he grows up. If he is immature, he will be disciplined like a younger child. If he creates an expensive loss, he must pay for the damage. He must earn a certain amount of money before he can make purchases. Whether he likes it or not, he learns that there are limits. He learns that there are laws governing society, and there are police officers who enforce those laws.

Jason's parents agree not to take his side against teachers, unless a particular teacher clearly has been unfair. His parents and close relatives teach him that a family must maintain a certain level of courtesy and mutual respect. They do not give him money freely or pay the bills he accumulates. As time goes by, Jason learns that he cannot get away with using people. He learns that he must give if he hopes to receive. These basic social lessons can be learned if adults do not wait too late. However, because the underlying cause for irregular social behavior lies within brain structure, dyslogic syndrome (severe SELD) is impossible to change completely.

Becoming Independent

Being independent means that people can handle life alone without help. Without needing a supervisor, they can make personal decisions, plan ahead, work toward goals, and make choices based on commonsense reasoning. On their own, they can work toward establishing a comfortable life with occasional help from others. Being independent means that individuals may turn to friends or parents for opinions, but they do not require the approval of others to know what to do. As adults, they must "cut childhood roots" to a certain degree and replant their lives with new concepts that do not depend on what the mom or dad says or does. They must be able to read all of the signs and do what they say without having to ask an interpreter for help. An independent person enjoys talking things over with a trusted advisor, because being independent includes knowing the value of wisdom. Being independent means one can make decisions, change plans, establish new values, and start on new journeys without depending on others.

It is difficult for persons with dyslexia to reach this level of independence. When SELD or NVLD also exist, it is doubly hard to become independent. During my four decades watching dyslexic children grow up, I have learned that they go one of four ways.

1. Replace Parental Supervision with Help from Someone Else

Most youngsters with LD gradually replace parent supervisors with a close friend, usually someone they are dating. As a special friendship or romantic relationship develops, teens who are LD become dependent on this new important person. Girls who are not LD often become supervisors for boys who are dyslexic. Occasionally a boy who is not LD becomes the supervisor for a girl who is. These relationships tend to become intensely emotional and usually are lopsided. The relationship actually becomes a parent–child situation with the supervisor taking the place of mom or dad. Although romance often is the basis for their relationship, these partners find themselves in conflict when one person gives advice and instructions while at the same time is the object of romantic affection. The partner with dyslexia often resents the parental role of the other, but he or she cannot get along without this help, even when it triggers stress. Not many teens are mature enough to comprehend all of the factors in these complex relationships. The strong bonding that occurs in romantic partnerships is in conflict with the nurturing bond that exists between parent and child. When dyslexic individuals fall in love with someone who does not have LD, it is difficult for them to work through the stress and frustrations that emerge from their unequal needs, unless they are willing to receive counseling.

Marriage

When individuals with dyslexia marry, usually they choose spouses who can fulfill the role of supervisor. The spouse keeps the budget, makes all the family lists, manages the money, takes care of family details, reminds the partner when and where to be, and so forth. The supervisory spouse writes all the letters, pays the bills, plans for gifts and birthday celebrations, keeps the family on schedule for holidays, and stays in touch with important relatives. Through today's computer-based correspondence, many persons with dyslexia learn how to communicate with certain relatives and friends through quick e-mail messages. Aside from this abbreviated form of communication, partners who are dyslexic seldom participate in communication that keeps a family functioning.

Obviously, this marriage style is not an equal relationship. The spouse with no LD must be both a marriage partner, with all that implies, and the "parent" who makes lists to keep the "child" on schedule. Solid, comfortable marriages can develop between a dyslexic adult and someone who is not. However, the spouse with dyslexia must be willing to delegate organizational chores to the other without feeling threatened, jealous, or diminished by this supervisory help. Meanwhile, the supervising spouse must be able to accept this dual role without complaint or resentment. Most marriages that include a partner with LD are marked by conflict, resentment, misunderstanding, too much criticism, and suspicion. Someone must be the organizer and manager of time and schedules, and the other must accept this help with grace and gratitude.

Having Children

The vastly important issue of having children often becomes a point of major disagreement within such a marriage. Most of the dyslexic adults I have known since they were children are reluctant to become parents. Countless times, I have heard this expression, mostly from men who are dyslexic: "I don't want to bring a child into this world to face all the problems I had as a kid." For intensely emotional reasons, they never have intended to have children. Most of these men carry heavy emotional baggage from childhood and adolescence that continually reminds them of unhappy struggle all their lives. Although they are in love with a wonderful person, they do not want to risk passing their LD misery on to a child.

This issue seldom is discussed during courtship. Most of these dyslexic men recoil from talking about such a powerful, intimate factor of their lives. In most instances, dating leads to marriage with the spouse unaware of how the dyslexic partner feels about having children. Most of these marriages fall apart when the issue of childbearing is made clear. "I don't want to have children!" the agitated husband reveals. "Why didn't you tell me this before we married?" his spouse wonders. "I can't talk about it!" he responds in an angry voice. At that point, counseling with someone whom the dyslexic partner trusts is required to enable the marriage to survive. Only a few of the marriages I have observed between a man who is dyslexic and a woman who is not have survived this entrenched refusal to father a child.

2. Stay with Parents for Safe Supervision

Not all young adults with dyslexia, NVLD, or SELD are ready to become independent of parents or supervisors when they reach adulthood. A growing trend in the United States is for young adults to continue to live with parents long after their peers are living independently. A similar growing trend is for adult children to move back home when they cannot succeed on their own. In most instances, this continuing dependence on parents occurs because the child with LD was not prepared over time to become an independent adult. The steps in teaching visible structure, described earlier in this chapter, were not taken during childhood and early adolescence. The level of fear within the child's feelings and emotions was not reduced through careful teaching over a long enough period of time. In many families, it was easier for the adults to do all of the planning and decision making without doing the work of teaching the child how to do so. Few of these adults who move back home were taught money management, how to perform on a job, nutrition and simple meal preparation, housekeeping skills, and time management. Away from parental supervision, their lives fall apart.

It requires never-ending patience for parents to prepare a child with dyslexia or social disability for independent adulthood. These children are like all others in that they mature at different rates. Many adolescents with dyslexia or SELD are late developers, reaching their late teens or early 20s with the physical maturity of most 14- or 15-year-olds. Young men with LD often do not shave or achieve full voice change until age 21. When their high school peers were dating and practicing romance, these late bloomers had no interest in such activity. As children, they were too immature to fit in with classmates in kindergarten and elementary school. In their early teens, they were too immature to take part successfully in middle school or high school social life. As young adults, they are several years behind schedule in being ready to live alone without supervision. Therefore, they continue to live with parents who do not know how to help them other than to provide safe shelter. Members of this special population struggle to find jobs at which they can make an independent living. When they work, it usually is for minimum wage, which does not provide enough net pay to support themselves separately.

3. Live Alone

Many individuals with dyslexia or NVLD find themselves living alone. They have not developed enough social flexibility to live successfully with a roommate or partner. Often they are shy by nature, never having felt comfortable with strangers or within a group. All their lives they have avoided social events, placing themselves outside the circle of their peers. These loners did not participate in sports, were not members of clubs, did not participate in religious youth groups, and did not "run around" with friends. As young adults, they are too uncomfortable socially to be part of typical adult society. As a rule, they earn a modest income that does not permit any form of luxury. Their lifestyle is reclusive, isolated, celibate, and alone. They choose the loneliness of solitary living because they cannot cope with the emotions and feelings of sharing life with a partner. They have virtually no concept of or experience with intimacy on any level. Each of these private, reclusive individuals has one or two friends with whom they spend time to do certain things, such as watch sports events together, attend a movie now and then, or share simple meals at low-cost restaurants. Sometimes they venture out for worship with a congregation that does not make demands for them to join. But these low-key social contacts are limited. These quiet loners go out of their way not to attract public attention. If they maintain family contact, those occasions are brief and seldom. They construct firm boundaries that enable them to feel safe within their solitary lifestyles.

4. Serve Time in Prison

Since the early 1970s, numerous studies were done of the learning patterns and levels of literacy among men and women in prison (Brier, 1989; Gilligan, 1996; Jordan, 1974, 1996a; Payne, 1994; Pollan & Williams, 1992; Weisel, 1992, 2001). These and other studies have documented the fact that learning disabilities are prevalent among adjudicated delinquent adolescents and convicted adult felons. Approximately three out of four adolescent and adult males serving time within the penal systems of the United States show significant signs of LD (dyslexia, ADHD or ADD, SELD). The average level of literacy skills among this prison population is below fourth grade. Virtually none of these males serving time were identified as being LD during their school years. Most of them were evaluated for the first time as they entered a correctional facility or during an adult education program within prison. It is well established that many dyslexic and SELD males in our culture forfeit their freedom through crime.

There are numerous reasons for this social problem. A majority of the incarcerated males with LD come from impoverished economic lifestyles where basic needs were not met during childhood and adolescence and in which education was unimportant. Often there was no stable supervisory parenting during their formative years. The critical factor in their becoming involved with criminal activity was their lack of literacy skills. They could not compete with better educated individuals in the job market, did not have the personal skills to cope successfully with marriage, could not handle the literacy requirements of society in order to establish stable lives, and had no trustworthy parenting models to follow in their efforts to be fathers and husbands. They entered adolescence and adulthood mostly illiterate, insecure, unstable, and unskilled. The question must be raised: How many of these men could have been saved had their LD patterns been identified and supervised when they were open to teaching and guidance? Society has paid a staggering price in the loss of these men who otherwise might have been guided toward productive lives.

Adults Who Have Overcome Dyslexia

9

N ot all persons with dyslexia are able to overcome their challenges and become successful. Many are too scarred by childhood experiences to have the necessary courage or inner strength to overcome their learning differences. For many, life circumstances overwhelm their ambitions, crushing hopes and dreams. Yet many who are dyslexic do break through the barriers that block their way. As they pass through adolescence and enter early adulthood, they find ways to compensate, bypass their LD patterns, and achieve victories that may have seemed impossible in early years. How does someone overcome such a deep-seated, life-saturating condition? Why do certain individuals emerge from years of struggle and near failure as happy, creative adults while classmates and peers with the same challenges do not?

This chapter presents intriguing stories of victorious adults who had the right support at right moments in their lives. They had the courage and tenacity to respond to the help, which enabled them to rise above the challenges that almost crushed them. The shame and despair of their early years were transformed into hope and success. As Gilligan's model (1996) illustrated in Chapter 7, their crushed self-esteem was resurrected into living hope that allowed them to transcend earlier struggles. Chapter 8 told the unfortunate stories of Eric and Joseph who could not overcome their childhood adversity. It is appropriate to counter those stories of lost opportunities by telling some exciting victory stories from adults who overcame their language dysfunctions in remarkable ways.

Thomas Alva Edison

Like many individuals with dyslexia, Thomas A. Edison barely survived the first years of childhood. His mother, Nancy Edison, was 37 when he was born. Already she had lost three children through miscarriage, and she was determined that this last child should survive. Her son was somewhat deformed at birth with an overly large head, and his early motor and language skills were very slow to emerge. Edison's biographer Maurice Josephson reported that Thomas's head was so large that the attending physician concluded that Edison might have brain fever. Physicians of that day advised the Edisons that this child always would be an "invalid." It is recorded that relatives, friends, neighbors, and professionals of that day counseled Nancy Edison to "put him away" and not hope that he would ever be normal (Josephson, 1959, p. 12).

When Thomas Edison was sent to school, he was diagnosed as mentally ill because he could not do the academic work expected at that time. When Thomas was 8 years old, he was enrolled in a one-room school. Later he recalled that it was impossible for him to learn the alphabet or arithmetic by rote. All his life, Edison learned by inventing his own multisensory strategies to build permanent memory for new information.

After attending school for 3 months, Edison overheard his teacher say, "That boy is addled." Mrs. Edison became enraged over that attitude toward her son. She withdrew him from school and vowed to teach him at home. When Edison was 7, he contracted scarlet fever, which set into motion the gradual deafness that destroyed his hearing by early adulthood.

During Edison's childhood, adults continued to call him "backward" and "addled." He strongly resented such labels, and he turned to his mother as his main source for knowledge and information. Mrs. Edison, who was a former teacher, developed ways to help her son learn. Mr. Edison became strongly disappointed in his "retarded son" and refused to pay for extra things. This determined mother and son were on their own to devise an educational program the best they could. From time to time, Edison returned to public school, but he never could fit into a classroom structure. In his later years he wrote, "I remember I used never to be able to get along in school. I was always at the foot of the class. . . . My father thought that I was stupid, and I almost decided that I was a dunce" (Josephson, 1959, p. 14).

Throughout his developmental years, Edison listened as his mother read to him. Through listening he absorbed great quantities of literature, history, science, philosophy, the Bible, and whatever else Mrs. Edison could supply. This home-school education nurtured the boy's literacy skills, but Edison struggled with spelling, grammar, and writing skills. At age 19, he wrote the following letter to his mother:

> Dear Mother. Started the Store several weeks. I have growed considerably I don't look much like a Boy now- How all the folk did you receive a Box of Books from Memphis that he prepared to send them-languages. You son Al. (Josephson, 1959, p. 22)

Edison kept a diary for most of his adult life. As he grew older, he developed a simple writing style that allowed him to express his thoughts clearly, but he always used simple words and short sentences. He avoided words that he could not spell. At age 67, he wrote an essay that revealed his deep, often bitter feelings toward public education:

> I am frequently asked about our system of education. I say that we have none. Our system is a relic of the past. It consists of parrot-like repetitions. It is a dull study of twenty-six hieroglyphs. Groups of hieroglyphs. That is what the young of this present day study. Here is an object. I place it in the hands of a child. I tell him to look at it. . . . Why should we make him take impressions of things through the ear when he may be able to see? . . . It is of the utmost importance that every faculty should meet the environment. What is the use of crowding the mind with facts which cannot be utilized by the child because the method of their acquisition is distasteful to him?
>
> I like the Montessori method. It teaches through play. It makes learning a pleasure. . . . That system of education will succeed which shows to those who learn the actual thing—not the ghost of it. I firmly believe that the motion picture is destined to bear an important part in the education of the future. (Josephson, 1959, pp. 112–113)

The fertile mind of Thomas Alva Edison, which gave the world so many life-changing inventions, realized the value of multisensory learning for children. He had achieved his knowledge by developing multisensory techniques and strategies that allowed him to connect several sensory pathways at the same time. He realized that rote memory was not the best way to teach children, especially those who struggle with traditional methods of silent learning.

Edison's writing displays numerous signs of dyslexia. What was the key to his success? Early in his life, he became angry, and his anger became the primary drive that allowed him to conquer his language dysfunctions. Edison's intuitive mother was able to channel that anger in productive ways so that her son did not waste his potential just being angry. He learned to move ahead in spite of being rejected by his father and being hideously labeled by his school. For Edison, anger turned the right way was the key to his future success. In his later years, he no longer needed that anger to drive him forward, but it was the essential ingredient that kept him moving ahead during his difficult formative years.

George S. Patton IV

George S. Patton IV, the famous general of World War II, had a most unusual childhood. His father was a strong, domineering man who reared the family in isolation on a ranch. The Patton children were forbidden to mix with other youngsters, and they did not attend school until their teen years. George Patton III strongly believed in the oral learning tradition. He thought that no child should learn to read until age 12. The Patton children were immersed in oral reading. Adults in the family took turns reading aloud from the classics and the Bible. George S. Patton IV spent his first 12 years in this isolated environment, absorbing oral literature the way he breathed air. He had an extraordinary memory for what he heard. After hearing an adult read or deliver a speech, he could recite it almost word by word without ever having seen the printed text. Patton developed a grand style of oratory, strutting about the ranch shouting long poems and literary passages by the hour. He brought great pride to his father, who probably had a reading disability himself and therefore had no regard for traditional literacy skills. By his 12th birthday,

Patton had the literary education of an adult, all of which he had learned orally.

At age 12, Patton was sent to a private school designed to prepare him to enter the U.S. Military Academy at West Point. At that time he could not read. He was an authority on world literature and he could write in a unique script, but he could not read. Entering the private preparatory school was a deep shock to his self-esteem. Suddenly he was transplanted from a home environment where he was adored as a "genius" to a school environment where he was regarded as ignorant. He compensated by getting information from classmates as well as quickly placing himself in the good favor of his instructors by keeping every rule better than anyone else. In the prep school, and later at West Point, Patton astonished his peers and leaders by his remarkable auditory memory. He could hear a lecture or sermon once, then repeat it verbatim days later.

Patton never became a fluent reader, which forced him to compensate through his oral retention skills. He developed irritating show-off habits of overwhelming his critics by his phonomenal memory. He was an avid student of the Bible, military history, poetry, and certain areas of literature, but his reading always was slow and labored. When he commanded armies during World War II, he often was seen alone, laboriously working through the Bible or some other reading material by muttering it aloud to himself as he slowly sounded out the words.

How did this brilliant man with dyslexia succeed? Critics have been harsh in describing Patton's arrogance and often haughty behavior. His enemies delighted in reminding the world of his famous outbursts of temper, as when he slapped a hospitalized soldier across the face for refusing to rejoin the front lines in combat. However, those who regarded Patton as a friend recognized that he had an extraordinary drive to succeed. He was a proud man who strongly held to certain principles. He had an abiding religious faith, which he was not ashamed to proclaim. He never resolved certain hostile feelings toward military leaders who made his life difficult, and he had a constant need to prove that he was as good or better than anyone else. Pride, ambition, and a brilliant capacity to absorb what he heard gave Patton the ability to overcome the language-processing difficulties that embarrassed him so deeply during his adolescent years.

Woodrow Wilson

It seems incredible that a person with language disabilities could become president of a prestigious university and then president of the United States. But that is the story of Woodrow Wilson. At the beginning of the 20th century, he was president of Princeton University. This man, who had been a child during the Civil War, was elected president of the United States in time to guide the nation through World War I.

Like so many others with dyslexic-like patterns, Wilson had been taught at home during his early school years. There he listened to many hours of oral reading from the Bible and classical literature, yet he did not learn the alphabet until age 9 and did not learn to read until age 11. He never did well in school. Those who have researched Wilson's life report that he always was considered to be a "mediocre student." Biographers have discovered family letters in which relatives thought it odd that "young Woodrow is so dull and backward." Those relatives expressed sorrow for the boy's parents (Thomson, 1971). Wilson tried to avoid subjects that required abstract reading. Instead, he excelled as a public speaker and in student debates. During his early adult years, he became known as a gifted orator.

Tommy, as Wilson was called by his family, was ill much of his life. As a result, he did not finish high school, and his college studies often were interrupted. He became fatally ill toward the end of his term in office as U.S. president. This lifelong tendency for illness, along with his language-processing difficulties, often forced him to drop out of school or change his plans. During his childhood, a major influence that enabled him to deal with these problems was his father, who was a minister. The Reverend Wilson spent long hours reading the Bible to his son, discussing doctrine, and helping Tommy to develop a deep sense of right and wrong. As an adult, Wilson carried this spiritual attitude into his career. He exhausted himself working for world peace and was a major force behind the creation of the League of Nations following World War I. In fact, he no doubt shortened his life as he pressed for his ideals for peace and world brotherhood. Wilson always needed help to express his ideas in writing. His outstanding speaking skills masked the underlying struggle he always had with reading and spelling.

What was the secret of Wilson's success? There is no evidence that he was angry, or that he sought to vindicate himself before his critics. His motivation came from deeply held spiritual values that his father had helped to instill. Wilson overcame his language handicaps and poor health in his drive to make the world a better, more peaceful place for future generations.

Albert Einstein

Of all the famous people within the last century, perhaps it is most surprising to find that Albert Einstein was considered to have a language disability. His son, Albert Einstein, Jr., gave a thoughtful summary of his famous father's early years: "He was even considered backward by his teachers. He told me that his teachers reported to his father that he was mentally slow, unsociable, and adrift forever in his foolish dreams" (Thomson, 1971). During his early years, Einstein had very poor speech. His oral language skills developed slowly, far behind the usual schedule for his age. His parents feared that their slow-developing son was "dull." At one point, Einstein was dismissed from school and called a "dunce" by exasperated teachers. Throughout his life, his speech was slow and labored, which caused him to appear shy. In his later years as a faculty member at Princeton University, Einstein spoke softly and was difficult to understand. In fact, he lost three teaching positions early in his career because he could not communicate adequately during lectures.

At age 12, Einstein could barely read, and his speech was awkward and difficult to understand. Yet his brilliance began to emerge in his mastery of mathematics and physics while he struggled to verbalize his astonishing mathematical concepts. His writings of that time are filled with poor spelling and dysgraphic patterns. His language skills always were poor, even while his skills in higher math soared beyond the understanding of all but a few of the world's scholars.

All his life, Einstein remained a private, very shy man who occasionally blossomed in a public way. During his tenure as professor at Princeton University, he appeared in commercial advertisements, and his unique personal appearance became known worldwide.

How could such a shy, sensitive, man with a language disability succeed? Einstein had to absorb enormous insults during the first third of his life. This gentle person had no way to hold his own in a competitive world in which success was measured by how well one could "defend his own territory." This soft-spoken individual saw within himself the ability to contribute new knowledge to the world, knowledge that would revolutionize civilization. Yet he never revealed the emotional pain he endured before his intelligence finally was recognized. Einstein succeeded in spite of language disabilities because he had a new dream, one that he strongly believed had to be recognized by the critical world in which he lived. There was no anger or driving ambition behind his success—just enormous strength that gave him the ability to absorb insult and keep on trying until finally he caught the attention of others.

Nelson A. Rockefeller

One of the most powerful political figures of the mid-1900s had severe dyslexia. Nelson Rockefeller was governor of New York for four terms, then was appointed vice president of the United States. He was a philanthropist who gave millions of dollars to improve the quality of life for people around the world. This talented, important man had a reading disability that was so severe he could not read speeches without elaborate accommodations. In fact, he employed full-time assistants to be with him at all times to help him cope with language situations made difficult by dyslexia. In 1976, Rockefeller published a brief autobiography to promote a nationally televised program about dyslexia. His own words are the best way to understand how this courageous man finally won success:

> Those watching the Public Broadcasting Service program on "The Puzzle Children" (October 19, 1976) will include a very interested Vice President of the United States. For I was one of the "puzzle children" myself—a dyslexic, or "reverse reader"— and I still have a hard time reading today. But after coping with this problem for more than 60 years, I have a message of encouragement for children with learning disabilities and their parents. Based upon my own experience, my message to dyslexic children is this:

Don't accept anyone's verdict that you are lazy, stupid, or retarded. You may very well be smarter than most other children your age. Just remember that Woodrow Wilson, Albert Einstein, and Leonardo da Vinci also had tough problems with their reading.

You can learn to cope with your problem and turn your so-called disability into a positive advantage. Dyslexia forced me to develop powers of concentration that have been invaluable thoughout my career in business, philanthropy, and public life. And I've done an enormous amount of public speaking, especially in the political campaigns for Governor of New York and President of the United States.

No one ever heard of dyslexia when I discovered as a boy, along about the third grade, that reading was such a difficult chore that I was in the bottom one-third of my class. None of the educational, medical, and psychological help available today for dyslexics was available in those days. We had no special teachers or tutors, no special classes or courses, no special methods of teaching—because nobody understood our problem. Along with an estimated 3 million other children, I just struggled to understand words that seemed to garble before my eyes, numbers that came out backwards, and sentences that were hard to grasp.

And so I accepted the verdict of the IQ tests that I wasn't as bright as most of the rest of my class. Fortunately for me, the school (though it never taught me to spell) was an experimental, progressive institution with the flexibility to let you develop your own interests and follow them. I had a wise and understanding counselor (Dr. Otis W. Caldwell). "Don't worry," he said, "just because you're in the lower third of the class. You've got the intelligence. If you just work harder and concentrate more, you can make it." So I learned through self-discipline to concentrate, which in my opinion is essential for a dyslexic. While I could speak French better than the teacher, I couldn't conjugate verbs. I did flunk Spanish—but now I speak it fluently because I learned it by ear. My best subject was mathematics. I understood the concepts well beyond my grade level. But it took only one reversed number in a column of figures to cause havoc.

When I came close to flunking out in the ninth grade—because I didn't work very hard that year—I decided that I had better follow Dr. Caldwell's advice if I wanted to go to college. I even told my high school girl friend that we would have to stop dating so I could spend the time studying in order to get into Dartmouth College. And I made it by the skin of my teeth. I made it simply by working harder and longer than the rest—eventually learning to concentrate sufficiently to compensate for my dyslexia in reading. I adopted a regimen of getting up at 5 a.m. to study, and studying without fail. And thanks to my concentration and the very competitive nature I was born with, I found my academic performance gradually improving. In my freshman year at Dartmouth, I was even admitted to a third-year physics course. And in the middle of my sophomore year, I received two A's and three B's for the first semester. My father's letters were filled with joy and astonishment.

I owe a great debt to my professors. Most of all, however, I think I owe my academic improvement to my roommate, Johnny French. Johnny and I were exact opposites. He was reticent and had the highest IQ in the class. To me, he was that maddening type who got straight A's with only occasional reference to books or classes. He was absolutely disgusted with my study habits—anybody who got up at 5 in the morning to hit the books was, well, peculiar. Inevitably, Johnny made Phi Beta Kappa in our junior year, but my competitive instincts kept me going. We were both elected to senior fellowships and I made Phi Beta Kappa in my senior. Johnny, of course, had the last word. He announced that he would never wear his PBK key again—that it had lost all meaning.

Looking back over the years, I remember vividly the pain and mortification I felt as a boy of 8 when I was assigned to read a short passage of Scripture at a vesper service—and did a thoroughly miserable job of it. I know what a dyslexic child goes through—the frustration of not being able to do what other children do easily, the humiliation of being thought not too bright when such is not the case at all. My personal discoveries as to what is required to cope with dyslexia could be summarized in these admonitions to the individual dyslexic:

Accept the fact that you have a problem. Don't just try to hide it.

Refuse to feel sorry for yourself. Realize that you don't have an excuse. You have a challenge.

Face the challenge.

Work harder and learn mental discipline, the capacity for total concentration.

Never quit.

If it helps a dyslexic child to know I went through the same thing . . .

> BUT I can conduct press conferences in three languages
>
> AND I can read a speech on television—IF I rehearse it six times, with my script in large type, and my sentences broken into segments, and long words into syllables
>
> AND I learned to read and communicate well enough to be elected Governor of New York four times
>
> AND I won Congressional confirmation as Vice President of the United States

then I hope the telling of story as a dyslexic will be an inspiration to the "puzzle children," for that is what I really care about.

(Reprinted with permission from *TV Guide Magazine.* Copyright 1976 by Triangle Publications, Inc., Radnor, Pennsylvania.)

What was the key to Nelson Rockefeller's success in spite of having dyslexia? He was fiercely competitive. Instead of getting his feelings hurt when adults and roommates criticized him, he was determined to show them that he was just as smart as anyone else. This overachievement brought him all kinds of honors that did not seem possible for a person with his learning difficulty. Rockefeller wanted to win badly enough to sacrifice pleasure, convenience, and comfort to reach his goals.

Stephen J. Cannell

Not everyone has heard the name Stephen J. Cannell, but since 1966, millions of people around the world have enjoyed his television programs, which include *The Rockford Files, Hardcastle and McCormick, Riptide, The A-Team, Hawkeye, Silk Stalkings,* and *Renegade.* The writer and producer of these successful television shows has dyslexia. Cannell remembers his struggle in getting through school. "When I was in junior high school," his biographer reports, "people used to say to me, 'Stephen, can't you look at that word and see it's not right?' But every time I looked at the word, it looked fine" (Cannell Studios, 1998). Throughout his public school years and college studies, this kind of pressure from teachers and friends often got him down. Sometimes

Cannell thought he could not do anything right. "Dyslexics tend to be pretty poor students," he said. "But it has nothing to do with intellience. The biggest problem with dyslexic kids is that they get down on themselves. They can feel that they aren't smart in some ways, that they're retarded, and of course they aren't."

Cannell recalls that when he was growing up, dyslexia was still a mystery. No one understood it well enough to explain the problem to the children who had it or to parents and teachers. However, Cannell decided to become a writer, even though he could not spell well or write without mistakes. To accomplish his goal, he developed strict habits for studying. He was up early every morning, not allowing himself to sleep late or to put off the task of getting to his work. In college he did a lot of writing. He recalled that his professors would say, "Stephen, your writing is very interesting," but they gave him F's because of poor spelling. Still, he knew that his ideas were good enough to put on paper. He developed a method for enrolling in college courses—he would ask each instructor what his or her policy was regarding misspellings. In this way he found professors who would overlook poor spelling and give him credit for the value of his ideas and concepts. One instructor became intrigued with Cannell's vivid storytelling ability and taught him how to express his ideas in clear writing. He learned how to polish his visual imagination, which can be seen in the 47 popular television shows and movies he has developed or produced.

For 35 years, Cannell has followed a strict routine of starting work by 6:00 a.m. every day, writing steadily at his keyboard until 11:00 a.m. "My secretary has learned to figure out my mistakes," he explained. "What happens is that I tend to mirror-read and reverse letters. I am absolutely unaware that I'm doing it. It slows me down as a reader and makes me a horrible speller because no word really looks right to me." Through discussing his dyslexia publicly, Cannell hopes to be a good role model for youngsters who are dyslexic. "I hope they are saying, 'Gee, here's a guy who couldn't even read and now he's making a living as a successful, famous writer.'"

What was the key to Stephen Cannell's ability to overcome his dyslexia? He developed strong self-discipline and learned to write at a keyboard, letting someone else worry about correct spelling, good grammar, and accurate punctuation. He learned not to feel sorry for himself. Cannell developed an attitude that let him turn loose the worry and frustration of having dyslexia and allowed his mind to soar with ideas.

Phil Troyer

Few people have heard of Phil Troyer. Dyslexia almost destroyed his life before he found a source of love, acceptance, and guidance in overcoming his deep fear of failure. In 1986, Troyer published a novel titled *Father Bede's Misfit,* a story about his personal struggles to overcome his language disability. Troyer was reared by a father who considered it a weakness for men to show emotion or affection. As a child, Phil Troyer had severe dyslexia, but his language difficulties were not diagnosed. His family had no idea why their son struggled so hard yet achieved so little in academic learning. This deeply sensitive boy, who grew up without enough support to develop good self-esteem, was crushed by the experience of being laughed at by classmates because he could not read, write, or spell. His parents and teachers were unsympathetic when he turned to them for help. As he described in his novel, he grew up fearing that he was "dumb" and defective. During his teen years he was desperately insecure, lonely, and frightened, and there was no help available to relieve this deep misery.

In his early adult years, Troyer discovered a small monastery in New Mexico where he was taken in by compassionate monks. Father Bede became especially interested in this broken young man and helped him become part of the monastic community. At the point of emotional breakdown, Troyer began counseling with a psychiatrist, who provided a diagnosis of dyslexia. As part of his recovery therapy, Troyer began to write. Over a period of time he produced a novel that is a slightly fictionalized account of his life, telling the story of a man with dyslexia who almost did not survive. Troyer then began writing a second novel about his reconciliation with his father, who before his death, learned to express his love for his son.

How did Troyer overcome dyslexia? When he was at the lowest possible level of depression and confusion, a loving counselor and mentor came into his life and became a strong friend who believed in Troyer at a time when he could not believe in himself. An unexpected demonstration of love and confidence awakened the life that had almost slipped away through despair. With the support of this mentor and a community of dedicated friends, Troyer came back to life. With guidance and therapy he was able to rebuild his lost self-esteem and discover talent and intelligence within himself.

Josef Sanders

One of the most courageous men I have ever known is Dr. Josef Sanders. Although he has dyslexia, he founded a successful publishing company, Modern Education Corporation, that has produced excellent educational materials for more than 20 years. Like thousands of children with dyslexia, Sanders was almost a casualty in his early years. In an unusually candid essay, he told his life story in the following words:

> I was LD before it was popular to be LD. I was born prematurely and weighed only 3 pounds, 2 ounces. In those days, it was tough dealing with premature babies. My development was fairly normal until it was time to speak. I began to stutter at age 3 and continued stuttering until age 5. I used my left hand more than my right hand, and my parents were told to tie my left hand to my side to force me to be right-handed. My kindergarten teacher discovered that I had difficulty concentrating, and I talked a lot in class. I was never a discipline problem, but I was always restless in structured situations. I was told to wear glasses, but I hid them under my bed because I felt ugly wearing them.
>
> By the time I was in second grade, my learning problems were becoming obvious. I had difficulty learning to deal with symbols, both letters and numbers. My writing was very poor, and I had trouble following the teacher's directions. During second grade I realized that learning was becoming very difficult for me and that I was not catching on like my classmates. My teacher that year was frustrated with me. That was the first time I perceived myself as not being as good or as smart as other students. The teacher tied colored yarn to my wrists so I could tell the difference between right and left. I had great difficulty copying from the board. I severely reversed words (was/saw, on/no), and I had a hard time with b, d, and p. I could not write the alphabet without melody (singing the alphabet song).
>
> By the time I entered fourth grade, I was so far behind the others the principal called my parents in for a conference. They

were told that I appeared to be mentally retarded, and they were advised to place me in a special school for mentally retarded children. I will never forget coming home from school and seeing my mother crying. I asked what was wrong, and she said that the principal had told her that I needed to go to Sunshine School. My first response was that it sounded like a nice place. Sunshine School sounded pleasant and pretty. I will never forget how this caused my mother to sob. Finally she told me that Sunshine School was for mentally retarded children. She explained that my school thought I was mentally retarded and needed special education. The tone of my mother's voice struck fear into me. Suddenly I knew why she had been crying. All at once I realized that I was a different student. That moment was a major turning point in my life. I felt like a lost child with no sense of direction.

A few days later, I discovered that I was a very fortunate person. My mother became intensely angry about what the principal had said. She vowed not to send me to that school for retarded children. She declared that she would work with me herself every day until I could read, write, spell, and do math like other kids my age. This was an awful, painful period for me and my family.

As I struggled with my learning disabilities, I learned to escape from school frustration by playing by myself and using my imagination. I would create my own toys. My parents had very little money, and they could not buy things for me. So I created my own playthings. I learned to be grateful for being able to create things for myself. If I had a choice of playing or studying with my mother, I naturally chose to play outdoors. I did not like school and could not concentrate longer than a few minutes at a time. Half an hour of study with my mother was like an overweight 50-year-old man trying to run the Boston Marathon. It was difficult and very painful. My mind would wander, and I would cause my mother to become so frustrated. I just wanted to get out of the kitchen and play outdoors. Mother made me read aloud to her every day, and I hated it. Reading aloud is still a traumatic experience for me. I had so much trouble reading aloud in class or with my mother, I developed psychosomatic illnesses. The thought of reading aloud made me want to die. I was overwhelmed by extreme fear. My eyes could not track along the lines of the page. I stuttered and sounded like a little child just learning to read in first grade. I hated those times in reading circle or with my mother when I had to read aloud because my disability was always "found out."

I sounded so dumb! To this day, all of those old feelings come back if I am asked to read aloud in public. Recently I turned down a prestigious part in a worship service at my synagogue because of this old phobia toward oral reading. (Personal communication, 1988)

Sanders struggled through high school, finally earning his diploma. Then he joined the military service, where he began to discover new skills within himself. Like most low-birthweight boys, he was very late reaching important developmental milestones. Sanders is a classic example of a late bloomer who began to blossom during his early 20s. Eventually he earned a bachelor's degree, a doctorate in educational psychology, and his credentials as a speech therapist. He worked for several years as a highly successful speech therapist, then entered private practice, working with frustrated youngsters who were struggling with language difficulties. In the 1960s, Sanders founded Modern Education Corporation in Tulsa, Oklahoma, and began to market helpful materials for the field of special education.

What gave Josef Sanders the ability to overcome dyslexia? It was his unquenchable courage. No matter how difficult his life became through the pain of arthritis, the frustration of having dyslexia, and the anxiety of surviving the uncertain economics of private practice and running a business, he never gave up. His deep religious orientation has given him a sense of purpose. He believes that he is on this earth for a reason and that he will receive the strength he needs to function day to day. Sanders' courage has enabled him to overcome dyslexia.

How Do Persons with Dyslexia Achieve Success?

These heroic examples of achievement by individuals with dyslexia contain important wisdom for those who struggle with learning differences. What does it take to cope successfully with the hidden language-processing challenge called dyslexia? As we have seen in these brief glimpses into the lives of past and present persons with dyslexia, certain factors must exist to enable frightened, frustrated, and often overwhelmed individuals to come to grips with their language differences. The following characteristics seem to be necessary to allow dyslexic strugglers to overcome the challenges of their language difficulties.

Anger

The role of anger in overcoming dyslexia must be understood carefully. Of itself, anger usually is a destructive force that distorts reality and blocks the person's ability to deal with issues clearly. To be angry is to be deeply upset. To feel anger is to see an enemy who must be attacked and conquered. Anger is an explosion of the feelings that usually destroys objective thinking and distorts the intentions of others. To stay angry very long triggers a cascade of destructive forces within one's body and personality. As a rule, therefore, it is wise to avoid being angry.

The kind of anger that actually helps individuals with dyslexia overcome their difficulties takes the form of righteous indignation. For example, being indignant over injustice can be a constructive feeling and emotion. Indignation played a powerful role in Edison's eventual victory. He would not accept the verdict that he was defective, retarded, or unworthy. His pride was wounded by the treatment he received from the schools of his day, and he vowed never to submit to that kind of insult. Within Edison the young man was a burning indignation that smoldered like a carefully banked fire. He was angry at being treated in such a thoughtless fashion, and he simply would not permit it. That simmering resentment over the injustice of being wrongly labeled was the driving force that gave Edison the power to compensate for and eventually to overcome the disabling effects of dyslexia. Although his writing always contained poor spelling and limited language expression, he honed his skills to prove to the world that he was worthy of respect and admiration. Without that fire of anger, Edison, the right-brain genius, would never have emerged, and the world would have lost his vital contributions.

Fortunately, Edison had the devoted support of a mother who believed in him and pledged with him to beat the odds. She molded his anger into a constructive force, helping him develop strategies of success. With her assistance, Edison learned how to channel his anger and not waste his strength in useless battles against events and attitudes he could not change or control.

Edison's first motivation was to prove himself to a critical, skeptical world that did not care whether he lived or died.

Unfortunately, many persons with dyslexia are taught to believe themselves to be undesirable and unattractive. Edison, for example, was rejected by his own father and pushed from the educational system of his day. He experienced failure at numerous jobs during his early years, but he learned how to turn his hostility into strength. Constructive anger is essential for many individuals who are dyslexic. This kind of anger often is described by these persons as a motivating force for success. Those who overcome dyslexia do not allow their anger to make them overly bitter or resentful. Instead, they gain the wisdom to reflect on early struggles with the eye of a philosopher—an angry one, to be sure, but not a bitter one. The right form of anger can help open the door to success for individuals with or without dyslexia.

Pride

Like anger, pride often is the downfall of those who feel its intoxicating power. In its usual form, pride does indeed make tyrants and arrogant braggarts of us all. Raw pride is an ugly force that steps all over others and brags of its own worth. Unrefined pride struts and postures while claiming rights it does not deserve to have. In most religions, excessive human pride is regarded as sin, a feeling to be avoided, not cultivated among our children. Pride is the root of all sorts of difficulties in human relationships, perhaps because a proud person seldom is attractive. Of itself, pride is to be avoided and brought under control.

Yet pride can be the key to success for many persons with dyslexia. For example, Patton overcame his dyslexia through pride, even though he was not fully successful in taking the raw edge off that characteristic. History records many moments when he behaved in an arrogant fashion that disappointed his friends and created embarrassment for himself. However, Patton survived his reading disability exactly because of that strong confidence in himself. When pride takes the form of self-confidence, it energizes the person to keep on trying. Pride must exist to a certain degree before a healthy self-image can evolve. Being sure of one's own worth is vital if any kind of victory over adversity is to be achieved. This is especially true for individuals with dyslexia.

Often underlying the stories of successful persons with dyslexia is the quiet theme of pride. Conquering a language disability must involve a certain degree of pride because the struggling reader, speller, or writer must feel worthy of learning in order to do difficult work better. Overcoming the disabling aspects of dyslexia requires pride in its positive form. In Chapter 8, the unfortunate effects of arrogance and self-centeredness were displayed in Joseph's pathetic story. His kind of pride cannot help the person with dyslexia to break free. But quiet, calm, low-key pride continually reassures the person: "I am worthy of success. I am worth what it costs to overcome this present condition. I have a worthwhile contribution to make in the years ahead. I am valuable. I am intelligent. I deserve an opportunity to prove myself."

Faith

Having faith is such a simple thing, yet it does not always exist in the individuals who surround children who are dyslexic. Several of the success stories in this chapter have included the element of faith: A mother believed in her child when other relatives did not; parents believed when school leaders did not; the person with dyslexia believed, even when everyone else did not. Struggling individuals believed beyond doubt in a Creator who had a purpose for their lives. Faith could be considered the most "blind" of all human feelings, for it knows even when there is nothing tangible to see or to provide a foundation for knowing.

Faith is the most optimistic of all of our attitudes because it insists that substance exists where only emptiness appears. Faith is based on hope, and hope believes far beyond facts and scientific data. Faith says that this struggling person is not mentally retarded, even when standard test scores indicate otherwise. Faith looks beneath the surface of life and sees undeveloped potential that cannot be seen by casual observers. It could be compared to the person who, when all others see random bits and pieces, immediately perceives a finished mosaic. Critics see only useless fragments that should be swept away. Faith looks at a child with learning differences and sees beauty in the soul and strength in the unbloomed intelligence. Faith does not give up when leadership wants to end the relationship and send the struggler away.

Faith, that invisible, rather foolish, unscientific, often irrational force, is absolutely essential if persons with language processing dysfunctions are to overcome their struggles. Those of us who build our relationships on faith continually hear suffering people say, "I could not have made it without you. You are the only person who still believes in me." We who do intervention counseling with individuals on the verge of suicide often hear, "You are the only reason I'm still alive. If it weren't for you, I wouldn't be alive today." It is impossible for a child to survive the earlier years of dyslexic struggle without someone's faith. Someone must be able to see beyond test scores or classroom behavior and recognize the potential that can be developed through patient care. That person must teach the discouraged child that he or she is worthy of being loved, that he or she has value, and why that value must be preserved for the future. Without faith, there is no hope. Without hope, there is no reason to endure the endless challenges that must be overcome if individuals with dyslexia are to succeed.

Inner Strength

Individuals who overcome disabilities have an inner strength that does not always display itself on the surface. The stories about Wilson and Einstein tell of two men with language disabilities who at first seemed too weak to overcome their handicaps. They did not have the blustering self-confidence of Patton or the fiery anger of Edison. However, as their lives slowly developed, Wilson and Einstein demonstrated enormous inner strength that allowed them to overcome their language dysfunctions. Wilson was able to be become a successful speaker who could convince world audiences of the merit of his concepts of peace. Einstein did not learn to speak or write fluently, but he manifested a relentless spirit that produced the revolutionary formula $E = MC^2$, which changed the course of human life forever. Individuals who overcome dyslexia must have an inner strength that is as tough as an old oak tree whose roots anchor it firmly against hurricanes and tornadoes. These quiet ones must absorb insult without breaking apart. They must bend beneath the force of attacks against their integrity, then come back to a standing position still unbroken and intact. Overcoming life's extra challenges involves having an inner structure as tough as iron.

The quality of inner strength includes the ability to absorb enormous insult without retaliating. The teachings of Jesus include the challenging concept of going the extra mile, doing more than is required, and surprising adversaries by unexpected acts of kindness. Adults with dyslexia often need this quality, this capacity to stand still in the face of powerful forces, to know not to fight every battle that comes along. A certain degree of meekness—that ability to turn the other cheek in the face of confrontation—is required at times. In their quest to overcome their differences, persons who are dyslexic must control the urge to gain revenge. If they react to conflict on that level, they will be unable to overcome their limitations successfully.

Competitive Spirit

As was seen in the stories of Einstein and Wilson, not all individuals with dyslexia succeed through competition. Josef Sanders did not need to defeat his critics in order to climb to the top of his profession. On the other hand, individuals such as Rockefeller did find their victory through competition. For them, the urge to compete is the key to opening up the future. There is a heady quality in competition that triggers an adrenaline flow that kicks the person's skills into overdrive. Those who have such a spirit are lost when there is no challenge. They need a clearly defined adversary to overcome.

This spirit of competition can easily get out of control, of course. Most of us recoil from fiercely competitive people who thrive on challenge. Overly aggressive persons who live for competition often are very uncomfortable to be with. Like prancing, high-spirited colts in a stockade, aggressive individuals cause others to feel unsafe. In fact, making others feel ill at ease is an effective strategy for taking control of situations and of others. But the competitive spirit that enables dyslexic individuals to overcome challenges is a more disciplined attitude that does not involve an intent to dominate or subdue others while achieving one's goals.

For competitive adults such as Rockefeller, the key difference is an underlying theme of thoughtfulness and concern for others. Chapter 8 describes NVLD and SELD, unfortunate behavior patterns called social disability. These "socially dyslexic" lifestyles include self-centeredness, which is a universally unpleasant characteristic. The competitive spirit described in Rockefeller's story is a compassionate attitude, not an aggressive desire to have one's own way. Persons like Rockefeller need the challenge of someone such as his roommate, Johnny. The spirit of competition cannot see itself except by looking into the mirror of challenge. Once competitiveness sees its counterpart in the mirror, it is able to focus energy toward specific, well-defined goals. Without this focus through challenge, individuals who are dyslexic do not have a clear enough vision to know how to move ahead succcessfully. As we have seen, individuals like Albert Einstein, Josef Sanders, and Woodrow Wilson are able to see themselves clearly without standing before the mirror of challenge. If so, then the spirit of competition need not be part of their lives. However, the competitive spirit is essential for those who cannot define themselves any other way.

Self-Discipline

To succeed, every person who is dyslexic must be self-disciplined. This characteristic is the glue that holds all the other ingredients of success together. Each person must learn how to say no to things that would distract them from their main goals. Everyone who succeeds must be able to start early, as Rockefeller and Cannell explained, instead of taking it easy. Dyslexic individuals who succeed must be able to ignore pain, inconvenience, disappointment, frustration, depression, and all of the other voices that clamor for attention. Being self-disciplined means being able to make one's own plans, manage one's own time, meet one's own obligations on schedule, control desires that would consume scarce resources, and so forth.

Cultivating self-discipline is probably the least appealing activity anyone is asked to do. If human characteristics were given colors, self-discipline no doubt would be dull gray. Staying in control of self is a parental role. One cannot romp as a carefree youngster and be self-disciplined. One cannot always take second helpings or have rich desserts or satisfy strong cravings the moment they arise. Self-discipline is like a parent having to say no to a clamoring child. Staying in charge of oneself is not always a pleasant activity. When everyone else is goofing off, out at the lake, or on a holiday, self-discipline sternly says, "No, you have to stay home and work." Sooner or later, everyone gets tired of doing one's duty. Everyone wants to take a break at some point. The self-disciplined person must do one's duty and keep on with chores until important goals are accomplished.

As Rockefeller explained, self-discipline is the structure that holds the dyslexic pieces in place. When the loose pieces of dyslexia are carefully organized into a solid mosaic, self-discipline is the glue that makes the picture stay together. Persons with dyslexia who fail are those who never develop the structure of self-discipline. They go through life with too many pieces missing from the mosaic. Those who overcome are the ones who learn how to say no when the inner self clamors for satisfaction.

Loving Support

Chapter 7 presents Gilligan's model (1996) of how lack of love (affection) crushes an individual's self-esteem through overwhelming shame that often leads to violent behavior. Through his therapy with violent prisoners, Gilligan has demonstrated that through replacing lifelong shame with love and affection, crushed self-esteem can be "resurrected" into a new life of success. Those who work with discouraged individuals do not require validated studies to know that love is an essential part of overcoming challenges. Troyer's story brings this quickly to mind. As Chapter 7 described, lack of love during their developmental years created disabling guilt in the lives of Julian and Daniel. During the past 40 years, I have known many dyslexic individuals who did not receive enough loving support to sustain them. Professionals who counsel persons struggling with LD, SELD, or NVLD continually deal with torn feelings, emotions, and moods that destroy self-esteem because the person has no one to whom he or she can turn for love and reassurance. Every success story is about loving support from some important source. I always am grieved to hear a sorrowing person say, "You are the only one who still loves me after the mess I've made of everything." When loving support is taken away by those who lose faith, there may be nothing left on which the person with a disability can depend. Many attempts at suicide are triggered when the struggling individual believes that no one cares.

Loving support always is evident in victory stories of individuals who are dyslexic. As a rule, this support comes more from mothers than from fathers. I have seen many grandparents or an aunt or uncle assume this role. Youngsters continually find loving support within their extended families of religious leaders, scout leaders, coaches, and teachers. Teenagers with dyslexia often form their own support groups, finding among their peers the nonjudgmental acceptance they cannot find elsewhere.

Frequently I discover caring support behind prison walls where we least expect to find it. Often one sees a bond of loving support within sports teams for those who struggle with academic learning. It is impossible to overcome dyslexia if one is all alone.

As was seen in several of the stories in this chapter, the presence of loving support was a healing agent for an embattled child. To spend a day struggling through school, as Sanders described, is to suffer emotional bruises and wounds. To have dyslexia within a high-achieving family often inflicts battle scars on the ego structure of a vulnerable child. To have dyslexia in a competitive world where everyone else earns praise is to expose oneself to constant danger of emotional injury. The vulnerable child must have a source of healing from day to day. Loving support is the healing medicine for these battle-weary strugglers.

A Friendly Advocate

Every individual, but especially someone who is dyslexic, needs a person to be on his or her side. This goes beyond loving support because it also involves playing the role of advocate, speaking out on the struggler's behalf, and arguing his or her case when words fail. Someone must be there who believes, who cares, and who will come to the defense of the individual with dyslexia. This advocate usually is the mother, although when matters become serious, many fathers do step in for a while. Teachers frequently intervene on behalf of a struggling learner, and school counselors forever are trying to change a teacher's mind regarding a low-achieving student. Individuals with dyslexia often can go a while managing fairly well, if their lives are well structured. However, at some point they must have a friendly advocate to speak for them.

As I look back over the past four decades of working with dyslexic learners, I remember many who failed. In almost every case, there was no one to intervene. In the highly competitive arena of fluent speech, these individuals with language dysfunctions cannot find the necessary words to defend themselves against articulate, aggressive authority. Occasionally, stubbornness that emerges in some individuals who are dyslexic can defeat the efforts of friendly advocates. Usually, however, failure occurs because there is no one to take a stand on the individual's behalf. Conversely, all of the dyslexic individuals I have known to succeed had at least one forceful advocate. Edison, Sanders,

Einstein, and Troyer would not have survived without courageous advocates who took charge of their troubles and guided
them safely through their times of crisis. In these four cases, parents played this vital role of safeguarding their beloved children.

Courage

Repeatedly I have been astonished by the level of courage I have
seen in individuals who struggle to learn. Because of my own
moderate dyslexia, I have needed a certain degree of courage in
my own life. Yet I never have faced the enormous daily problems
faced by individuals with severe dyslexia. In the competitive
language-based cultures of the Western world, it is impossible for
dyslexic individuals to survive without courage. As dyslexic children struggle through school years, they often do not realize that
their level of struggle is unusual. They often assume that everyone must work just as hard. They are amazed when they learn
that their classroom struggle actually is unique among their
peers. How can a rational person face certain daily failure without becoming mentally ill? How can children with LD endure the
constant threat of failure and disappointment without at least
becoming neurotic? How do people who cannot read, write, spell,
or do math computation survive mainstream education where
busy teachers often have no idea how to meet their needs? Individuals with dyslexia who succeed exhibit persistent courage and
emotional toughness. They do not become neurotic or mentally ill.
Those who do not possess enough courage will go under.

During the 1980s, Sandra Jernigan at the Menninger Foundation began to map certain forms of mental illness that often
emerge during the middle teen years with the dyslexic population (Jernigan, 1985). The Menninger Foundation research discovered that eating disorders, especially anorexia nervosa and
bulimia, appear more frequently among dyslexic individuals
than among those who are not dyslexic. Certain forms of schizophrenia also occur more frequently among adolescents who are
dyslexic. As earlier chapters in this book have explained, severe
emotional damage is caused during childhood when dyslexic
children are labled "lazy." Self-esteem is crushed when adults
claim hard-working LD youngsters "just won't try." Youngsters
with LD are shamed by smart-aleck remarks from peers about
"going to the dummy class" when they leave the classroom to go

elsewhere for special help. When an inflexible or incompetent psychological examiner reports a low IQ score from a timed, standard test, how does the dyslexic child handle the shocking conclusion that he or she is "moderately retarded"? When classmates win praise and have their better work displayed, how does the child with dysgraphia cope with public shame? When everyone else is telling good stories about academic success, what does the struggling learner say? To survive 12 or 13 years in a generally hostile environment should produce several million emotionally disturbed children, but it does not.

Like Sanders, Einstein, and Edison, these children survive because they have courage. They have a built-in toughness that enables them to deal successfully with chronic near-failure, although not happily, not joyfully, and often with much pain. If they have courage, they make it through those destructive years with only old scars left to show their conflict.

No Self-Pity

A person with dyslexia cannot overcome those differences if he or she wallows in self-pity. To feel sorry for self is to look inward: "Poor little me! Look at my misfortune! Life is not fair! Everyone else is to blame! Look, everyone, look at me! Poor, pitiful little me!" This pathetic litany cannot be within the vocabulary of individuals with dyslexia if they are to overcome their language-processing challenges. As Chapter 7 describes, feeling sorry for oneself cripples the personality, leaving no strength for forward movement. Self-pity drains away vital emotional energy that is needed to sustain courage. Wallowing in the dark pool of self-pity submerges the person in a sticky emotional mess that quickly snuffs out any beauty. No one has much sympathy for someone who shows self-pity, but this is especially true for individuals with dyslexia.

The antidote for self-pity is a sense of humor, at least to some degree. No one can laugh very much at true misfortune, and there certainly is nothing to chuckle over when one is in pain. But the attitude of good humor must flourish strongly enough to enable a person to break free when self-pity reaches out to take control. It is impossible to overcome dyslexia if this defeatist feeling is an active part of one's life.

Appendix A
Jordan Scotopic Sensitivity Assessment Scale

	Never 0	Sometimes 1	Usually 2	Always 3
1. Do your eyes sting, burn, or water under bright light?	____	____	____	____
2. Do your eyes become sleepy and want to close after reading or writing for a while?	____	____	____	____
3. Do you start to yawn after reading for a while?	____	____	____	____
4. Do you skip words as you read or copy?	____	____	____	____
5. Do you skip lines as your eyes move down the page?	____	____	____	____
6. Does your mind start to wander as you read?	____	____	____	____
7. Do your eyes want to quit looking at the page after a few minutes?	____	____	____	____
8. Do you prefer to read in low or indirect light?	____	____	____	____
9. If you could, would you want to turn off bright light when you read or do your work?	____	____	____	____
10. Do you have to run your finger or hold a marker under each line to keep your place on the page?	____	____	____	____
11. Is there too much glare from white paper?	____	____	____	____

	Never 0	Sometimes 1	Usually 2	Always 3
12. Do lines move up and down on the page?	____	____	____	____
13. Do words smudge together, then move apart?	____	____	____	____
14. Do things on the page blink or flash or sparkle?	____	____	____	____
15. Do you ever see the fade-out/ fade-in effect in Figure A.1?	____	____	____	____
16. Do you ever see the halo (ghost) effect in Figure A.2?	____	____	____	____
17. Do you ever see the rivers effect in Figure A.3?	____	____	____	____
18. Do you ever see the swirl effect in Figure A.4?	____	____	____	____
19. Do you ever see the blurred effect in Figure A.5?	____	____	____	____
20. Do you ever see the up-and-down ripple effect in Figure A.6?	____	____	____	____
21. Do you ever see the smudged effect in Figure A.7?	____	____	____	____
22. Do things ever seem to fall off the edge of the page?	____	____	____	____
23. Do you feel dizzy or sick when you ride in a moving vehicle?	____	____	____	____
24. Do you go to sleep soon after you start riding in a vehicle?	____	____	____	____
25. Do things come up toward your face, then go back down?	____	____	____	____
26. Do things startle you from the side, as if something is coming at you?	____	____	____	____
27. Do you feel dizzy or afraid of falling when you look down from high places?	____	____	____	____

	Never	Sometimes	Usually	Always
	0	**1**	**2**	**3**
28. Do you flinch or jerk back when you try to catch a ball?	____	____	____	____
29. Do you bump into doorways or furniture as you move around?	____	____	____	____
30. Do you accidentally hit or knock things over as you reach across the dining table or work space?	____	____	____	____
Subscore	____	____	____	____

TOTAL SCORE _____

Scoring

1. Add all the checks in each column to find the Subscore for each column. Each check in the Never column equals 0. Each check in the Sometimes column equals 1. Each check in the Usually column equals 2. Each check in the Always column equals 3.

2. Add the Subscores to find the TOTAL SCORE.

3. Enter the TOTAL SCORE in the appropriate place on the following Scotopic Sensitivity Profile page.

Scotopic Sensitivity Profile
Rating Scale

Mild 0–10	Low Moderate 11–25	Moderate 26–35	High Moderate 36–45	Severe 46–55	Critical Above 55
____	0–10	*Not enough vision problems to need correction.* Person compensates naturally.			
____	11–25	*Enough vision problems to embarrass or cause difficulties in reading, copying, or working at a computer screen.* Can compensate by using a marker, touching the page, shading eyes, having extra time, working in low or indirect light.			

_____ 26–35 *Enough vision problems to cause difficulty in reading, writing, or using a computer screen.* Person is clumsy getting around and handling classroom or workplace materials. Needs modified light. Must think about next moves to avoid accidents. Should be referred to developmental optometrist for examination of eye tracking and eye teaming. Should be assessed by a trained Irlen procedure screener to find appropriate color application. Requires extended time for reading, copying, and writing. Must do visual work in short segments with breaks to let eyes rest. Must hear/say/see/touch to keep the place and process words correctly.

_____ 36–45 *Major problems reading, writing, and using a computer screen.* Has many small accidents with much clumsiness moving about and handling things. Must have a vision examination for eye teaming/eye tracking. Must have extra time to take breaks to rest eyes. Must do multimodality processing (say/see/hear/touch). Should work with a study partner. Requires oral testing and a trial at listening to books on tape to see if that would be effective.

_____ 46–55 *Severe problems with any vision task.* Person is handicapped in reading, writing, and working at a computer screen. Is accident prone in eye/hand coordination tasks (handling tools, placing things, using silverware, driving, operating machinery). Has severe struggle to function in any visual task that requires seeing small details. Must have Irlen screening to find appropriate color application. Must read and work under reduced light.

_____ Above 55 *Visual perception is nonfunctional for reading.* Person is noted for poor eye/hand coordination and clumsiness. Has noticeable difficulty driving a vehicle or operating machinery safely. Behavior may appear "weird" or eccentric because of how much compensation is required to get through life. Literacy skills and workplace skills are severely handicapped without correction for eye teaming and eye tracking, along with appropriate color application.

Finally the long journey was over. Luis and Maria held hands tightly as the airliner floated downward toward the runway. At last they were coming to their new home in this land of freedom. Their journey had started 12 years ago. For 12 long years Luis and Maria had worked beyond exhaustion, saving every peso they could earn. They had gone without new clothes. They had eaten only the least expensive food. They had worked at every extra job they could find. They had waited to have children. How many times had Maria cried herself to sleep whispering: "I am so tired. Oh, Luis, I am so tired. Will we ever be able to rest again?"

Luis squeezed Maria's hand as they felt the airplane dip downward for the last time. Together they held their breath waiting for the squeal of tires against the runway. Suddenly they felt the landing bump. Then the engines roared with a mighty backward push. The airplane slowed its race down the runway. Through their tears of joy Luis and Maria heard the voice of the cabin attendant saying: "Welcome to Dallas/Fort Worth. Please remain seated until the aircraft has come to a complete stop at the terminal. Have a good day in the Dallas area, or wherever your travel may take you."

Figure A.1. Fade-out/fade-in effect. *Note.* From *Jordan Dyslexia Assessment/Reading Program,* by D. R. Jordan, 2000, Austin, TX: PRO-ED. Copyright 2000 by PRO-ED. Reprinted with permission.

Figure A.2. The halo effect. *Note.* From *Jordan Dyslexia Assessment / Reading Program,* by D. R. Jordan, 2000, Austin, TX: PRO-ED. Copyright 2000 by PRO-ED. Reprinted with permission.

Finally the longjourney   wasover.Luis   andMari   aheld
tightly as theairliner   floateddown   wardtoward   the
runway. At lastthey   werecomingt   otheirnewhome   in
this landoffreedom.   Theirjourneyh   adstarted12yea   r
ago. For12long year   sLuisandMaria   hadworked beyon
exhaustion,savingevery   pesotheyco   uldearn.They   h
gonewithoutnew clothes.   Theyhad   eatenonlythe   lea
expensivefood.Theyha   dworkedate   everyextra   job
theycould find.They   hadwaitedtohave   children.How
manytimeshadMaria   criedeerselftosleep   whisper   ing
"Iamsotired.Oh, Luis,   I amsotired.Will we   everbeable
torestagain?"

Luis squeezed   Maria'shandasthey   felttheairplanedip
downwardfor   thelasttime.Together   theyheldtheir
breathwait   ingforthesqueal of tir   esagainstthe   runw
Suddenlythey   feltthelandingbump.   Thentheengi   nes
roaredwithamig   htybackward push.   Theairplaneslow
itsracedowntherun   way.Throughthe   irtearsofjoy   Luis
andMariaheard   thevoiceofthecabin   attendantsaying
"WelcometoDal   las/Fort Worth.Plea   seremainseated
untiltheaircr   afthascometoacom   pletestopatthe   ga
Haveagood   dayintheDallasarea,or   whereveryour   trav
maytake   you."

Figure A.3. The rivers effect. *Note.* From *Jordan Dyslexia Assessment / Reading Program,* by D. R. Jordan, 2000, Austin, TX: PRO-ED. Copyright 2000 by PRO-ED. Reprinted with permission.

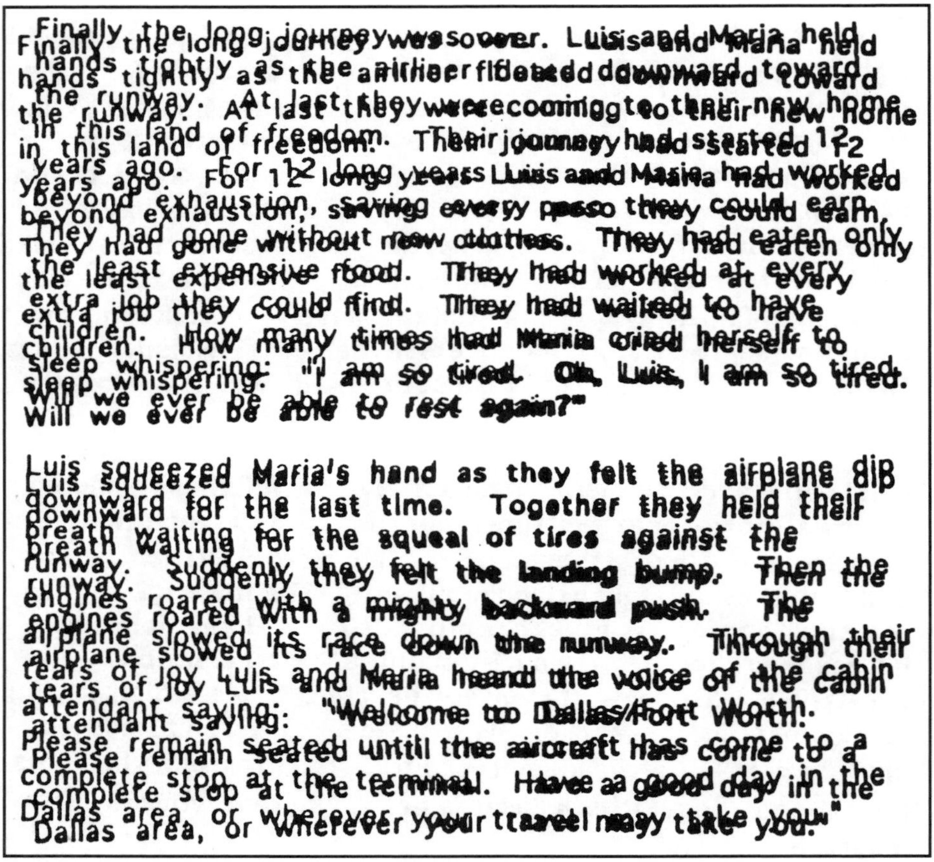

Finally the long journey was over. Luis and Maria held
hands tightly as the airliner floated downward toward
the runway. At last they were coming to their new home
in this land of freedom. Their journey had started 12
years ago. For 12 long years Luis and Maria had worked
beyond exhaustion, saving every peso they could earn.
They had gone without new clothes. They had eaten only
the least expensive food. They had worked at every
extra job they could find. They had waited to have
children. How many times had Maria cried herself to
sleep whispering: "I am so tired. Oh, Luis, I am so tired.
Will we ever be able to rest again?"

Luis squeezed Maria's hand as they felt the airplane dip
downward for the last time. Together they held their
breath waiting for the squeal of tires against the
runway. Suddenly they felt the landing bump. Then the
engines roared with a mighty backward push. The
airplane slowed its race down the runway. Through their
tears of joy Luis and Maria heard the voice of the cabin
attendant saying: "Welcome to Dallas/Fort Worth.
Please remain seated until the aircraft has come to a
complete stop at the terminal. Have a good day in the
Dallas area, or wherever your travel may take you."

Figure A.4. The swirl effect. *Note.* From *Jordan Dyslexia Assessment/Reading Program,* by D. R. Jordan, 2000, Austin, TX: PRO-ED. Copyright 2000 by PRO-ED. Reprinted with permission.

Finally the long journey was over. Luis and Maria held hands tightly as the airliner floated downward toward the runway. At last they were coming to their new home in this land of freedom. Their journey had started 12 years ago. For 12 long years Luis and Maria had worked beyond exhaustion, saving every peso they could earn. They had gone without new clothes. They had eaten only the least expensive food. They had worked at every extra job they could find. They had waited to have children. How many times had Maria cried herself to sleep whispering: "I am so tired. Oh, Luis, I am so tired. Will we ever be able to rest again?"

Luis squeezed Maria's hand as they felt the airplane dip downward for the last time. Together they held their breath waiting for the squeal of tires against the runway. Suddenly they felt the landing bump. Then the engines roared with a mighty backward push. The airplane slowed its race down the runway. Through their tears of joy Luis and Maria heard the voice of the cabin attendant saying: "Welcome to Dallas/Fort Worth. Please remain seated until the aircraft has come to a complete stop at the terminal. Have a good day in the Dallas area, or wherever your travel may take you."

Figure A.5. The blurry effect. *Note.* From *Jordan Dyslexia Assessment / Reading Program,* by D. R. Jordan, 2000, Austin, TX: PRO-ED. Copyright 2000 by PRO-ED. Reprinted with permission.

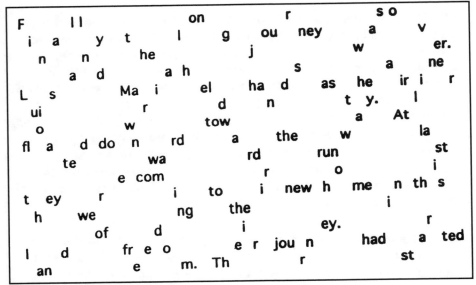

Figure A.6. The ripple effect. *Note.* From *Jordan Dyslexia Assessment / Reading Program,* by D. R. Jordan, 2000, Austin, TX: PRO-ED. Copyright 2000 by PRO-ED. Reprinted with permission.

Finally the long journey was over. Luis and Maria held hands tightly as the airliner floated downward toward the runway. At last they were coming to their new home in this land of freedom. Their journey had started 12 years ago. For 12 long years Luis and Maria had worked beyond exhaustion, saving every peso they could earn. They had gone without new clothes. They had eaten only the least expensive food. They had worked at every extra job they could find. They had waited to have children. How many times had Maria cried herself to sleep whispering: "I am so tired. Oh, Luis, I am so tired. Will we ever be able to rest again?"

Luis squeezed Maria's hand as they felt the airplane dip downward for the last time. Together they held their breath waiting for the squeal of tires against the runway. Suddenly they felt the landing bump. Then the engines roared with a mighty backward push. The airplane slowed its race down the runway. Through their tears of joy Luis and Maria heard the voice of the cabin attendant saying: "Welcome to Dallas/Fort Worth. Please remain seated until the aircraft has come to a complete stop at the terminal. Have a good day in the Dallas area, or wherever your travel may take you."

Figure A.7. The smudged effect. *Note.* From *Jordan Dyslexia Assessment / Reading Program,* by D. R. Jordan, 2000, Austin, TX: PRO-ED. Copyright 2000 by PRO-ED. Reprinted with permission.

Appendix B
Jordan Attention Deficit Scale

	Never	Sometimes	Usually	Always
	0	1	2	3

1. *Hyperactivity*
   Excessive body activity. Cannot ignore what goes on nearby. Cannot say "no" to impulses. Cannot leave others alone. Cannot spend time alone without feeling nervous or left out. Cannot leave things alone. Cannot keep still or stay quiet.

2. *Passive Behavior*
   Below normal level of body activity. Is reluctant to become involved with group activity. Tries not to be involved in group discussion. Avoids answering questions or giving oral responses. Does not volunteer information. Prefers to stay alone in play situations. Avoids being included in games. Spends long periods of time off in own private world doing make-believe/fantasy thinking. Uses fewest possible words when required to talk.

3. *Short Attention*
   Cannot keep thoughts concentrated longer than 60 to 90 seconds. Is continually off on mental rabbit trails. Must continually be called back to tasks. Attention drifts or darts away from task before finishing.

	Never	Sometimes	Usually	Always
	0	1	2	3

4. *Loose Thought Patterns*
Cannot maintain organized
mental images. Continually
loses important details. Cannot
do a series of things without
starting to make mistakes. Cannot remember a series of events,
facts, or details. Must have continual help to tell what has happened. Cannot remember a series of instructions. Cannot
remember assignments over a
period of time. Cannot remember rules of games. Keeps forgetting names of people and things.

5. *Poor Organization*
Cannot keep life organized without help. Continually loses
things. Cannot stay on schedule
without supervision. Lives in a
cluttered space. Cannot tidy up
a room or work space without
help. Cannot do homework without supervision.

6. *Change of First Impressions*
First impressions do not stay the
same. Mental images immediately change. Continually erases
and changes as writing is done.
Has impression that others are
"playing tricks" because things
seem to shift and change. Is continually surprised or startled as
mental images change. Word
patterns, spelling patterns, math
problems seem to change.

	Never	Sometimes	Usually	Always
	0	1	2	3

7. *Poor Listening Comprehension*
Cannot get the full meaning of
what others say. Continually
says "What?" or "Huh?" or "What
do you mean?" Does not get the
full meaning without hearing
it again. Needs oral information
to be repeated and explained
again. Does not keep on listening. Attention drifts or fades
away before speaker finishes
speaking. Later insists, "You
didn't say that" or "I didn't hear
you say that." Cannot remember
later what a speaker said.

8. *Time Lag*
Long pauses before person reacts. Does not start assignments
without being pushed or guided
to start. Long periods of time go
by with no work done. Long
pauses while he or she searches
memory for information. Continually falls behind the pace of
group activities. Does not stay
on set schedules.

9. *Overly Sensitive*
Is immediately defensive toward
criticism or correction. Blames
others. Spends much emotional
energy defending self or blaming
others. Flies into tantrums when
criticized. Jumps the gun, does
not wait to receive all of the information before becoming angry
or defensive. Leaders must spend
a lot of time restoring calm and
soothing hurt feelings.

	Never 0	Sometimes 1	Usually 2	Always 3
10. *Leaves Tasks Unfinished* Does not finish any task without supervision. Leaves several unfinished tasks scattered around. Thinks tasks are finished when they are not. Does not realize when more is yet to be done.	___	___	___	___
11. *Trouble Fitting in Socially* Cannot fit into groups without conflict. Whines or clamors for own way. Complains about rules not being fair. Storms out of games when not winning. Wants to quit and do something else before others are finished. Is aggressive and domineering in order to get own way. Cannot carry on small talk as part of social events. Wanders about, avoiding personal involvement in social gatherings. Is insensitive to normal manners and social protocol. Tends to be abrupt, rude, impolite in expressing opinions. Is overly critical of how social events are managed. Keeps conflicts going over unimportant issues. Displays self-centered attitude instead of noticing needs of others.	___	___	___	___
12. *Easily Distracted* Attention continually darts or drifts to whatever is going on nearby. Cannot ignore what others are doing. Is overly aware of nearby sound, odor, movement. Cannot ignore own body sensations. Must scratch every itch, adjust clothing, touch or feel nearby objects.	___	___	___	___

	Never	Sometimes	Usually	Always
	0	1	2	3

13. *Immaturity*

Behavior is obviously less mature than expected for that age. Behaves like a much younger person. Cannot get along well with age-mates. Prefers to play or be with younger persons. Has interests and thought patterns of much younger individuals. Does not make effort to "grow up." Refuses to accept responsibility or to be responsible. Behavior is impulsive/compulsive. Acts on spur of the moment instead of thinking things through. Refuses long-range goals. Insists on immediate satisfaction of wishes and desires. Puts self ahead of others. Blames others for own mistakes. Triggers displeasure of companions. Often is disliked by others.

14. *Insatiability*

Desires never are satisfied fully. Clamors for more. Cannot leave others alone. Demands attention. Becomes bored quickly and wants something different. Complains that others get larger share. Drains emotions of those who must be involved with this person's life. Triggers desire in others to push this person away. Often is dreaded by others. Becomes target of rejection by others.

	Never 0	Sometimes 1	Usually 2	Always 3
15. *Impulsivity* Does not plan ahead. Acts on spur of the moment. Does whatever comes to mind. Shows no common sense in making decisions. Does not think of consequences. Demands immediate satisfaction of wishes and desires. Is a "now" person. Cannot put off desires or wishes.	____	____	____	____
16. *Disruptiveness* Is a disruptive influence in a group. Keeps things stirred up. Triggers conflicts within group. Disturbs neighbors during study time. Causes others to complain about how this person is behaving. Others are relieved when this person is absent.	____	____	____	____
17. *Body Energy Overflow* Some part of the body is in continual motion. Cannot sit still. Cannot be quiet. Can hold body motions under control briefly, but energy overflow starts again soon. Fingers fiddle with things. Feet scrub the floor and bump furniture. Body squirms around. Mouth continually makes irritating sounds.	____	____	____	____
18. *Emotional Overflow* Emotions always are near the surface. Cries too easily. Laughs too loudly. Squeals too much. Giggles too often. Protests too frequently. Clamors in an emotional way. Is triggered easily into a state of hysteria. Tantrums always are near the surface.	____	____	____	____

	Never	Sometimes	Usually	Always
	0	1	2	3

19. *Lack of Continuity*
Lifestyle has no continuity.
This person's life is lived in unconnected segments. One event
does not flow into the next.
Must have supervision and
guidance to stay with a course
of action. In this person's mind,
a present activity is not connected with what happened
previously or what will follow.
Daily patterns and routines do
not register. Continually, this
person is surprised by each
task requirement, no matter
how many times this routine
has been done.

20. *Poor Telling and Describing*
Stumbles over words, names,
and specific details while telling.
Speech jumps around without
following an organized theme.
Speech is made of fragments instead of whole statements.

Subscore ‗‗‗‗ ‗‗‗‗ ‗‗‗‗ ‗‗‗‗

TOTAL SCORE ‗‗‗‗‗‗‗‗‗‗‗‗‗‗‗‗‗‗‗

Scoring

1. Add all the checks in each column to find the Subscore for each column. Each check in the Never column equals 0. Each check in the Sometimes column equals 1. Each check in the Usually column equals 2. Each check in the Always column equals 3.

2. Add the Subscores to find the TOTAL SCORE.

3. Enter the TOTAL SCORE in the appropriate place on the following Attention Deficit Profile page.

Attention Deficit Profile

<u>   </u>   0–25

Borderline Attention Deficit
This individual can be managed in a mainstream classroom by giving extra attention to keep him or her on schedule. Make sure that all oral information has been understood. Frequently remind him or her to be sure each task is completed. Life partners, parents, and workplace supervisors must do consistent reminding, supervising, and repeating of oral information. Individual tutoring is required from time to time to fill in gaps in basic skills.

<u>   </u>   26–35

Moderate Attention Deficit
This person requires a system that provides enough supervision to keep him or her on task. He or she must be reminded continually about observing details. Oral information must be given in segments, then repeated, to make sure it is comprehended. This "loose thinker" must have help keeping track of materials in the classroom, at home, and in the workplace. Someone in his or her private life must be a "supervisor" to monitor forgetfulness, remind of important deadlines, and help organize his or her life so that attention deficit habits do not sabotage success. This person cannot function effectively alone. He or she can be successful with consistent help.

<u>   </u>   Above 35

Severe Attention Deficit
This individual cannot function in traditional classrooms or most workplace situations unless special intervention and supervision are provided. Severe attention deficit disorder requires cortical stimulant medication to bring neurotransmitters into balance. Without medication, his or her feelings and emotions are filled with chaos, conflict, and confusion. With medication, modifications must be made in classroom and workplace expectations. This individual must have written guidelines to review frequently. He or she must have study buddies and work partners who remind them to slow down, think about it first, and review finished work for mistakes. This person must have one-to-one instruction because he or she is too distractible to function even in small groups.

Appendix C
Jordan Test for Visual Dyslexia

Part 1: Write the Alphabet, Days, and Months

Give students a sheet of lined writing paper and ask them to write the alphabet, the days of the week, and the months of the year from memory. The room should not have posters or other printed information from which students can glean clues. Individuals who are dyslexic usually have trouble starting this task. Often they ask, "Do we print or write cursy?" They may ask, "Do we write big or little letters?" They may ask, "Do we start here?" while pointing to a certain place. Be patient and work slowly as you guide insecure students through these preliminary questions. Remember that the midbrain must make sure that each new event is safe. Growing up dyslexic has implanted many fearful feelings and emotions in individuals who struggle to read, write, and spell. Assure uncertain students that it does not matter how they write this assignment. Tell them to write naturally, and assure them that this is not a spelling test. It is an activity to see how well they remember the alphabet, days, and months.

Most students who are dyslexic ask if they may abbreviate the days or months. If you have seen a major struggle writing the alphabet, you may choose to let individuals abbreviate. First, however, ask if they remember how to spell Sunday. Let them practice orally to see if they can recall how to spell Sunday. Most dyslexic individuals realize that they can write Sunday, even if it is mispelled. Use this method of encouragement until students settle into writing the days. Those who struggle to write the alphabet and days seldom can write the months. If so, let them abbreviate or write the first letter of the months they recall.

Watch closely for any of these dyslexic signals as this work is done. Check the symptoms you observe. Make notes of unusual behavior to remind yourself later.

Assessment Checklist

_____ Letters written backwards.

_____ Reversed loops on certain letters.

_____ Loss of sequence after remembering the first part correctly.

_____ Humming or singing the alphabet song.

_____ Going back to the beginning and repeating the sequence in order to remember what comes next.

_____ Mixing capital and lowercase letters.

_____ Mixing cursive and printing.

_____ Continual erasing and changing.

_____ Constant whispering or talking to self while remembering.

_____ Spelling phonetically (how words sound) instead of following spelling rules.

_____ Working very slowly with long pauses to think things through.

_____ Writing is barely legible or is illegible.

_____ Heavy pressure on the pencil or pen.

_____ Continual head turning from side to side, looking from different angles to see the page.

_____ Right-handed persons turn the pencil back toward the body in an awkward pencil grip.

_____ Lays the head down on left arm or on the elevated left wrist while looking sideways at pencil.

_____ Frustration signals, such as heavy breathing, feet scrubbing the floor, kicking the table leg, squirming about in the chair, muttering or complaining about "this is hard," breaking the pencil point from too heavy pressure, tears about to spill over.

_____ Reaches burnout point when the brain gives up trying to finish the task.

_____ Shows signs of eye strain: rubbing at eyes, rubbing inside corner of one eye, eyes watering, eyes growing red.

_____ Signs of light sensitivity: leaning over the page to shade it from overhead light, wearing baseball cap with bill pulled down over eyes, squinting at brightness of overhead light or glare from the page.

_____ Writing is too large for the line spaces.

_____ Writing cuts downward through the line, then floats above the line.

_____ Spacing is so poor that letters or words jam against each other, or are too far away from each other.

_____ Gives up and refuses to finish the task.

_____ Shows signs of anger or resentment at having to do this task.

Count the Number of Checks You Made

_____ 1–5
Mild Problems Writing from Memory
This person may not be dyslexic, unless you find dyslexic symptoms on other parts of this test, or on other writing tasks.

_____ 6–10
Low Moderate Visual Dyslexia
This individual must work hard to meet classroom or workplace writing expectations. He or she requires help to produce fully correct writing.

_____ 11–15
Moderate Visual Dyslexia
In every activity that requires memory for details, this individual struggles to keep details in sequence. He or she never is sure that his or her memory has correctly recalled information in the right order or sequence.

_____ 16–20
High Moderate Visual Dyslexia
This individual faces constant struggle to read successfully, write correctly, and remember things in the right sequence. This person must have a lot of one-to-one help to meet classroom or workplace literacy expectations.

_____ More than 20
Severe Visual Dyslexia
This is deep dyslexia that does not improve with age. All his or her life, this person will struggle with reading, writing, and spelling skills below fourth-grade level. This person must learn to write through a keyboard. Doing handwritten projects will be impossible.

Part 2: Copying from the Board

Print the following story on a wall chart or on the chalkboard:

Bob and Dan

Bob and Dan saw Sam Watts on the dock. The three men stopped. "See the big ship?" asked Sam.

"Sure did," Dan and Bob said. "Must be a mile long."

Bob and Dan saw Sam was in a hurry. "Got to run," Sam said. "See you."

"Sure," said Bob and Dan. "See you, Sam."

Ask students to copy this story onto lined writing paper. Have them sit across the room from the board or wall chart, as far away as they can yet still see the print comfortably. If individuals cannot see clearly, let them move close enough to see well. Make a note of how close he or she must sit to see clearly. Check the following behaviors you observe as this copying is done:

Assessment Checklist

_____ Must sit close to the board or chart to see clearly.

_____ Leans forward and squints to see the print clearly.

_____ Writes letters backwards.

_____ Turns letters upside down.

_____ Scrambles the sequence of letters while copying.

_____ Writes words backwards.

_____ Fails to copy punctuation marks.

_____ Fails to copy capital letters.

_____ Continually loses the place and has to find it again.

_____ Points pencil or finger at the story to find the place.

_____ Frequently erases and changes errors.

_____ Fails to notice or correct errors.

_____ Continually whispers while copying.

_____ Places heavy pressure on pencil or pen.

_____ Writing is barely legible or illegible.

_____ Writing cuts downward through the line, or floats above the line.

_____ Frequently stops to shake out muscle cramps in fingers.

_____ Continually turns head to see the story from different angles.

_____ Shows increasing frustration as copying continues (heavy breathing, signs of irritation or anger, impatience, hurries to get through without doing his or her best).

_____ Refuses to try or to continue after starting.

Count the Number of Checks You Made

_____ 1–5 _Mild Problems with Copying_
This person may not be dyslexic, unless you find dyslexic symptoms in other parts of this test or on other writing tasks.

_____ 6–10 _Moderate Visual Dyslexia_
This individual may have eyesight deficits that will appear on other tests for eye tracking and ability to focus from far to near. If so, correcting vision problems may remove most of the dyslexic-like patterns you see here.

_____ 11–15 _High Moderate Visual Dyslexia_
This individual likely has undiagnosed vision problems. Correcting vision deficits will leave a layer of visual dyslexia that continues to cause reversals, reading backwards, and scrambling sequence.

_____ 16–20 _Severe Visual Dyslexia_
This individual probably has severe vision problems. If so, correcting his or her vision is critically important. This person cannot make progress in literacy skills until vision deficits have been corrected. Beneath any vision problems lies lifelong dyslexia that makes classroom learning very difficult. This individual must have a lot of help at work and in the classroom to interpret printed information.

Part 3: Word Matching

Print the following words on cards, but do not capitalize any letters: *barn, tops, silver, trap, must, reverse, sheep, trash, wash.* Give students the worksheet for this activity (page 368). Instruct them to mark the word that is just like the word on each card. Allow all the time these individuals need to study the card before searching for the matching word.

Some dyslexic individuals must touch the card and finger-trace each letter to build a mental image of the word. Assure students that there is no pressure to hurry. When they are comfortable and feel safe with this matching activity, show the first card (*barn*) until students indicate they are ready. Then point to line 1 on the worksheet and remind them to find the word that matches what they just saw on the card. Some individuals may ask how you want them to mark their words. Explain that they can circle, underline, make a check mark, or draw an X across the word. If a student says that there are two (or more) words just alike, say that he or she is to mark all the words that are same. If an individual shows frustration and wants to see the card again, show it a second time, but make a note to remind yourself later of this sign of poor short-term memory.

Assessment Checklist

_____ Must touch the card or trace the word with a finger.

_____ Must whisper over and over to learn and remember.

_____ Sees two or more that are like the word on the card.

_____ Reverses letters.

_____ Turns letters upside down.

_____ Reads words backwards.

_____ Scrambles the sequence of letters inside words.

_____ Changes his or her way of marking from line to line.

_____ Makes backward circular strokes (clockwise).

_____ Has delayed recognition. Goes back to correct mistakes.

Count the Number of Checks You Made

_____ 1–3 *Mild Visual Dyslexia*
This individual may have poor reading vision. Correcting vision problems may remove word recognition mistakes that look like dyslexia.

_____ 4–6 *Moderate Visual Dyslexia*
If vision problems are corrected, this person will continue to stumble over which way symbols turn and how to keep details in sequence. He or she must have help spotting and correcting dyslexic glitches.

_____ 7–10 *Severe Visual Dyslexia*
If vision problems are corrected, this person will continue to stumble over printed symbols. Reading always will be slow and somewhat labored. This person cannot cope with time-limited reading activities or exams.

Part 4: Student Worksheet

Mark the word just like you saw on the card.

1. bran   pran   puar   bnar   narb   uarp   barn

2. spot   tobs   tops   stop   stob   sbot   tods

3. sliver   silver   vilser   revils   revlis   selvir   verlis

4. trad   brat   rapt   part   prat   bart   trap

5. tums   tsum   smut   swnt   tsuw   must   wnst

6. severe   esrever   reverse   eversen   servere   neverse   nervese

7. sheeb   speeh   sheed   sdeey   sheep   speey   peehs

8. tarsh   shraf   farsh   shart   trash   frash   sharf

9. mash   sham   wash   shaw   whas   hsaw   sahw

Appendix D
Jordan Auditory Dyslexia Test

Part 1: Repeating What Is Heard

As you do this activity, be sure to have eye contact with the individual, unless his or her culture disapproves of eye contact with an authority figure or with persons of the opposite sex. Explain that you will say some words, and the person is to repeat exactly what you say. Individuals with severe tone deafness to soft/slow speech sounds might ask you to repeat each statement several times. If so, suggest that you say it again three times. Be sure to speak slowly and distinctly. Then ask the student to repeat what he or she heard you say. Use the Assessment Worksheet to jot down exactly what the student repeats.

1. olives in vinegar
2. aluminum animal
3. suddenly suspicious
4. curiosity seekers
5. announced candidacy
6. conscientious maneuver

Next, explain that you will say a complete sentence. The person is to repeat it exactly as you say it. Say each segment slowly and distinctly, pause for a moment, then say the next segment. It is important to pause where the sentences are segmented. Individuals who are tone deaf may clamor for you to say it again. If so, repeat the sentence to reduce the person's frustration. Make a note of this on the Assessment Worksheet.

7. Three men—raced down the hill—to the boat—in the river.
8. After dark one night—he gave the money—to his best friend.

Finally, ask the student to give a rhyming word for each of the 10 words you say from the Rhyming portion of the Assessment Worksheet. Write exactly what the student says as he or she tries to rhyme. Check items on the following Assessment Checklist to develop a profile of auditory dyslexic patterns from Part 1.

Assessment Checklist

_____ Cannot maintain eye contact. (If eye contact is culturally inappropriate, disregard this item.)

_____ Cannot keep on listening without losing mental image or becoming distracted.

_____ Leaves out chunks when repeating.

_____ Tongue-twists parts of words while repeating.

_____ Asks to hear it again before repeating.

_____ Reverses word sequence while repeating.

_____ Scrambles word sequence while repeating.

_____ Shows excessive frustration during this activity.

_____ Shows increasing nervousness or irritability in this activity.

_____ Gives up trying to listen and repeat, or refuses to try.

_____ Is tone deaf (cannot hear) to soft/slow vowels or consonant.

_____ Cannot give exactly rhyming words.

_____ Is puzzled or confused regardless of how clearly you explain.

_____ Seems unsure whether answers are correct.

_____ Changes response, as if mental image has changed and he or she is searching for correct response.

Count all the checks you made _____

Part 2: Matching Oral Words with Printed Words

Give each person the Student Matching Worksheet for matching what they hear with what they see. Explain that you will say a word, then the person is to mark that same word on the worksheet. Remind them to scan left to right, not top to bottom. Be sure to say the number of each line: "Number One—wish. Number Two—every," and so forth. Pause a moment after you say each number before you say the word to make sure that you do not speak faster than students can process.

Watch for individuals who lose the place and must be guided to stay on the line, or who skip lines as they move down the page. Have some card markers available for those who cannot keep their place on the page. Tone-deaf individuals will ask to hear the word again. Repeat the word until everyone seems sure enough to look for the matching printed word. If someone asks you to use the word in a sentence, do so to reduce frustration. Make a note of which students need this reinforcement. Make sure that everyone is ready before you pronounce the following words:

Number One—wish

Number Two—every

Number Three—shine

Number Four—prior

Number Five—riot

Number Six—bark

Number Seven—quit

Number Eight—scorch

Number Nine—valve

Number Ten—madge

Number Eleven—singer

Number Twelve—part

Assessment Checklist

_____ Asks to hear words repeated.

_____ Asks to hear words used in a sentence.

_____ Cannot understand the words you say.

_____ Leaves out chunks when marking words (*ever* for *every, val* for *valve, sinner* for *singer*).

_____ Reverses inside parts of words (*scratch* for *scorch, prat* for *part*).

_____ Reverses letters (*dark* for *bark, quart* for *part*).

_____ Must whisper over and over to be sure.

_____ Must see/say/hear/touch to do this activity.

_____ Erases and changes first choices.

_____ Shows frustration or irritation doing this activity.

Count all the checks you made _____

Part 3: Writing from Dictation

Give each person the Student Spelling Worksheet for the 39 spelling words you will dictate. Explain that you will give them plenty of time before moving on to the next word. Make sure that everyone writes on the correct numbered lines. Pronounce each word distinctly and slowly, and repeat each word as many times as individuals ask to hear them again.

1. dig	14. pig	27. big
2. ate	15. rode	28. goes
3. play	16. please	29. toes
4. duck	17. buck	30. track
5. party	18. pretty	31. try
6. brown	19. born	32. for
7. barn	20. brand	33. from
8. girl	21. bird	34. stop
9. saw	22. was	35. post
10. kind	23. king	36. slat
11. city	24. cent	37. salt
12. this	25. think	38. how
13. on	26. no	39. who

Assessment Checklist

_____ Spells phonetically (how words sound) instead of by rules.

_____ Reverses letters (*b/d, p/g*).

_____ Reverses letter sequence inside words (*bran/barn, slat/salt, from/form, gril/girl, brid/bird, paly/play, gose/goes*).

_____ Cannot hear differences between who and how.

_____ Writes words backwards (*was/saw, on/no*).

_____ Mixes capital and lowercase letters.

_____ Mixes cursive and print writing.

_____ Misconnects sounds with letters (*sity/city, sent/cent*).

_____ Cannot tell the difference between similar words (*party/pretty, born/barn*).

_____ Leaves out letters or sound chunks (*gos/goes, prty/party*).

_____ Asks to hear words again.
_____ Asks to hear words used in a sentence.
_____ Shows increasing frustration partway through this activity.
_____ Stops trying or refuses to try.
_____ Frequently erases and changes first response.

Count all the checks you made _____

Scoring

Summary Scores

Part 1 _____

Part 2 _____

Part 3 _____

TOTAL TEST SCORE _____

Scoring Summary Page

_____ 1–7   *Borderline Auditory Dyslexia*
This person may not be dyslexic, unless you find dyslexic patterns in reading and other writing activities.

_____ 8–15   *Low Moderate Auditory Dyslexia*
This person has continual difficulty hearing speech sounds and words correctly, remembering how to spell, and matching oral words with printed words. Must have extra time with freedom to see/say/hear/touch while doing assignments. Should be referred for hearing evaluation to make sure that hearing ability is normal.

_____ 16–23   *Moderate Auditory Dyslexia*
This person faces constant struggle to spell correctly, understand oral information, sound out words in reading, and produce acceptable written assignments. Must hear important information again. Must have plenty of time to do assignments. Must work part of the time with a study partner to clarify oral information and to understand instructions. Must be referred for hearing evaluation to make sure that hearing ability is normal.

_____ 24–31   *High Moderate Auditory Dyslexia*
This person cannot cope with listening activities without help. Must have study partners to interpret oral information. Cannot be expected to spell correctly or read well without help. Must have a complete hearing evaluation to make sure no hearing loss exists.

_____ Above 31   *Severe Auditory Dyslexia*
This person cannot cope with spelling, reading, listening, and writing tasks without special accommodations. Must have study partners who provide patient guidance in doing assignments. Must have modified assignments that do not require accurate encoding and decoding skills.

PART 1
Assessment Worksheet

Student Repeats What You Say

1. olives in vinegar _____

2. aluminum animal _____

3. suddenly suspicious _____

4. curiosity seekers _____

5. announced candidacy _____

6. conscientious maneuver _____

7. Three men—raced down the hill—to the boat—in the river.

_____

_____

8. After dark one night—he gave the money—to his best friend.

_____

_____

Rhyming

1. take _____

2. hot _____

3. said _____

4. seat _____

5. crowd _____

6. maker _____

7. brother _____

8. preacher _____

9. sure _____

10. whistle _____

PART 2
Student Matching Worksheet

1.	wish	which	witch	with
2.	every	ever	very	even
3.	chime	shin	shine	chin
4.	prior	prayer	pry	priory
5.	write	right	rite	riot
6.	bark	brake	back	dark
7.	quit	quiet	quite	quid
8.	scratch	scarce	scorch	source
9.	vowel	val	valve	value
10.	mash	madge	match	mad
11.	sinker	singer	sinner	seen
12.	prat	part	quart	brat

PART 3
Student Spelling Worksheet

1. _____ 14. _____ 27. _____

2. _____ 15. _____ 28. _____

3. _____ 16. _____ 29. _____

4. _____ 17. _____ 30. _____

5. _____ 18. _____ 31. _____

6. _____ 19. _____ 32. _____

7. _____ 20. _____ 33. _____

8. _____ 21. _____ 34. _____

9. _____ 22. _____ 35. _____

10. _____ 23. _____ 36. _____

11. _____ 24. _____ 37. _____

12. _____ 25. _____ 38. _____

13. _____ 26. _____ 39. _____

Appendix E
Jordan Asperger's Syndrome Scale
Nonverbal LD (NVLD)

An irregular, disruptive lifestyle is seen frequently in persons who have difficulty fitting into mainstream classroom and workplace situations. This irregular behavior first was called *nonverbal LD* (NVLD). Recently this socially disruptive lifestyle has also been called *Asperger's syndrome*. This physically and socially awkward lifestyle is a subtype of autism that is caused when axon pathways fail to connect vital regions of the higher brain and midbrain. In severe autism, so many neuronal links are missing that regions of the higher brain are isolated so that vision does not connect to hearing, touch does not integrate with sight, and so forth.

Very high-functioning autism, or Asperger's syndrome, allows enough brain regions to communicate with each other to let the individual's intelligence become usable in restricted ways. A person with Asperger's syndrome usually is highly intelligent, reads well, and shows no signs of dyslexia or attention deficit disorder. However, the individual's behavior is so different from normal that he or she is labeled "weird" by most others. Many persons with Asperger's syndrome have master's or doctoral degrees, yet their social habits and personality differences are so eccentric that it is difficult for them to find a job within their field of education.

The Jordan Asperger's Syndrome Scale is designed to reveal ranges of severity in Asperger's behavior. Knowledge of this unique type of behavior allows instructors and workplace leaders to understand why a well-educated individual is so strange. Knowing about the neurological basis for Asperger's syndrome removes blaming individuals for behaviors they cannot change.

Jordan Asperger's Syndrome Scale

	Never 0	Sometimes 1	Usually 2	Always 3
1. *Is Noticeably Awkward in Gross Motor Activity* Lifelong awkwardness in walking, running, skipping, hopping, standing, playing games, catching balls.	___	___	___	___
2. *Speaks in a Monotone Voice* Speech is slow and deliberate like giving a boring lecture. Voice does not relax into natural rhythms during conversation.	___	___	___	___
3. *Has Toneless Voice* Voice is flat with no rise or fall in tonation. Voice has no vocal coloration or inflection.	___	___	___	___
4. *Is Very Slow Responding to Conversation* Cannot think of anything to say at parties or when introduced to new people. Struggles to turn personal knowledge into social conversation.	___	___	___	___
5. *Has Very Limited Sense of Humor* Does not get the point of jokes or friendly teasing. Takes everything literally. Bristles when teased, believing that he or she has been criticized. Cannot repeat or tell jokes effectively.	___	___	___	___
6. *Has Awkward, Stiff Body Posture* Body does not relax when person stands or sits. Always seems to be stiffly awkward in standing around or sitting down.	___	___	___	___
7. *Has Extraordinary Recall of Trivial Details* Is a specialist in one or two narrow areas of expertise. Drones on and on to others about trivial details that do not interest others.	___	___	___	___

	Never	Sometimes	Usually	Always
	0	1	2	3

8. *Has Extremely Narrow Range of Interests*
   Lives and breathes one or two topics that he or she works to death. Does not expand personal interest to new issues.

9. *Has Irritating Habit of Hair Splitting*
   Overanalyzes everything he or she sees and hears. Cannot let loose ends go by without correcting them. Constantly splits, then splits the splits. Corrects others when they fail to do or say exactly correct things.

10. *Is Dreaded by Others*
    Others try to avoid interaction or conversation with this person. Others make excuses not to be involved with this person.

11. *Has Extremely Boring Personality*
    Nothing is socially appealing about this person. Others soon glance at the time and make excuses to get away.

12. *Displays Inappropriate Social Behavior*
    Personal habits embarrass others. Eating habits and poor personal hygiene are obnoxious. Does not learn better manners. Does not change inappropriate habits or behaviors.

13. *Lives a Ritualized, Eccentric Lifestyle*
    This person lives by rigid rituals. Others call him or her "weird." Is inflexible and obsessive in protecting lifestyle rituals. Cannot stop doing same eccentric things over and over.

	Never	Sometimes	Usually	Always
	0	**1**	**2**	**3**
14. *Cannot Read Social Signals* Is "socially dyslexic." Does not read social signals to "back off," "leave me alone," "give me a break," "not now." Barges in when others want to be left alone.	_____	_____	_____	_____
15. *Lives by Controlling Others* Uses wide range of control strategies to coerce others into doing things his or her way. Is a poor member of groups, commit- tees, and work teams. Has poor sense of deferring to needs or wishes of others. Tries to isolate certain persons to keep them away from influence of others.	_____	_____	_____	_____
16. *Rationalizes Automatically* Automatically explains away own mistakes and poor judg- ment. Blames others. Sets oth- ers up to take the blame when things go wrong.	_____	_____	_____	_____
17. *Works Best When Alone in Highly Structured Tasks* Is totally frustrated by changes in job or social routines. Does best in activities that do not change, can be controlled, and do not involve opinions of others.	_____	_____	_____	_____
18. *Is Highly Creative Within Narrow Range of Interests* Has reputation of being "an ec- centric genius" if left alone in his or her own territory or work space. Often is the best in- formed person within a busi- ness or educational institution.	_____	_____	_____	_____

	Never	Sometimes	Usually	Always
	0	**1**	**2**	**3**

19. *Does Not Know When to Stop*
Talks or writes on and on and
on. Does not recognize normal
stopping places or when enough
has been said or expressed in
writing. ___ ___ ___ ___

20. *Holds Unrealistic, Grandiose
Hopes for Fame or Success*
Talks endlessly about writing
the great novel, producing sen-
sational screenplays, making
a million dollars, or becoming
world famous. ___ ___ ___ ___

21. *Is Excessively Stubborn and
Inflexible*
Clings stubbornly to ritualized
beliefs and habits. Refuses to
change. Argues against change.
Often sabotages change in
workplace. ___ ___ ___ ___

Subscore ___ ___ ___ ___

TOTAL SCORE _____

Scoring

1. Add all the checks in each column to find the Subscore for each column. Each
   check in the Never column equals 0. Each check in the Sometimes column
   equals 1. Each Check in the Usually column equals 2. Each check in the Always
   column equals 3.

2. Add Subscores to find the TOTAL SCORE.

3. Enter the TOTAL SCORE in the appropriate place on the following Asperger's
   Syndrome Profile page.

Asperger's Syndrome Profile

None 0–11	Mild 12–25	Moderate 26–40	Moderately Severe 41–45	Severe Above 55

	0–11	Not enough habits to be called Asperger's syndrome.

	12–25	*Mild Asperger's Syndrome*

Is noticeably boring in conversation. Social behavior is noticeably awkward as if this person has not been taught good social manners. Is noticeably self-focused. Talks about self and own interests more than he or she pays attention to others. Lives within a very narrow range of interests, but can briefly pay attention to interests of others if reminded to do so. Can work with others if team leader is firm and patient. Prefers to work alone in own private space. Has peculiar sets of ritualized habits that are seldom replaced by new routines. Has noticeably good recall for details within narrow range of personal interests. Quickly irritates classmates, work partners, and new acquaintances. Droning, flat, monotone voice immediately irritates others.

	26–40	*Moderate Asperger's Syndrome*

Has reputation of being "weird," but can be tolerated briefly by most others. Is boring in all situations. Is acknowledged to be highly competent in one or two areas. Launches into boring, droning monologues whenever he or she is alone with anyone. Social manners are noticeably crude, irregular, and "strange." Lifestyle is highly ritualized and inflexible with habits repeated over and over without change. Body posture and movements are stiff and awkward. This person has very little sense of humor. Efforts to tell jokes are embarrassing to others. Effort to make small talk is often painful for others to watch.

This person resists attempts by others to change behaviors or to expand range of interests. Resists any change that would involve modifying rituals and habits. Argues against change. Blames others for own mistakes or poor judgment. Puts more time and energy into rationalizing than into developing new skills or procedures. Becomes offended by advice from supervisors or colleagues about changing habits or modifying behavior.

| | 41–55 | *Moderately Severe Asperger's Syndrome* |

This individual is distinctly "weird" in general behavior. Cannot carry on conversations without launching into self-centered, overbearing monologues about one or two very narrow topics. This person's flat, droning voice quickly annoys others who dread to be with this individual. Others plot ahead how to avoid this person. He or she is a controller and manipulator. Lifestyle is rigidly ritualized with many eccentric behaviors. Is rigidly inflexible toward change. Spouts streams of trivial information that bore and exasperate others. Is a poor member of teams or committees because of rigid, inflexible attitudes. Automatically blames others for own mistakes. Loses much valuable time arguing and splitting hairs over unimportant issues.

Openly resists or sabotages efforts to upgrade, change, or modify job procedures. Cannot be relied on to follow through on new procedures. Social manners are generally obnoxious and unpleasant. Flat, monotonous voice is a major source of irritable responses from others. Triggers much conflict and contention within work groups, study groups, and classrooms.

Rarely responds to counseling or other efforts to bring about change. Is extremely sensitive, often paranoid, toward constructive criticism. Is a very poor risk for behavior modification.

| | Above 55 | *Severe Asperger's Syndrome* |

Asperger's patterns are overwhelming to others. Impossible for this person to fit into social groups. Is seldom possible for this individual to succeed in work groups. Behavior is so rigid, irregular, obnoxious, "weird," that others shun and avoid. Personal habits are offensive. Has virtually no tact or social amenities. Is completely self-focused and blind to needs or interests of others. Is hostile toward change. Is surly and rude when others suggest that he or she should change. Automatically blames others for own mistakes. Devotes much time to blaming others. Rarely apologizes unless it is apparent that an apology will give him or her additional control.

Struggles to find employment. Cannot do job interviews successfully. May be well educated with advanced degrees, but is too irregular and offensive to be employed. May do satisfactory work in a highly structured job in a private space away from others.

Is actively resistant to and suspicious of counseling or guidance. There is virtually no hope that counseling might modify or improve this level of Asperger's patterns and behaviors.

What To Do for Asperger's Syndrome

1. Set Clear Limits
It is possible to get along with individuals with Asperger's syndrome if boundaries are defined and limits are clearly stated. The foundational problem of this disorder is that the brain interprets the world literally. There is no imagination outside the individual's narrow range of specialization. The Asperger's brain does not recognize nuance, variation in word usage, or figures of speech. Therefore, instructors, family members, and workplace supervisors must be sure to speak precisely.

Setting limits must be done orally and in writing so that the individual with Asperger's syndrome has a written outline of what is discussed. With this list of boundaries, the supervisor speaks directly to the point, regardless of how cruel this straight talk seems. For example, the boundary list might include these limits:

1. When I hold up my hand, that means that you are too close. You must step back two paces.

2. When I frown at you and pinch my nose, it means you forgot to take a shower and wear fresh clothes.

3. When I shake my head, it means that you must stop what you are doing without any argument.

4. When I tap my watch, it means that your time is up and you are to leave me alone for half an hour.

2. Replace Old Rituals with New Ones
Regardless of counseling or good advice from others, individuals with Asperger's syndrome cannot stop doing their rituals. However, they sometimes learn to replace an obnoxious old ritual with a better new one. Occasionally an individual with Asperger's syndrome asks a trusted friend,

"Why don't people like me? Why don't they ever invite me to parties or call me at home?" Such intimate questions open the door for a trusted one (often a teacher) to make some suggestions.

The process begins by having the person with Asperger's syndrome make a list of times when he or she was rejected or left out of a situation. This list should be a column down the left side of a page. Then the friend asks leading questions: "Can you think of any reasons why you might not have been included? Did you perhaps forget to take a shower and change your socks and underwear that week? Is it possible you forgot to use deodorant or brush your teeth that week? Did you wear the same shirt (or blouse) several days without washing it? Did you keep on talking too much without letting others have a turn? Did you go on and on about yourself too much without asking others about themselves?"

These leading questions are specific enough for the literal, unimaginative Asperger's brain to use logic in thinking through these situations. The person with Asperger's syndrome invariably replies, "What does not bathing every day have to do with it?" Sometimes the blunt response "Because it makes you stink" is enough to start the process of self-appraisal.

At this point, the friend suggests that the person with Asperger's syndrome try an experiment for 30 days. On another page a new lifestyle ritual is outlined:

1. Take a shower every day.

2. Use deodorant every day.

3. Brush teeth twice a day.

4. Change to a fresh shirt (or blouse) each day.

5. Change socks and underwear every day.

6. Don't talk more than 2 minutes. Then stop so others can have their turn to talk.

7. Make sure to ask others about what they think, then give them time to tell their ideas.

Individuals with Asperger's syndrome can learn to substitute a new tidy ritual for an old untidy one that was part of the reason for social rejection. When they change from being smelly and untidy to being clean, fresh smelling, and neat, a definite change will result in how they are accepted by associates. When an individual with Asperger's syndrome memorizes some new social skills, such as making an effort not to talk too much and not to talk about self all the time, he or she can fit into social groups better. Replacing old antisocial rituals with new socially acceptable ones can be practiced in many ways.

For example, most persons with Asperger's syndrome are sharply critical of others. When others do things differently, they automatically try to "straighten them out" by preaching at them or criticizing them. Individuals with Asperger's syndrome can learn to control this criticism by saying it silently to themselves but not aloud. They can learn to "button their lips" (most of the time) instead of butting into conversations of others. These new rituals will become as rigidly inflexible as old routines, but socially acceptable rituals trigger much less rejection.

Appendix F
Jordan Scale for Social–Emotional LD (SELD)

The Jordan Scale for Social–Emotional LD is designed to focus your attention on specific types of disruptive behavior in a person's lifestyle. Occasionally it is possible to use this checklist in an interview, if the SELD individual trusts you enough to be candid. The value of this assessment is that it summarizes in a nonjudgmental format the various ways in which an individual's habits are disruptive to society and within groups. Often this information helps parents, instructors, lifemates, and workplace supervisors understand why certain bright individuals are so difficult to be with, live with, or work beside.

Jordan Scale for Social–Emotional LD

	Never 0	Sometimes 1	Usually 2	Always 3
1. *Follows Irregular Lifestyle* Style of living flies in the face of tradition. Lifestyle has little or no relationship to what society regards as being valuable, sacred, or morally important.	___	___	___	___
2. *Behavior Defies Logic* Does not live by logic or common sense. Decisions are not guided by logical thinking. Is unaware of what logical thinking is or why it is important.	___	___	___	___

	Never 0	Sometimes 1	Usually 2	Always 3
3. *Has No Concern for Consequences* Does not think in terms of consequences. Choices and decisions are unrelated to what might happen as a result of this behavior.	____	____	____	____
4. *Is Self-Focused* Lives for self. First consideration is what he or she can get out of this relationship or situation. All conscious thought revolves around self. Uses others to get what he or she wants for self.	____	____	____	____
5. *Lives by Impulse* Lives by impulse with no effort to put off wishes or desires. Lifestyle is "I want what I want when I want it."	____	____	____	____
6. *Is Insatiable* Lives by consuming, not giving or sharing with others. Personal needs, desires, and wishes are never fully satisfied. Clamors for more, blames others for not being fair, complains about not getting his or her fair share.	____	____	____	____
7. *Is Insensitive to Needs of Others* Does not see or perceive needs of others. Is blind to the signals that others present.	____	____	____	____
8. *Has Explosive Temper* Explodes at anyone or any event that gets in his or her way. Any criticism is met with a tantrum. Any effort by parents, partners, instructors, colleagues, or boss to give constructive criticism triggers a temper tantrum.	____	____	____	____

	Never 0	Sometimes 1	Usually 2	Always 3
9. *Is Always on the Defensive* Lives in a defensive attitude. Has hair-trigger response that blames others, makes excuses, rationalizes away all mistakes.	___	___	___	___
10. *Has Short Job Tenure* Impossible for this prickly, self-focused, immature person to hold a job. Triggers too much conflict to be worth keeping as an employee.	___	___	___	___
11. *Does Not Learn from Mistakes* Does not change behavior because of mistakes. Lifestyle is immune to the normal process of learning from mistakes.	___	___	___	___
12. *Does Not Respond to Counseling* Is too defensive and hot tempered to learn from counseling. Cannot drop automatic defenses long enough to hear or heed what is suggested.	___	___	___	___
13. *Has Shallow Lifestyle* Has no spiritual, moral, or emotional depth. Is too self-focused to relate to any outside influence that would deepen or enrich the lifestyle.	___	___	___	___
14. *Has No Loyalty to Family Values* Is loyal only to own needs and wishes. Often is intensely loyal to peer group who also are SELD because these peers do not judge or criticize this person's choices and decisions. Feels no guilt for violating family values and standards.	___	___	___	___

	Never	Sometimes	Usually	Always
	0	1	2	3

15. *Is Irresponsible*
Displays no social responsibility.
Takes no responsibility for the
disruptive example his or her
lifestyle presents. Feels no responsibility to pay bills on time,
be punctual, avoid pregnancy or
disease, or follow through on
promises and committments.

Subscore _____ _____ _____ _____

TOTAL SCORE _____

Scoring

1. Add all the checks in each column to find the Subscore for each column. Each check in the Never column equals 0. Each check in the Sometimes column equals 1. Each check in the Usually column equals 2. Each check in the Always column equals 3.

2. Add the Subscores to find the TOTAL SCORE.

3. Enter the TOTAL SCORE in the appropriate place on the following SELD Profile page.

SELD Profile Rating Scale

Mild 1–7	Low Moderate 8–14	Moderate 15–21	High Moderate 22–28	Severe 29–35	Critical Above 35
_____	1–7	*Mild* This person would not be diagnosed as SELD. However, his or her social behavior is noticeably disruptive, often rude or thoughtless, and frequently angry for no apparent reason. This person can respond to guidance and counseling to learn how to control urges that turn into disruptive behavior.			

——— 8–14

Low Moderate SELD

This individual is a difficult person to live with, work with, or be with. Others must overlook flashes of temper, self-centered attitude, lack of social sensitivity, and overall irritability toward rules and limitations. This person continually tests boundaries to see if the rules can be bent or broken without getting into trouble. At this level, counseling and guidance can be helpful if counseling is specific enough to pinpoint areas where behavior triggers conflict. Low dosage strength SSRI or MAO medication would be appropriate to assist the limbic system in controlling surges of strong emotions and impulses.

——— 15–21

Moderate SELD

This individual is a difficult member of any group. Supervisors and instructors spend much time restoring order when SELD outbursts trigger conflict. This person is regarded as selfish and hot tempered, and rarely is sensitive to the needs of others unless those needs benefit him or her in some way. This individual continually tests authority and tries to change boundaries set by authority figures. This person's lifestyle is irregular in dress, personal interests, choice of friends, forms of recreation, and ritualized habits. This individual lives on the edge of being removed from the workplace, social situations, or educational programs. He or she rejects counseling, or refuses to cooperate if forced into counseling. Lifestyle is disobedient, oppositional, defiant, and arrogant toward rules and limitations. SSRI or MAO medication is required to lower the level of aggression and oppositional reflexes.

——— 22–28

High Moderate SELD

This person cannot function in traditional classroom, social, or workplace environments. Behavior is so disruptive that he or she will be removed from traditional school attendance. He or she likely will drop out of formal schooling. This person is at high risk of failure in all personal relationships and will be fired time after time from the workplace. This individual has abandoned family values to become part of a "separate tribe" that refuses to conform or obey. He or she is intensely loyal to the "separate tribe" that has replaced family, school, and childhood religion. This person is out of control in situations that require obedience to authority. Lifestyle is closely guarded against intrusion by parents or other relatives. This individual is attracted to bizarre Web sites and chat rooms on the Internet. This lifestyle brings the individual close to danger through disregard of consequences. Often this person is one step away from borderline criminal behavior. He or she thrives on high-risk, thrill-seeking adventures.

_____ 29–35 *Severe SELD*
This person has severed ties to traditional family values and civility toward society. Lifestyle is aggressive, often violent, usually angry, and borderline paranoid in believing that others get a larger, better share. This individual is committed to the often outrageous dress and behavior of the "separate tribe." Conscious effort is made to shock society through bizarre hairstyle, body piercing, outrageous clothing, and obnoxious habits. Much time is spent on Internet search for bizarre Web sites and chat rooms that promote issues related to hate, racial superiority, deviant sex, or methods of killing people and destroying property. Lifestyle is devoted to rebellion against tradition and authority. If necessary to survive or to buy special things, this person works part-time to earn enough to satisfy a certain wish. He or she is indifferent to family needs, but is devoted to needs of the "separate tribe." This individual suffers from bouts of deep depression and often thinks of suicide. He or she may write secret volumes of poetry or song lyrics that reflect the chaos and emptiness of this alien lifestyle. A major underlying component of this lifestyle is deep, painful shame that is tied to death of self-esteem. This individual refuses medication and counseling.

_____ Above 35 *Critical SELD*
The lifestyle of this person is beyond civil control. He or she has severed all meaningful ties to traditions of society, family, and religion. This person frequently joins cult-like groups devoted to rebellion and to creating chaos in the rest of society. Often persons at this critical level of SELD become dangerous by acting out fantasies of killing others, bombing public property, and "getting even" for perceived rejection by family, school, the workplace, and governmental agencies. This level of SELD includes bizarre and dangerous practices, such as self-mutilation or autoerotic

asphyxiation. This lifestyle is built on paranoid suspicions that often involve membership in secret militaristic groups who believe in pending catastrophy. The major themes of this lifestyle are paranoid perceptions, rage against society, self-preoccupation, racial hatred, and eliminating perceived enemies. Suicidal thinking is very active for these individuals, along with plots to kill classmates or workplace colleagues who have snubbed or offended them. This critical level of SELD is a form of mental illness that often poses a dangerous social threat.

What To Do for SELD

1. *Do not attempt to force this person into traditional educational and social programs.* Because oppositional defiant disorder is strongly involved in social–emotional LD, these individuals cannot function or thrive in traditional classrooms, social situations, or highly structured workplace positions. Persons who are SELD must be approached through nontraditional strategies that do not trigger underlying phobias or fears. First of all, programs for SELD persons must be safe and emotionally comfortable for them.

2. *Discover multiple intelligences within SELD individuals.* Traditional views of intelligence have no meaning for individuals who are SELD. Instead, they must be seen through the lens of multiple intelligence that gives value to right-brain intuition, creativity, nonacademic interests, and alternative forms of spirituality.

3. *Develop action-centered learning programs based on SELD strengths.* SELD individuals present a "pathology of superiority" that can be directed into positive productivity if personal strengths form the foundation for further learning. Bias against SELD differences must be removed. These individuals must not be expected to become traditional. By identifying personal strengths in intuition and creativity, new knowledge and individual special interests can be honed for the workplace. Few SELD persons ever fit well into traditional workplace situations. However, they have the potential to become successful entrepreneurs.

4. *Replace shame and crushed self-esteem with success and new self-confidence.* Beneath SELD behavior lies deep shame and loss of self-esteem that rarely is defined for these restless individuals.

The most direct remedy is through step-by-step success that comes through discovery of strengths the individual did not know that he or she had.

5. *Provide talking therapy that avoids judgment.* SELD individuals are deeply hungry for acceptance and for understanding from others. Few SELD adolescents have ever known an adult who practiced unconditional affection with no strings attached. The most effective healing process for SELD is through talking at length with an intelligent, nonjudgmental adult who knows how to listen actively without interrupting.

6. *Provide medication that stabilizes dopamine, serotonin, and norepinephrine.* A wide variety of SSRI and MAO medications are available to stabilize neurotransmitters that are out of balance in SELD, such as Prozac, Zoloft, Welbutrin, Paxil, Catepres, BuSpar, Pamelor, Tofranil, Anafranil, Effexor, Luvox, Serzone, Ritalin, and Adderall.

References

Adolphs, R., & Damasio, A. R. (1998). The human amygdala in social judgment. *Nature, 393,* 470–474.

American Psychiatric Association. (1994). *Diagnostic and statistical manual of mental disorders* (4th ed.). Washington, DC: Author.

Ardrey, R. (1961). *African genesis.* New York: Macmillan.

Ardrey, R. (1972). *The territorial imperative.* New York: Macmillan.

Armstrong, T. (1995). *The myth of the A.D.D. child.* New York: Penguin Putnam Inc.

Atkinson, J. (1984). Human visual development over the first 6 months of life: A review and a hypothesis. *Human Neurobiology, 3,* 61–74.

Aubert, H., & Foerster, M. (1857). Beitraege zur Kenntnisse der indirecten Sehens. *Graefes Archiv für Ophthalmologie, 3*(2), 1–37.

Bandler, R., & Shipley, M. T. (1994). Columnar organization in the midbrain periaqueductal gray: Modules for emotional expression? *Trends in Neurosciences, 17,* 379–389.

Barkley, R. A. (1990). *Attention-deficit hyperactivity disorder: A handbook for diagnosis and treatment.* New York: Guilford.

Barkley, R. A. (1995). *Taking charge of ADHD: The complete, authoritative guide for parents.* New York: Guilford.

Barnard, K. E., & Brazelton, T. B. (Eds.). (1990). *Touch, the foundation of experience.* Madison, CT: International Universities.

Bastian, C. H. (1869). On various forms of loss of speech in cerebral disease. *The British Medico-Chirurgical Review, 43,* 209–236, 470–494.

Berlin, R. (1884). Über dyslexie [About dyslexia]. *Archiv für Psychiatrie, 15,* 276–278.

Berlin, R. (1887). *Einebosondere art der wortblindheit: Dyslexie* [A special type of wordblindness: Dyslexia]. Wiesbaden: J. F. Bergmann.

Birren, J. E., & Shaie, K. W. (Eds.). (1990). *Handbook of the psychology of aging* (3rd ed.). San Diego, CA: Academic Press.

Block, N., Flanagan, O., & Guzeldere, G. (Eds.). (1997). *The nature of consciousness: Philosophical debates.* Cambridge, MA: MIT Press.

Branstetter, Z. (2000, March 12). Running scared from the police. *Tulsa World,* pp. A1–4.

Bredburg, G. (1985). The anatomy of the developing ear. In S. E. Trehub & B. Schneider (Eds.), *Auditory development in infancy* (pp. 3–20). New York: Plenum.

Brier, N. (1989). The relationship between learning disability and delinquency: A review and reappraisal. *Journal of Learning Disabilities, 2,* 546–583.

Broadbent, W. H. (1872). On the cerebral mechanism of speech and thought. *Transactions of the Royal Medical and Chirurgical Society, 15,* 145–194.

Brody, B. A. (1987). Sequence of central nervous system myelination in human infancy: 1. An autopsy study of myelination. *Journal of Neuropathology and Experimental Neurology, 46,* 282–301.

Brothers, L. (1997). *Friday's footprint: How society shapes the human mind.* New York: Oxford University Press.

Calvin, W. H., & Ojemann, G. A. (1980). *Inside the brain.* New York: New American Library.

Cannell Studios. (1998). *About Stephen.* Universal City, CA: Author.

Carlson, B. M. (1994). *Human embryology and developmental biology.* St. Louis, MO: Mosby.

Charness, N., & Bosman, E. A. (1992). *The handbook of aging and cognition.* Hillsdale, NJ: Erlbaum.

Chugani, H. T. (1999). Metabolic imaging: A window on brain development and plasticity. *Neuroscientist 5,* 29–40.

Copeland, E. D. (1991). *Medications for attention disorders (ADHD/ADD) and related medical problems.* Atlanta: 3 C's of Childhood.

Craik, F. I. M., & Salthouse, T. A. (Eds.). (1992). *The handbook of aging and cognition.* Hillsdale, NJ: Erlbaum.

Damasio, A. R. (1994). *Descartes' error: Emotion, reason, and the human brain.* New York: Avon Books.

Damasio, A. R. (1995, September 9). Sex hormones key in brain development. *Tulsa World,* p. A7.

Damasio, A. R. (1999). *The feeling of what happens: Body and emotion in the making of consciousness.* New York: Harcourt Brace.

Dechesne, C. J. (1992). The development of vestibular sensory organs in humans. In R. Romand (Ed.), *Development of auditory and vestibular systems* (Vol. 2; pp. 192–197). New York: Elsevier.

DeFries, J. C., Olson, R. K., Pennington, B. F., & Smith, S. D. (1991). Colorado reading project: An update. In D. D. Duane & B. D. Gray (Eds.), *The reading brain: The biological basis of dyslexia* (pp. 302–312). Parkton, MD: York Press.

Denckla, M. B. (1972). Clinical syndromes in learning disabilities. The case for "splitting" versus "lumping." *Journal of Learning Disabilities, 5,* 405–406.

Denckla, M. B. (1978). Minimal brain dysfunction. In J. S. Chall & A. F. Mirshy (Eds.), *Education and the brain* (pp. 223–268). Chicago: University of Chicago Press.

Denckla, M. B. (1985). Issues of overlap and heterogeneity in dyslexia. In D. B. Gray & J. F. Kavanaugh (Eds.), *Biobehavioral measures of dyslexia* (pp. 41–46). Parkton, MD: York Press.

Denckla, M. B. (1991a). Academic and extracurricular aspects of nonverbal learning disabilities. *Psychiatric Annals, 21,* 717–724.

Denckla, M. B. (1991b, March). *The neurology of social competence.* Paper presented at the Learning Disabilities Association national conference, Chicago.

Denckla, M. B. (1993). The child with developmental disabilities grown up: Adult residua of childhood disorders. *Behavioral Neurology, 11(1),* 105–125.

Dennett, D. (1991). *Consciousness explained.* Boston: Little, Brown.

Duane, D. (1985, March). *Psychiatric implications of neurological difficulties.* Paper presented at symposium conducted at the Menninger Foundation, Topeka, KS.

Duane, D. (1987, November). *The anatomy of dyslexia and neurobiology of human aptitude.* Paper presented at symposium conducted by the Orton Dyslexia Society, San Francisco.

Eden, G. E. (1996, November). *Visualizing vision in dyslexic brains.* Paper presented at symposium conducted by the Society for Neuroscience, San Francisco.

Education for All Handicapped Children Act of 1975, 20 U.S.C. 1400 *et seq.*

Ekman, P. (1992). Facial expressions of emotions: New findings, new questions. *Psychological Science 3,* 34–38.

Eliot, L. (1999). *What's going on in there: How the brain and mind develop in the first five years of life.* New York: Bantam.

Fisher, B. (1992). Successful aging and life satisfaction: A pilot study for conceptual clarification. *Journal of Aging Studies, 6,* 191–202.

Galaburda, A. M. (1983). Developmental dyslexia: Current anatomical research [Proceedings of the 33rd annual conference of the Orton Dyslexia Society]. *Annals of Dyslexia, 33,* 41–45.

Galaburda, A. M. (1986, November). *Neuroendocrinology and dyslexia.* Paper presented at the Neuroendocrinology Symposium conducted by the Association for Children and Adults with Learning Disabilities, New York.

Galaburda, A. M., Sherman, G. F., Rosen, G. D., Aboitiz, F., & Geschwind, N. (1985). Developmental dyslexia: Four consecutive patients with cortical anomalies. *Annals of Neurology, 18,* 222–233.

Geiger, G., & Lettvin, J. Y. (1987). Peripheral vision in persons with dyslexia. *New England Journal of Medicine, 316,* 1238–1243.

Geschwind, N. (1972). Anatomical evolution and the human brain. *Bulletin of the Orton Society, 22,* 7–13.

Geschwind, N. (1982). Why Orton was right. *Annals of Dyslexia, 32,* 13–30.

Geschwind, N. (1984). The biology of dyslexia: The after-dinner speech. In D. B. Gray & J. F. Kavanaugh (Eds.), *Biobehavioral measures of dyslexia* (pp. 1–19). Parkton, MD: York Press.

Geschwind, N., & Levitsky, W. (1968). Human brain: Right-left asymmetries in temporal speech region. *Science, 161,* 186–187.

Gilligan, J. (1996). *Violence: Reflections on a national epidemic.* New York: Vintage Books.

Goodale, M. A., & Milner, A. D. (1992). Separate visual pathways for perception and actions. *Trends in Neuroscience, 15,* 20–25.

Gottfried, A. W. (1990). Touch as an organizer of development and learning. In K. E. Barnard & T. B. Brazelton (Eds.), *Touch: The foundation of experience* (pp. 349–361). Madison, CT: International Universities.

Grimm, V. (1986, November). *Neuroendocrinology and fetal development.* Paper presented at the Neuroendocrinology Symposium conducted by the Association for Children and Adults with Learning Disabilities, New York.

Hallowell, E. M., & Ratey, J. J. (1994a). *Answers to distraction.* New York: Pantheon.

Hallowell, E. M., & Ratey, J. J. (1994b). *Driven to distraction.* New York: Pantheon.

Hammill, D. D., & Bryant, B. R. (2000). *Learning disabilities diagnostic inventory.* Austin, TX: PRO-ED.

Hampton-Turner, C. (1981). *Maps of the mind.* New York: Macmillan.

Hardman, P. K., & Rennick, R. A. (2000). *Removing the barriers to employment for disabled welfare to work clients.* Tallahassee, FL: Dyslexia Research Institute.

Hendrickson, A. E. (1993). Morphological development of the primate retina. In K. Simons (Ed.), *Early visual development: Normal and abnormal* (pp. 287–295). New York: Oxford University Press.

Hepper, P. G., & Shahidullah, B. S. (1994). Development of fetal hearing. *Archives of Disease in Childhood, 71,* F81–F87.

Hill, D. L., & Mistretta, C. M. (1990). Developmental neurobiology of salt taste sensation. *Trends in Neuroscience, 13,* 188–195.

Hinshelwood, J. (1896). A case of dyslexia: A peculiar form of word blindness. *Lancet,* 1451–1454.

Hinshelwood, J. (1900). Congenital word-blindness. *Lancet, 1,* 1506–1508.

Hooker, K. (1992). Possible selves and perceived health in older adults and college students. *Journal of Gerontology: Psychological Sciences, 47,* 85–95.

Huttenlocher, P. R. (1990). Morphometric study of human cerebral cortex development. *Neuropsychologia, 28,* 517–527.

Individuals with Disabilities Education Act of 1990, 20 U.S.C.1400 *et seq.*

Inhelder, B., & Piaget, J. (1974). *The early growth of logic in the child.* New York: Harper & Row.

Irlen, H. (1991). *Reading by the colors: Overcoming dyslexia and other reading disabilities through the Irlen method.* Garden City, NY: Avery.

Jacobson, M. (1991). *Developmental neurobiology* (3rd ed.). New York: Plenum.

Jernigan, S. (1985, November). *Measures of brain function: Understanding the influence of brain dysfunction on behavior and learning problems.* Symposium conducted by The Menninger Foundation, Topeka, KS.

Johnson, D. J., & Myklebust, H. R. (1971). *Learning disabilities.* New York: Grune & Stratton.

Johnson, M. H. (1990). Cortical maturation and the development of visual attention in early infancy. *Journal of Cognitive Neuroscience, 2,* 81–95.

Johnson, M. H. (1994). Brain and cognitive development in infancy. *Current Opinion in Neurobiology, 4,* 218–225.

Jordan, D. R. (1972). *Dyslexia in the classroom.* Columbus, OH: Merrill.

Jordan, D. R. (1974). *Learning disabilities and predelinquent behavior of juveniles.* Oklahoma City: Oklahoma Association of Children with Learning Disabilities.

Jordan, D. R. (1989a). *Jordan prescriptive/tutorial reading program for moderate and severe dyslexia.* Austin, TX: PRO-ED.

Jordan, D. R. (1989b). *Overcoming dyslexia in children, adolescents, and adults.* Austin, TX: PRO-ED.

Jordan, D. R. (1996a). *Overcoming dyslexia in children, adolescents, and adults* (2nd ed.). Austin, TX: PRO-ED.

Jordan, D. R. (1996b). *Teaching adults with learning disabilities.* Malabar, FL: Krieger.

Jordan, D. R. (1998). *Attention deficit disorder: ADHD and ADD syndromes* (3rd ed.). Austin, TX: PRO-ED.

Jordan, D. R. (2000a). *Jordan dyslexia assessment/reading program* (2nd ed.). Austin, TX: PRO-ED.

Jordan, D. R. (2000b). *Understanding and managing learning disabilities in adults.* Malabar, FL: Krieger.

Joseph, R. (1988). The right cerebral hemisphere: Emotion, music, visual-spatial skills, body image, dreams, and awareness. *Journal of Clinical Psychology, 44,* 632–673.

Josephson, M. (1959). *Edison, a biography.* New York: McGraw-Hill.

Khan, A. A. (1994). Development of human lateral geniculate nucleus: An electron microscopic study. *International Journal of Developmental Neuroscience, 12,* 661–672.

Killackey, H. P. (1995). The formation of a cortical somatosensory map. *Trends in Neuroscience, 18,* 402–407.

King, D. (1985). *The Diana King method of touch typing.* Groton, VT: Author.

Kirsch, I. W., Jungeblut, A., & Campbell, A. (1992). *Beyond school doors: The literacy needs of job seekers served by the U.S. Department of Labor.* Princeton, NJ: Educational Testing Service.

Kogan, N. (1990). Personality and aging. In J. E. Birren & K. W. Shaie (Eds.), *Handbook of the psychology of aging* (3rd ed., pp. 330–346). New York: Academic Press.

Larsen, W. J. (1993). *Human embryology.* New York: Churchill Livingstone.

Lehmkuhle, S., Garzia, R. P., Turner, L., Hash, T., & Baro, J. A. (1993). A defective visual pathway in children with reading disability. *New England Journal of Medicine, 328,* 898–996.

Levine, M. (1990). *Keeping ahead in school.* Cambridge, MA: Educators Publishing Service.

Levine, M. (1993). *All kinds of minds*. Cambridge, MA: Educators Publishing Service.

Levine, M. (1999, February 12). Pediatrician shares ideas about brain functions in young: Brain wiring key to learning needs. *Tulsa World*, p. A14.

Lichteim, L. (1885). On aphasia. *Brain, 7*, 432–484.

Lindamood, P. C., Bell, N., & Lindamood, P. (1992). Issues in phonological awareness assessment. *Annals of Dyslexia, 42*, 242–259.

Livingstone, M. S., Rosen, G. D., Drislane, F. W., & Galaburda, A. M. (1991). Physiological and anatomical evidence for a magnicellular deficit in developmental dyslexia. *Proceedings of the National Academy of Sciences, USA, 88*, 7943–7947.

Llinas, R. (1993). Coherent 40-Hz oscillation characterizes dream state in humans. *Proceedings of the National Academy of Sciences, USA, 90*, 2078–2081.

Lous, J. (1995). Otitis media and reading achievement: A review. *International Journal of Pediatric Otorhinolaryngology, 32*, 105–121.

Lyon, G. R. (2000, January/February). Why reading is not a natural process. *LDA Newsbriefs, 35*(19), 12–17.

Malcomesius, N. (2000). *Specific Language Disability Test*. Cambridge, MA: Educators Publishing Service.

McGinn, C. (1991). *The problem of consciousness*. Oxford: Basil Blackwell.

McGuinness, D. (1997). *Why our children can't read*. New York: Touchstone.

Merzenich, M. M., Jenkins, W. M., Miller, S. L., Schreiner, C., & Tallal, P. (1996). Temporal processing deficits of language-learning impaired children ameliorated by training. *Science, 271*, 77–81.

Missildine, W. H., & Galton, L. (1972). *Your inner child of the past*. New York: Simon & Schuster.

Moses, M. (1998, September). *Dyslexia and related disorders: Texas state law, state board of education rule, and the revised procedures concerning dyslexia*. Austin, TX: Texas Education Agency.

Muller, K., & Homberg, V. (1992). Development of speed of repetitive movements in children is determined by structural changes in cortisospinal efferents. *Neuroscience Letters, 144*, 57–60.

Nagarajan, S., Mahncke, H., Salz, T., Tallal, P., Roberts, T., & Merzenich, M. (1999, May 25). Cortical auditory signal processing in poor readers. *PNAS Online, 96*(11), 6483–6488.

National Institute of Child Health and Human Development. *Study of early childhood care* (NIH Pub. #98-4318). Washington, DC: Author.

O'Rahilly, R., & Muller, F. (1996). Neurolation in the normal human embryo. In G. Bock & J. Marsh (Eds.), *Neural tube defects* (pp. 70–89). CIBA Foundation, Symposium 181. Chichester, England: Wiley.

Orton, S. T. (1925). "Word-blindness" in school children. *Archives of Neurology and Psychiatry, 14*, 581–615.

Orton, S. T. (1928). Specific reading disability—strephosymbolia. *Journal of the American Medical Association, 90,* 1095–1099.

Orton, S. T. (1937). *Reading, writing and speech problems in children.* Armenia, NY: Academy of Orton-Gillingham Practitioners and Educators.

Osman, B. B., & Blinder, H. (1982). *Nobody to play with: The social side of learning disabilities.* New York: Random House.

Park, D. C. (1992). Applied cognitive aging research. In F. I. M. Craik & T. A. Salthouse (Eds.), *The handbook of aging and cognition* (pp. 449–493). Hillsdale, NJ: Erlbaum.

Parker, H. C. (1989). *The ADD hyperactivity workbook for parents, teachers, and kids.* Plantation, FL: Impact Publications.

Payne, N. (1994). [Learning disabilities in the workplace]. Unpublished raw data.

Peck, J. E. (1995). Development of hearing: Part III. Postnatal development. *Journal of American Academy of Audiology, 6,* 113–123.

Pennington, B. F., Gilger, J. W., Paul, D., Smith, S. A., Smith, S. D., & DeFries, J. C. (1991). Evidence for major gene transmission of developmental dyslexia. *Journal of the American Medical Association, 266*(11), 1527–1534.

Penrose, R. (1994). *The shadows of the mind.* New York: Oxford University Press.

Pollan, C., & Williams, D. (1992). [Learning disabilities in adolescent and young adult school dropouts]. Unpublished raw data.

Pujol, R. (1990). Physiological correlates of development of the human cochlea. *Seminars in Perinatology, 14,* 275–280.

Purves, D., & Lichtman, J. W. (1985). *Principles of neural development.* Sunderland, MA: Sinauer.

Ramachandrian, V. S. (1993). Behavioral and magnetoencephalographic correlates of plasticity in the adult human brain. *Proceedings of the National Academy of Sciences, USA, 90,* 10413–10420.

Ratey, J. J., & Johnson, C. (1997). *Shadow syndromes.* New York: Pantheon.

Rawson, M. B. (1988). *The many faces of dyslexia.* Baltimore: The Orton Dyslexia Society.

Rockefeller, N. A. (1976, June). The puzzle children. *TV Guide Magazine.*

Rogan, W. J., & Gladen, B. C. (1993). Breast-feeding and cognitive development. *Early Human Development, 31,* 181–193.

Romand R. (Ed.). (1992). *Development of auditory and vestibular systems* (Vol. 2). New York: Elsevier.

Rutter, M., & Yule, W. (1975). The concept of specific reading retardation. *Journal of Child Psychology and Psychiatry, 16,* 181–197.

Schacter, D. L. (1996). *Searching for memory.* New York: Basic Books.

Schieber, F. (1992). Aging and senses. In J. E. Birren, K. W. Sloane, & G. D. Cohen (Eds.), *Handbook of mental health and aging* (2nd ed., pp. 252–306). San Diego, CA: Academic Press.

Searle, J. (1997). *The mystery of consciousness.* New York: New York Review of Books.

Semrud-Clikeman, M., & Hynd, G. W. (1990). Right hemispheric dysfunction in nonverbal learning disabilities: Social, academic, and adaptive functioning in adults and children. *Psychological Bulletin, 107,* 196–209.

Shaywitz, S. (1996, November). Dyslexia: A new model. *Scientific American,* pp. 2–8.

Silver, L. (1985, March). *The learning disabled child: Who is he? What is he?* Symposium conducted by The Menninger Foundation, Topeka, KS.

Slingerland, B. H. (1984). *Slingerland Screening Tests for Identifying Children with Specific Language Disability.* Cambridge, MA: Educators Publishing Service.

Stanovich, K. D. (1993). Dysrationalia: A new specific learning disability. *Journal of Learning Disabilities, 26*(8), 501–515.

Steeves, J. (1987, November). *Computers: Powerful tools for dyslexic children.* Symposium conducted by The Orton Dyslexia Society, San Francisco.

Sutherland, N. S. (1992). *Irrationality: The enemy within.* London: Constable.

Tallal, P., Miller, S., & Fitch, R. (1993). Neurobiological basis of speech: A case for the preeminence of temporal processing. *Annals of New York Academy of Sciences, 682*(6), 74–81.

Tallal, P., & Piercy, M. (1974). Developmental aphasia: Rate of auditory processing selective impairment of consonant perception. *Neuropsychologia, 12,* 83–93.

Tallal, P., & Stark, R. E. (1981). Speech acoustic-cue discrimination abilities of normally developing and language-impaired children. *Journal of the Acoustic Society of America, 69,* 568–574.

Tallal, P., Stark, R. E., & Mellitis, D. (1985). The relationship between auditory temporal analysis and receptive language development: Evidence from studies of developmental language disorder. *Neuropsychologia, 23,* 527–534.

Thomson, L. J. (1971). Language disabilities in men of emminence. *Journal of Learning Disabilities, 4*(1), 39–50.

Thurber, D. N. (1993). *D'Nealian handwriting* (3rd ed.). Glenview, IL: Scott Foresman.

Tranel, D., & Damasio, A. R. (1993). The covert learning of affective valence does not require structures in the hippocampal system or amygdala. *Journal of Cognitive Neuroscience, 5,* 79–88.

Tranel, D., Hall, L. E., Olson, S., & Tranel, N. N. (1987). Evidence for a right-hemisphere developmental disability. *Developmental Neuropsychology, 3,* 113–127.

Travis, J. (1996, February 17). Let the games begin. *Science News, 149,* 104–106.

Troyer, P. (1986). *Father Bede's misfit.* New York: York Press.

Ungerleider, L. G., & Haxby, J. V. (1994). "What" and "where" in the human brain. *Current Opinion in Neurology, 4,* 157–165.

van Essen, D. C., & Gallant, J. L. (1994). Neural mechanisms of form and motion processing in the primate visual system. *Neuron, 13,* 1–10.

Voeller, K. K. S. (1986). Right-hemisphere deficit syndrome in children. *American Journal of Psychiatry, 143,* 1004–1009.

Wacker, J. (1975). *The dyslogic syndrome.* Dallas: Texas Association for Children with Learning Disabilities.

Warren, P., & Capehart, J. (1995). *You and your A.D.D. child: How to understand and help kids with attention deficit disorder.* Nashville, TN: Thomas Nelson.

Wechsler, D. (1974). *Wechsler Intelligence Scale for Children, Revised.* San Antonio, TX: Psychological Corporation.

Wechsler, D. (1994a). *Wechsler Adult Intelligence Scale* (3rd ed.). San Antonio, TX: Psychological Corporation.

Wechsler, D. (1994b). *Wechsler Intelligence Scale for Children* (3rd ed.). San Antonio, TX: Psychological Corporation.

Weis, G., & Hechtmann, L. T. (1993). *Hyperactive children grown up* (2nd ed.). New York: Guilford.

Weisel, L. P. (1992). *POWERPath to adult basic education.* Columbus, OH: The TLP Group.

Weisel, L. P. (2001). *POWERPath to adult basic education* (2nd ed.). Columbus, OH: The TLP Group.

Weiss, L. (1992). *Attention deficit disorder in adults: A practical guide for sufferers and their spouses* (2nd ed.). Dallas, TX: Taylor.

Weiss, L. (1995). *ADD on the job: Making your ADD work for you.* Dallas, TX: Taylor.

Zaidel, E., & Zaidel, D. (1979). Self-recognition and social awareness in the disconnected minor hemisphere. *Neuropsychologia, 8,* 41–55.

Author Index

Subject Index

Date Due

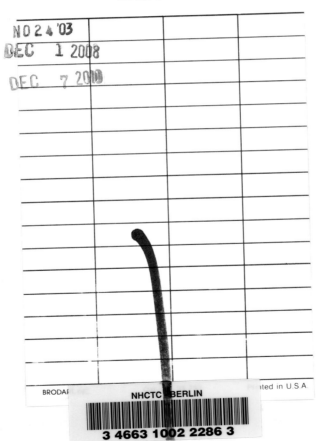

NO 2 4 '03			
DEC 1 2008			
DEC 7 2010			